Breast Cancer

Tibor Tot

Editor

Breast Cancer

A Lobar Disease

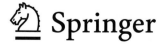 Springer

Editor
Tibor Tot
Department of Pathology and Clinical
Cytology
Central Hospital Falun
Falun
Sweden

ISBN 978-1-84996-313-8   e-ISBN 978-1-84996-314-5
DOI 10.1007/978-1-84996-314-5
Springer London Dordrecht Heidelberg New York

British Library Cataloguing in Publication Data
A catalogue record for this book is available from the British Library

Library of Congress Control Number: 2010936641

Printed on acid-free paper

Springer is part of Springer Science+Business Media (www.springer.com)

Foreword

To the women of my life: my wife Mária, my mother Zsuzsanna, my sister Jolán, and to the future generation: my daughters Boglárka and Emese.

FOREWORD

Preface

Speaking on the topic of the sick lobe theory on many occasions, I always watch the reaction of the audience. A new theory awakes three types of reaction: a (very) small minority will accept it as being new and revolutionary; the skeptics will argue against it and will do everything to prove that it is incorrect. But the vast majority will tell you that the theory is correct but not a new one, they have been aware of it for decades.

And the majority is always right. "The theory of the sick lobe and the theory of biological timing are new concepts but have their roots in previous observations and studies." But "The theory of the sick lobe and the theory of biological timing connect the process of carcinogenesis to an existing and well defined anatomic structure, a breast lobe, and provide a possible explanation for the progressive character and morphological heterogeneity of breast carcinoma. These theories are more than a description of morphological patterns. They put these patterns into a unifying concept with genetic, developmental, and morphological perspectives of understanding breast carcinoma as a process that develops over time under endogenous and exogenous influences, not like a photo, but like a life-long movie" (Tot, Chap. 1). "The 'sick lobe' hypothesis asks questions about the development of breast cancer in time and space, and observes that concentrating on events in a few cubic millimetres of tissue is not enough" (Going, Chap. 2). And the originality of the concept can be easily proved with a simple PubMed search.

I presented the sick lobe theory for the first time in Winnipeg Canada, on The First Workshop on Alternatives to Mammography 2004. The body of evidence, pro and contra, generated during the last years will be presented in this book in ten chapters on different subjects. Epidemiological evidence supports the facts that "...the genetic mutations or epigenetic abnormalities involved in breast cancer development are more likely to be perpetuated by cells undergoing continuous branching and ramification while the lobe is being formed, rather than originating within the terminal ductal-lobular units, the majority of which are not developed before birth" (Xue and Michels, Chap. 3). Genetic analysis aiming at "...topographical mapping revealed that the genetic changes were clustered in a segmental distribution in some of the breast samples. The study provided further evidence that a field of genetic instability can exist around a tumour and that this size was greater than one terminal duct-lobular unit" (Smart et al., Chap. 4).

Modern radiology, especially in multimodality approach, gives evidence for the complex and variable morphology of breast carcinoma which will be richly illustrated in this book. "Detecting breast cancer at an earlier phase in its development and at a smaller tumor size is, however, no guarantee that the disease will be localized to a small, confined volume in every case. In fact, multifocal and/or diffuse breast cancers comprise the majority of breast cancers in every size range" (Tabar et al., Chap. 7). Morphological evidence exists that the components of the cancer and pre-cancerous changes occupy a lobe-like space in the breast and "a more widespread use of large sections in routine pathology will give more accurate knowledge on extent and growth patterns of breast in situ neoplasms" (Foschini and Eusebi, Chap. 6). Ductal endoscopy also showed that "Whether unifocal or multifocal, breast cancers seem to arise within only a single ductal tree" (Dooley, Chap. 9), supporting the morphological data. A special ultrasound approach, ductal echography, provides further evidence for the lobar nature of breast carcinoma, not only scientific but based on everyday diagnostic routine, motivating Dr Dominique Amy to state: "It seems to us that the 'sick lobe theory' ...reflects the reality we daily observe 'in vivo'" (Amy, Chap. 8).

These theories have practical diagnostic and therapeutic implications. "The century old magic bullet approach to cancer has not served us well. It became part of the hegemony of biochemistry and later molecular biology, genomics and a massive pharmaceuticals industry with an attitude that there is a drug for every malady. In parallel, over the past century, x-ray and other forms of imaging developed and improved. These are now ready to overtake magic bullets precisely because they are nonspecific, i.e., potentially capable of detecting all tumors" (Gordon, Chap. 10). In addition to radiological imaging, "basic knowledge of the ductal/lobar systems intra-ductal approach to breast cancer would appear to be essential if the treatment and prevention of breast cancer is to evolve and to be applied in a more logical and less invasive way" (Love and Mills, Chap. 5). On the other hand, data also "suggest that sufficient tissue must be removed at surgery to avoid local recurrence and raises questions about whether such alterations could account for some cases of local recurrence after apparent 'complete excision' of the tumor" (Smart et al., Chap. 4).

Speaking about reactions of the audience, a leading breast surgeon told me after one of my presentations that there is no such thing as correct theory, but some of the theories may be useful. I hope that this book will be useful and stimulate the readers to rethink the established views and to develop new and more efficient approaches in diagnosing and treating breast carcinoma.

Tibor Tot
Falun, Sweden

Contents

Dominique Amy, MD Centre de Radiologie, Aix-En-Provence, France

Peter B. Dean, MD, PhD Diagnostic Radiology Department, Faculty of Medicine, University of Turku, Turku, Finland

William C. Dooley, MD Division of Surgical Oncology, Department of Surgery, The University of Oklahoma Health Sciences Center, Oklahoma City, OK, USA

Vincenzo Eusebi, MD, FRC Path Department of Hematology and Oncology, Section of Pathology "M. Malpighi" University of Bologna at Bellaria Hospital, Bologna, Italy

Maria P. Foschini, MD Department of Hematology and Oncology, Section of Pathology "M. Malpighi" University of Bologna at Bellaria Hospital, Bologna, Italy

James J. Going, MB, PhD Institute of Cancer Sciences, Glasgow University and Pathology Department, Glasgow Royal Infirmary, Glasgow, UK

Richard Gordon, PhD Department of Radiology, University of Manitoba, Winnipeg Manitoba, Canada

Mats Ingvarsson, MD Department of Mammography, Central Hospital Falun, Falun, Sweden

Sunil R. Lakhani, BSc, MBBS, MD, FRC Path, FRCPA University of Queensland Centre for Clinical Research, School of Medicine, and Pathology Queensland, The Royal Brisbane & Women's Hospital, Brisbane, Queensland, Australia

Nadja Lindhe, MD Department of Mammography, Central Hospital of Falun, Falun, Sweden

Susan M. Love, MD, MBA President, Dr. Susan Love Research Foundation, Santa Monica, CA, USA

Karin B. Michels, ScD, PhD Obstetrics and Gynecology Epidemiology Division, Department of Obstetrics, Gynecology and Reproductive Biology, Brigham and Women's Hospital, Harvard Medical School, Boston, MA, USA; and Department of Epidemiology, Harvard School of Public Health, Boston, MA, USA

Dixie J. Mills, MD Medical Director, Dr. Susan Love Research Foundation, Santa Monica, Boston, CA, USA

Peter T. Simpson, BSc University of Queensland Centre for Clinical Research, Brisbane, Queensland, Australia

Chanel E. Smart, BSc, PhD Molecular & Cellular Pathology Department, University of Queensland Centre for Clinical Research, Brisbane, Queensland, Australia

László K. Tabár, MD, PhD Department of Mammography, Central Hospital of Falun, Falun, Sweden

Tibor Tot, MD, PhD Department of Pathology and Clinical Cytology, Central Hospital Falun, Falun, Sweden

Ana Cristina Vargas, MD University of Queensland Centre for Clinical Research, Brisbane, Queensland, Australia

Fei Xue, MD, MS, ScD Obstetrics and Gynecology Epidemiology Division, Department of Obstetrics, Gynecology and Reproductive Biology, Brigham and Women's Hospital, Harvard Medical School, Boston, MA, USA and Department of Epidemiology, Harvard School of Public Health, Boston, MA, USA

Amy Ming-Fang Yen, PhD School of Oral Hygiene, Oral Medicine of College, Taipei Medical University, Taipei, Taiwan

The Theory of the Sick Lobe

Tibor Tot

1

1.1 Introduction

1.1.1 The Dimensions of the Problem

Breast carcinoma is among the most frequent malignant diseases in the world and is the leading cause of premature death among younger women in developed countries. Currently, every tenth to every seventh woman in these countries will have the disease in their lifetime (Boyle and Ferlay 2005). Since 1940, the incidence of breast carcinoma has gradually increased at a rate of approximately 1% per year in Western countries (Harris et al. 1992). On the other hand, mortality from breast cancer has declined in countries with organized population-based mammography screening (Smith et al. 2004; The Swedish Organized Service Screening Evaluation Group 2006), and new efficient therapeutic regimes have led to prolonged survival of patients with improved quality of life (Hortobagyi 2005). These interventions have considerably increased the number of breast cancer survivors, and a further increase of 31% is expected in the decennium from 2005 to 2015 (De Angelis et al. 2009). Although a decreased incidence has been observed in some industrial countries over the last few years, other countries, among them China and India with their very large populations, experience a continuous and constant increase in incidence (Kawamura and Sobue 2005). An increase of 30% in the number of detected cases between 2010 and 2030 was estimated in the US based on current

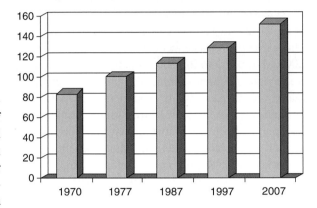

Fig. 1.1 The number of newly diagnosed breast carcinoma cases a year per 100,000 inhabitants in Sweden based on data from the Swedish Board of Welfare at www.sos.se, Accessed 2 May 2009

epidemiological trends, with a 57% increase for women older than 65 years (Smith et al. 2009). This increase may result in every fourth or every third woman in these countries carrying a risk of breast carcinoma in their lifetime (Fig. 1.1). Screening, diagnosis, and treatment will place an ever growing burden on the health care system, in addition to the psycho-social consequences for the women of coming generations. Obviously, a paradigm shift in understanding the natural history of breast carcinoma is needed to develop new and more efficient preventive, diagnostic, and therapeutic alternatives and break the negative trend.

1.1.2 Endogenous and Exogenous Risk Factors

The etiology of breast carcinoma remains unknown, though a number of risk factors have been identified. The female sex is the most powerful risk factor,

T. Tot
Department of Pathology and Clinical Cytology,
Central Hospital Falun, Falun,
Sweden
e-mail: tibor.tot@ltdalarna.se

T. Tot (ed.), *Breast Cancer*, DOI: 10.1007/978-1-84996-314-5_1,
© Springer-Verlag London Limited 2011

resulting in a roughly 100-fold higher incidence rate than in men. The risk of getting breast carcinoma increases with increasing age. Geographical influences are also evident as the disease is far more frequent in North America, Western Europe, Scandinavia, Australia, and New Zealand than in Asian and African countries (Kawamura and Sobue 2005). Daughters of women who migrate from low-incidence to high-incidence countries acquire the breast cancer risk of the new country (Buell 1973), indicating that local environmental factors and lifestyle also influence risk. Higher socioeconomic status and a higher level of education are also recognized risk factors (Clarke et al. 2002). In addition, race and ethnicity seem to play a role in breast cancer development (Harper et al. 2009). Exposure to ionizing radiation and some environmental synthetic chemicals may also represent major risk factors (Wolff et al. 1996). Prenatal and perinatal factors, including birth weight, birth length, and parental age at delivery, may also predispose women to breast cancer in adulthood (Xue and Michels 2007). Reproductive factors related to hormonal regulation of the ovaries in females are also important and may manifest in well-known risk factors, such as null parity, late first full-time pregnancy, early menarche, and late menopause. Restricted use of hormone replacement therapy was considered to be a major cause of the recently observed decreased incidence in the US and some other countries, indicating that exogenous estrogens may promote and antiestrogen therapy may counteract breast cancer development (Fisher et al. 1998).

A family history of breast and/or ovarian cancer is also an important risk factor, indicating that the inherited genetic background of the individual plays a crucial role in breast cancer development in up to 27% of patients (Hill et al. 1997). Carriers of mutated BRCA1 and BRCA2 genes are at a very high risk of getting breast carcinoma, but they represent only a small proportion of women with this disease (Ford et al. 1994; Easton et al. 1997).

Breast tissue composition affects the radiological density of the breast tissue on the mammogram (Tot et al. 2000). Increased mammographic breast density is associated with an increased risk of breast carcinoma. On the other hand, breast density is related to genetic, hormonal, constitutional (weight, height), and environmental factors; hormone replacement therapy also influences breast density (Tabár et al. 2007).

Being a woman, living in a high-incidence country, carrying a mutated gene, and all of the other risk factors listed above have a common feature: they affect the entire organism, all of the individual cells of the organism, and all of the cells in both breasts. On the other hand, breast cancer develops most often in a single quadrant of one of the breasts, indicating the presence of risk tissue there, a structure that is more sensitive to the effects of the endogenous or exogenous oncogenic stimuli than the other structures in the human body. Our hypothesis is that this risk tissue corresponds to a sick breast lobe that was malconstructed during its embryonic development.

Many of the listed risk factors are present from the very beginning of the life of the individual who develops breast carcinoma as an adult or in old age. If the sick lobe is present with its potentially malignant cells from embryonic life, a period of several decades is required for complete malignant transformation. We hypothesize that the necessary steps leading to malignant transformation are genetically determined in the potentially malignant cells and their clones. Potentially malignant cells at different points of the sick lobe may go through these steps synchronously, as well as asynchronously. The time needed for malignant transformation is also influenced by exogenous and endogenous factors. For example, women exposed to radiation for extended periods show an increased incidence of breast carcinoma, often occurring 30 years or more after exposure (Little and Boice 1999). Carriers of BRCA1 and BRCA2 gene mutations, on the other hand, get breast carcinoma at a much younger age than noncarriers.

These data are fundamental for the concept we termed the theory of biological timing.

1.2 Theoretical Background

1.2.1 Anatomy and Embryology

Breast is a glandular organ with lobar organization. A typical breast lobe is comprised of a single lactiferous duct opening at the nipple, branching into several segmental and subsegmental ducts, and ending in hundreds and thousands of terminal ducts and lobules, the last two comprising terminal ductal-lobular units (TDLUs). The epithelial structures of a lobe are tree-like with a trunk and branches, and the TDLUs correspond to leaves. Together with the stromal structures, the epithelial structures occupy a pyramid-like tissue space with a tip in the nipple and a wide base toward the pectoralis fascia. With the exception of a single study that demonstrated rare interlobar connections (Ohtake et al. 1995), the lobes are considered to be individual units with no connections between them. The number of lobes seems to be constant during a woman's lifetime, but their size and form varies considerably as a result of progressive and regressive morphological processes that depend on age and hormonal status, resulting in changes in the number and size of the lobules and smaller ducts.

The normal human breast arises from a primary ectodermal outgrowth (primary bud) in the second trimester of embryonic life. The primary bud is considered the primordium nipple, and the remaining breast tissue develops from the primary bud via the formation of secondary buds projecting into the underlying mesenchyme during the 21st—25th week of gestation (Howard and Gustersson 2000; Jolicoeur et al. 2003). Other investigators have determined week 8 to be the gestational age of the budding stage (Russo and Russo 2004). Thus, the lobes are initiated early during intrauterine life as secondary projections of the primary bud. All of the secondary projections from the primary bud represent the initiation of a potential breast lobe, but some are probably abortive and may disappear during intrauterine life.

Ductal morphogenesis continues during fetal life with the formation of new projections ending with the so-called end vesicle. The developing breast exhibits dual-cell architecture from a very early stage; the central cells in the projections coexpress cytokeratins (CKs) 19 and 14, whereas the peripheral (basal) cells gradually loose CK19 expression. Lobules may be present at the time of birth, but they are usually few or absent.

In addition to the changes in the parenchymal compartment of the breast tissue, the embryonic mesenchyme surrounding the mammary buds and projections exhibit important changes in the developing breast. For example, overexpression of tenascin C is considered to be a sensitive indicator of mesenchyme remodeling into a more specific periductal stroma (Sakakura et al. 1991). Thus, tenascin C overexpression may represent an indicator of active budding and branching during embryonic and fetal life, a sign of active arborization within a breast lobe. Tenascin C overexpression in the

stroma of some in situ carcinomas indicates that new duct formation may also appear in adults as part of cancer progression (Tabár et al. 2004).

The infant breast undergoes involution after being removed from the influences of maternal hormones. The prepubertal breast consists almost exclusively of ducts. During puberty, the breast enlarges, mainly due to the growth of stromal elements, but also due to further ramification of the ductal tree and lobule formation (Wellings et al. 1975). Lateral budding from existing ducts has also been described (Rudland 1991).

During the reproductive period, the female breast undergoes cyclical changes related to the menstrual cycle. Increased proliferation of the cells in the ducts and lobules, which appears mainly in the luteal phase, leads to increased epithelial cell number and an increased number of acini per lobule; new bud formation from the terminal ducts increases the number of lobules. At the end of the menstrual cycle, genetically programmed cell death (apoptosis) appears in the epithelial and myoepithelial cells, and the process reverts to a status similar to the status at the beginning of the previous menstrual cycle (Ramakrishnan et al. 2002).

The mammary gland attains its full development in pregnancy when a substantial increase in the lobule number, lobule size, and number of acini per lobules is observed. These increases are a result of lateral budding from existing ducts, branching of the subsegmental ducts, and branching of the terminal ducts into numerous acini. After lactation, the mammary gland regresses via collapse of the acini and small ducts, apoptosis of their epithelium and myoepithelium, and regeneration of the elements of the interlobular stroma. However, the postlactational parous breast never returns to prepregnancy status and the breasts of parous women differ from those of nulliparous in morphology (more glandular tissue) and at the molecular and genetic levels (Russo and Russo 2004).

During and after menopause, the mammary gland undergoes involution, a process similar to regression after lactation or the end of a menstrual cycle, but more pronounced. Involution of the parenchyma results in a diminished number of lobules, acini per remaining lobules, and terminal and segmental-subsegmental ducts. Importantly, the number of lactiferous ducts and, consequently, the number of lobes remains constant during the woman's lifetime. Parallel with parenchymal involution, stromal involution occurs, resulting in the replacement of the specialized intralobular and periductal stroma with fatty tissue, so-called fatty involution, or with collagen-rich fibrous tissue, so-called fibrous involution. The interlobular stroma is also affected by this process (Tot et al. 2002).

We consider the processes of initialization, arborization, and lobularization to be distinct phases of mammary gland development. Initialization is a process that occurs early during intrauterine life and leads to the appearance of a number of initial lobes. Arborization, the branching of the initial projection into duct-like structures of decreasing caliber, characterizes the fetal as well as prepubertal mammary gland, but may also happen during the entire life of the woman depending on adequate hormonal stimuli. Lobularization appears in the fetal breast, but mainly characterizes the pubertal and mature (especially the lactating) breast. Similarly, malignant transformation may also target these processes; low-grade in situ carcinomas tend to alter the normal process of lobularization, whereas a high-grade in situ tumor may also affect the process of arborization. Aberrations at the level of lobe initialization may lead to the development of a sick lobe (Tot 2005b).

1.2.2 The Progenitor Cell Concept

The actual morphology of a tissue is the result of a balance between renewal and loss of cellular and noncellular elements. Tissue-specific stem cells are defined by their ability to self-renew and produce differentiated cells. There are three basic types of stem cells: embryonic, from the blastocyst, representing the origin of all cells in the organism; germinal, the origin of the male and female reproductive cells; and somatic, for the renewal of normal tissue (Gudjonsson and Magnusson 2005). Differentiated cells tend to have a short life, whereas stem cells persist and reproduce themselves throughout the entire life of the organism. The division of a stem cell may result in two similar stem cells, in two more differentiated so-called progenitor cells, or more often in one stem cell and one progenitor cell. Stem cells and progenitor cells are capable of differentiating and are often pluripotent, giving rise to the different mature cells of an organ. The microenvironment of the actual stem cell plays a crucial role in determining the direction of this differentiation. Cells with stem cell properties correspond to

a small proportion of the cells in most mature organs (Liu et al. 2008).

Regarding normal breast tissue, the existence of self-renewing multipotent stem cells was first suggested several decades ago by Deome et al. (1959), who demonstrated that an entire mammary gland can be generated from serially transplanted random fragments of breast epithelium. The luminal and myoepithelial cells of mature breast tissue seem to originate from a common stem or progenitor cell (Boecker and Burger 2003). There is growing evidence for the existence of three distinct epithelial progenitor cell populations in the breast: one capable of producing all epithelial cells in the breast and two others capable of producing either secretory lobules or branching ducts (Smith and Boulanger 2003). During the embryonic development of the mammary gland, the stem cells undergo stepwise differentiation (commitment) (Villadsen 2005); the final steps of differentiation lead to the appearance of the two mature cell populations, the luminal population expressing CK18 and the myoepithelial ("basal") cells expressing CK14. Villadsen et al. (2007) demonstrated that stem cells in the breast reside in ducts and those with a capacity for clonal growth and self-renewal are derived only from ducts. Lobules may contain progenitor cells. Liu et al. (2008) reported evidence that the breast of BRCA1 mutation carriers is altered and show similar changes to those in the subsequent carcinoma. Stem cells/progenitor cells in the normal tissue were specifically stained and shown to be much more frequent in the lobules of BRCA1 mutation carriers than healthy controls. Clarke (2005) suggested the existence of two subtypes of mammary epithelial stem cells: one expressing estrogen receptor alpha and progesterone receptor, renewing the cells during the menstrual cycle, and the other not expressing these receptors, renewing the breast stem cell pool. Thus, the development and maintenance of the structures of the breast lobes seem to be a complex process with several types of stem cells/progenitor cells involved. The processes of arborization and lobularization may be, to a certain level, independent of one another.

For a cell to become neoplastic, a series of changes are needed to overcome the stringent controls of cell division. A malignant tumor represents a heterogeneous population of mutant cells that share some mutations but also vary in their genotype and phenotype. The original cancer cell(s) and its progeny exhibit stem cell properties (Reya et al. 2001; Al-Hajj et al. 2003). The cancer cells share their immortal character with tissue-specific stem cells; they are also slow-dividing, long-lived cells with a capacity for self-renewal and differentiation (Agelopoulos et al. 2008). Only a small proportion of the malignant cells has this unlimited proliferation potential and possesses the ability to lead to tumor formation, as in normal tissue. These cells are called cancer stem cells. The more differentiated cancer cells that account for the majority of the tumor cell population may have high, but not unlimited, proliferation potential.

The presence of cancer stem cells has been demonstrated in many types of tumors. During experiments with xenotransplantation of mammary carcinoma cells, cells expressing CD44 that did not express CD24 were isolated. The isolated cells did not express epithelial markers, but were more prone to develop breast cancer compared to other cell types (Al-Hajj et al. 2003). These CD44+/CD24− cells have been proposed to be breast cancer stem cells; however, they seem to be the origin of only a minority of breast cancer types, including the basal-like breast carcinomas and those associated with BRCA1 mutation (Honeth et al. 2008). In the model of stem cell hierarchy, cancer cells in the same tumor may originate from several stem cells, with some of these clones being more successful in the given microenvironment (Clarke et al. 2006b; Villadsen et al. 2007).

The origin of cancer stem cells is an area of ongoing research and probably varies in different tumors. Cancer stem cells may originate from either normal tissue stem cells or progenitor cells that have acquired the ability of self-renewal due to mutation (Al-Hajj et al. 2003). Stem cells and progenitor cells, as well as cancer stem cells, are slow-dividing, long-lived cells and, therefore, are exposed to the influences of damaging factors from their internal and/or external environment. The longevity of the cells makes them far more sensitive to mutagenic stimuli compared to mature cells. The accumulation of mutations may transform stems cells or progenitor cells into cancer cells according to the "multi-hit concept" of carcinogenesis. The first initiating genetic alteration determining the pathway to cancer development may occur as early as fetal life or the fertilized egg, but the accumulation of further genetic aberrations are needed, which may occur several decades later (Baik et al. 2004). This concept has been proposed for different malignant tumors (Wang et al. 2009) and is also fundamental to the sick lobe theory.

A mutated stem cell passes on its mutations to its daughter cells; thus, these mutations can be detected throughout the ducts and lobules of a lobe, in epithelial as well as myoepithelial cells, which are microscopically normal (Lakhani et al. 1999). If a mutation appears in a committed progenitor cell, it may result in a chimeric network of normal and mutated cells (Tsai et al. 1996), creating a field of genetic alterations in which malignant transformation may take place. Although the mutant cells in the genetic field share the same alteration(s), the next mutations are not necessarily identical in all committed progenitor cells within this field. Thus, these additional genetic hits may lead to development of independent and genetically different tumor foci within the same field (Agelopoulos et al. 2008). In our view, this field of genetic alterations corresponds to a sick breast lobe and is a result of mutation(s) in the stem cells at the phase of initialization of the fetal lobe. This concept, together with the well documented resistance of cancer stem cells to different therapeutic modalities (Donnenberg and Donnenberg 2005), defines the ideal target of therapeutic intervention at early stages of breast cancer development.

1.3 The Hypotheses

1.3.1 The Theory of the Sick Lobe

We hypothesize that breast carcinoma is a lobar disease in that the simultaneously or asynchronously appearing tumor foci develop within a single sick lobe. The sick lobe is characterized by the presence of a large number of potentially malignant cells corresponding to mutant stem cells/progenitor cells dispersed within the lobe and present in multiple sites, making the sick lobe more sensitive to the endogenous or exogenous oncogenic stimuli compared to other lobes of the same breast with no, much less, or less sensitive, potentially malignant cells. We termed this hypothesis the theory of the sick lobe (Tot 2005a, b, 2007a).

Taking into account the above-reviewed epidemiological data that roughly one in ten women in developed

Fig. 1.2 Schematic illustration of the occurrence of a sick breast lobe. The lobes are pyramid-like structures with a summit within the nipple and base resting on the pectoralis fascia. Theoretically, one of approximately every 500 lobes is malconstructed

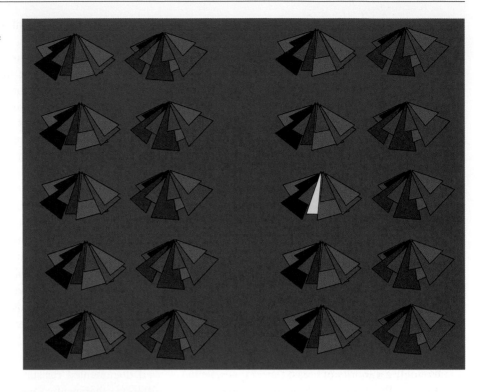

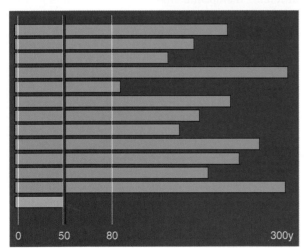

Fig. 1.3 Schematic illustration of the time needed for malignant transformation of the potentially malignant stem/progenitor cells within different lobes. The accumulation of genetic abnormalities would probably lead to malignant transformation of any of the lobes, but the time needed for it is substantially longer than the lifetime of the woman. The sick lobe is the exception because it is characterized by a greater number and/or increased sensitivity of these cells, and a much shorter time is needed for complete malignant transformation

of approximately 500 lobes are malconstructed the way we described (Fig. 1.2). Having a single sick lobe is a rule but not without exceptions. More than one sick lobe may also be present in the same woman on the rare occasion of multicentric or bilateral carcinomas. Several lobes of the same breast may be sensitive enough to develop carcinoma after a very long exposure to oncogenic stimuli, but the lifetime of most women is shorter. The prolonged average lifetime of women during the last century facilitated the appearance of breast carcinoma, even in sick lobes with relatively low sensitivity and with a very long period of biological timing (Fig. 1.3).

1.3.2 The Theory of Biological Timing

Potentially malignant cells may undergo malignant transformation under the influence of exogenous and endogenous oncogenic stimuli. The time of this transformation is determined by the number of required additional genetic alterations, which are mostly acquired during the division of these cells. If the oncogenic factors are of constant intensity, the time of malignant transformation is defined by the required number of replications of the mutant stem/progenitor cells in the

countries will get breast carcinoma during their life and the anatomical data that the median number of the largest ducts in one breast is 27 (Going and Moffat 2004; Going and Mohun 2006), we can conclude that only one

sick lobe and is dependent on the genetic construction of these cells and their progeny. Otherwise, the time of malignant transformation is also influenced by the changing intensity of exogenous or endogenous oncogenic stimuli. Malignant transformation may appear in a single locus within the sick lobe, more than one locus at the same time or with considerable time difference, or at a large number of loci. Thus, malignant transformation of the potentially malignant cells within the sick lobe is biologically timed, though this timing is not necessarily identical regarding all mutant stem/progenitor cell progeny. This hypothesis was termed the theory of biological timing.

As reviewed above, the lobes develop very early during embryonic life. The theory of the sick lobe implies that the sick lobe is already malconstructed from its initialization when the stem cells or progenitor cells acquire their first mutation(s), whereas the carcinoma within this lobe develops after the several decades of postnatal life necessary for the accumulation of additional genetic alterations. Thus, the biological timing may be valid for a very long period of time. Consequently, breast carcinoma is a lifelong disease that can be interrupted only by the elimination or destruction of the entire sick lobe.

1.3.3 Similar Concepts

The theory of the sick lobe and the theory of biological timing are new concepts, but have their roots in previous observations and studies. Similar formulations can be found in a 1921 article by Cheatle (1921). Dawson (1933), and later Wellings (Wellings et al. 1975; Cardiff and Wellings 1999), postulated that most breast carcinomas develop in the TDLUs within the breast. This partly incorrect concept has become a kind of dogma and influenced generations of breast specialists. Evidence that the ductal tree can also be the site of origin of carcinoma has been repeatedly reported, but these observations were overshadowed by the dogmatic approach. James Ewing stated in 1940, "DCIS grow in distended ducts over considerable segments of the breast" (Ewing 1940). Gallagher and Martin (1969) concluded, "Human mammary carcinoma is not a focal process but a disease which affects breast epithelia diffusely." Early observations of mammographically detected microcalcifications in cases of carcinoma in situ also indicated the localization of the process in a triangular area (Lanyi's triangle principle, Lányi 1977). Teboul, using large-field ultrasound, also recognized breast carcinoma as a malignant diffuse disease involving the whole epithelium of the affected lobe (Teboul and Halliwell 1995). Some surgeons advocated the "pyramidectomy concept," sector resection or segmental resection in other terminology, during the last few decades based on clinical experience that the excision of a pyramid (a lobe-like part) of the breast tissue provides better surgical results than a simple lumpectomy. The latest edition of the WHO book on breast tumors (Tavassoli and Devili 2003) states, "Segmentally distributed, ductal carcinoma in situ (DCIS) progression within the duct system is from its origin in the TDLU towards the nipple and into adjacent branches of the given segment of the duct system." Thus, an attempt, a compromise, was made to resolve the contradiction between the dogmatic approach and the radiological or clinical observations in that the cancer originates in the TDLU and spreads into the ducts of a segment. We shall critically address these points later in this chapter.

The influence of the intrauterine environment on the risk of getting breast carcinoma in adulthood was also hypothesized decades ago (Trichopoulos 1990).

1.4 Supporting Evidence

Cases in everyday routine diagnostic work with radiologically detected microcalcifications occupying a lobe-like space within the breast, a similar area on ultrasound (ductal echography), or similar enhancement on magnetic resonance imaging (Fig. 1.4a and b) are highly suggestive observations favoring the lobar location of the malignant process. Describing this pattern as "segmental distribution of the lesions," as it appears in the radiological literature, is confusing, however, as it does not reflect the underlying anatomy. The segment in this approach represents nothing else but a geometric term (part of a circle) and does not correspond to an anatomical segment (segmental branch of the lactiferous duct with lobules) but to an anatomical lobe (all of the structures belonging to a lactiferous duct). Interesting experience has been generated using ductal endoscopy, a relatively new method of endoscopic examination of the ductal system. As shown with this method, most of the malignant processes seem to belong to a single ductal tree, even if the lesions are distant from each other (Dooley 2003).

Fig. 1.4 (**a**) Magnetic resonance imaging of a case of high-grade in situ carcinoma, showing a lobe-like area of enhancement corresponding to a sick lobe (Tabár et al. 2008, Reprinted with permission). (**b**) Large-format histology section of a high-grade diffuse in situ carcinoma (with multiple invasive foci) occupying a lobe-like area

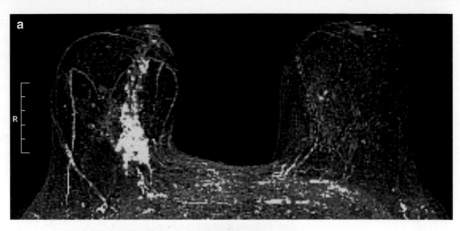

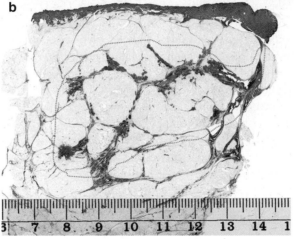

In addition to these observations, there is scientific evidence of the lobar nature of breast carcinoma from both morphological and genetic studies. On the other hand, supporting evidence for the theory of biological timing originates mainly from epidemiological investigations of the effects of prenatal and perinatal factors on the risk of developing breast cancer during adulthood. Furthermore, recent molecular genetic studies have also generated results concordant with our hypotheses.

1.4.1 Morphological Evidence

If an in situ carcinoma is present behind the nipple, it almost always involves only one of the lactiferous ducts. This observation is one of the most important pieces of supporting evidence for the sick lobe hypothesis. If the development of a cancer in the breast was not restricted to the structures of a single lobe, the involvement of more than one lactiferous duct could be expected. Going and his coworkers generated digitally reconstructed images of 1-mm-thick tissue slices proving the above described rule (James Going, 2007, personal communication). By paying attention to and regularly examining the nipple area, the involvement of a single lactiferous duct can be demonstrated in a large number of breast cancer cases exhibiting the lobar pattern of development. Such a case is illustrated in Fig. 1.5.

These observations are congruent with the findings of Mai et al. (2000), who demonstrated that the pattern of intraductal carcinoma spread within the breast has a pyramid-like shape with a summit toward the nipple (similar to a lobe). In their three-dimensional study using coronal giant sections, Mai observed that the detected in situ and invasive carcinoma foci, as well as the hyperplastic foci, were confined to the area of a single lactiferous duct in 27 of 30 mastectomy specimens.

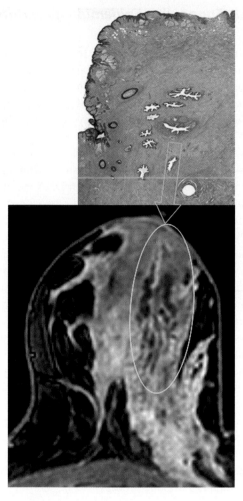

Fig. 1.5 Collage of a histology image of the nipple area (*upper*) and a magnetic resonance image of the same case (Courtesy of DR Mats Ingvarsson, Mammography Department, Central Hospital, Falun, Sweden). The in situ carcinoma involves only one of the lactiferous ducts; the others are free. The tumor exhibits a lobar subgross pattern involving the branches of the single ductal tree

Middleton et al. (2002) studied early stage synchronous multicentric carcinomas and found that they represent clonal proliferation of the same tumor in the majority of cases. A drawing that illustrated very well a lobe with diffuse continuous in situ carcinoma and two invasive foci belonging to this single breast lobe was included in that publication. However, they have not recognized this pattern as lobar.

Page and coworkers postulated that "ductal carcinoma in situ involves a single duct system," and the multifocal or multicentric appearance of this disease is related to fragmentation of the tissue during sampling for histological evaluation (Page et al. 2002). Although this study represents further recognition of the lobar nature of breast carcinoma (a single duct system is a major part of a lobe), the different patterns of malignant transformation within the duct system remained unrecognized.

1.4.2 Genetic Evidence

The theory of the sick lobe defines the risk tissue in the breast that has the potential of developing malignancy a long time before it happens in the other lobes. Simultaneous malignant transformation of all potentially malignant cells within the lobe is relatively rare; more often, only part(s) of the sick lobe appears to be transformed at the time of detection. This observation also means that the already malignant part(s) of the sick lobe is expected to be surrounded by the remaining nontransformed area of the risk tissue. At that point, the sick lobe theory is congruent with the ideas of several other research groups postulating the existence of a "genetic field" or "field of cancerization," or more recently, the "cancer-prone field" within the breast. Similar ideas and observations were presented by Slaughter et al. as early as 1953 (Slaughter et al. 1953) in relation to oral squamous cell carcinoma. As reviewed recently, a large series of publications indicate the correctness of this hypothesis (Heaphy et al. 2009).

The cells of in situ carcinomas exhibit similar or identical genetic changes as the invasive part of the tumor. This fact is not surprising because the invasive component develops from in situ lesions, which was already demonstrated in the middle 1990s regarding ductal carcinoma in situ (DCIS) using the method of demonstrating loss of heterozygosity (Stratton et al. 1995) and later using comparative genomic hybridization (Buerger et al. 1999), and regarding lobular carcinoma in situ (LCIS) (Lakhani et al. 1995a). Lakhani et al. (1995b) also demonstrated loss of heterozygosity in atypical ductal hyperplasia (ADH). Simpson et al. (2005) found identical alterations in columnar cell change (CCC) and the associated invasive cancer. DCIS, LCIS, ADH, and CCC are considered precursor lesions of invasive carcinomas; thus, sharing some genetic alterations with the invasive component was expected.

However, loss of heterozygosity was demonstrated by analyzing the cells of usual ductal epithelial hyperplasia in specimens containing breast carcinoma (Lakhani et al. 1996) and similar results were generated with comparative genomic hybridization (Jones et al. 2003). These results were more unexpected, because ductal hyperplasia is considered to be associated with an increased risk of developing cancer but not as being a direct precursor lesion.

Deng et al. (1996) found loss of heterozygosity in morphologically normal breast tissue surrounding invasive carcinoma; the results were later on confirmed by Meng et al. (2004). By cloning individual cells, Lakhani et al. (1999) demonstrated genetic changes in histologically normal breast tissue identical to those in invasive carcinoma, both close to and distant from the invasive tumor, and in breasts without morphological evidence of malignancy. Alterations were also shown to appear not only in the epithelial cells, but also in myoepithelial cells, indicating that the alterations occurred in a stem cell/progenitor cell lineage. These important observations were made by Clarke et al. (2006a), who demonstrated that genetic alterations at the single cell level may be clustered and extend to an area that consists of more than one TDLU, and that such clustering suggests that a change may have occurred in a precursor cell that gave rise to that area of the breast. In other words, they found that a field of genetic instability can exist around a tumor in a morphologically normal tissue, and it may exist before the tumor develops. By mapping geographic zones of "normal" breast tissue adjacent to primary breast carcinoma by DNA methylation changes, a field of these changes extending as far as 4 cm from the primary lesion was demonstrated (Yan et al. 2006). These findings are congruent with the average size of a sick lobe.

Cancer seems to be a stem cell/progenitor cell disease. As mentioned above, if a progenitor cell acquires a mutation, it can be passed on to all of its progeny, resulting in a chimeric network of normal and mutant cells. The mutant cells may be dispersed in the structures derived from the progenitor cells, explaining the susceptibility of this structure to oncogenic stimuli (Tsai et al. 1996; Cariati and Purushotham 2008). This idea was the basis of the so-called committed progenitor cell concept of Agelopoulos et al. (2008), a concept very close in its views to those of the sick lobe theory and the theory of biological timing.

1.4.3 Supporting Epidemiological Data

Additional evidence supporting the sick lobe theory was presented by recent epidemiological studies. A clear association between birth weight and other neonatal parameters and the risk of getting breast carcinoma as an adult was found by Xue and Michels (2007). The authors suggested that elevated levels of growth factors may increase the number of susceptible stem cells in the mammary gland during embryonic life and initiate tumors through DNA mutations. Birth weight was also found to be associated with mammographic breast density (Cerhan et al. 2005), which in turn is a strong risk factor for breast carcinoma, as discussed earlier in this chapter. Thus, we can conclude that experimental and epidemiological evidence supports the concept that the in utero environment influences the individuals' risk of breast carcinoma in adulthood.

As mentioned above, breast tissue is not fully differentiated until after the first full-time pregnancy. Consequently, the tissue seems to be more susceptible to carcinogenic influences during early life and adolescence. A positive relationship between breast cancer risk and birth weight, birth length, and adolescent height, and an inverse relationship with gestational age and childhood body mass index, has been suggested (Ruder et al. 2008), supporting the idea that breast carcinoma is a lifelong process.

1.5 Breast Cancer at Its Earliest Phase

1.5.1 Conditions for Perceiving Breast Carcinoma as a Lobar Disease

Several conditions have to be fulfilled to realize the lobar nature of breast carcinoma. Difficulties in perceiving breast cancer as a lobar disease are numerous and may prevent individuals, including those at the expert level, from seriously considering this possibility. Studying a fragment of an invasive carcinoma provides no opportunity for such a discovery. Nevertheless, the conventional fragmenting histopathology method is still a routine in most pathology laboratories diagnosing breast diseases and is advocated by most of the top experts in the field. Using this method, the pathologists examine the intact and sliced specimens macroscopically, localize the "dominant" mass, take samples from the mass and the surgical margins, and carefully cut out and throw away the surrounding tissue. This surrounding tissue corresponds, at least partly, to the risk tissue of the genetic field and often contains additional in situ and invasive tumor foci, foci of atypical hyperplasia, and minute monomorphic epithelial cell proliferations considered to be the source of some invasive carcinomas (Goldstein et al. 2007). Proper assessment of the focality of the in situ and invasive tumor components and proper judgment of the pattern of tumor development is not possible without thorough examination of the surrounding tissue. Nonfragmenting histology methods are necessary to facilitate the assessment of these important morphological features.

The routine use of large-format histology sections in diagnostic histopathology in connection with detailed and systematic radiological–pathological correlation in all cases provides the experience that facilitates the perception of the morphological growth pattern in breast cancer cases (Tot et al. 2002; Tabár et al. 2007). This approach also allows the careful observer to notice the tendency of the lesions to be concentrated in the area of a lobe-like space.

In addition, studying advanced cases provides no opportunity for realizing the lobar nature of breast carcinoma. Breast cancer is lobar at its origin, but propagates to the nearby tissue beyond the borders of the sick lobe when advanced, large, and overtly invasive. Carcinomas tend to be detected at their earlier phase in a mammographically screened population. We define early breast cancer as purely in situ tumors and tumors with invasive component of less than 15 mm. These tumors have a 10 year disease-specific survival of over 90%. This category of tumors comprised approximately 50% of all cases in a regularly screened population and approximately 70% of screen-detected cases in our subject pool (Tot 2007b).

1.5.2 Morphology of Breast Cancer at Its Earliest Phase

The two hypotheses described in the present chapter are based on our experience with a series of more than 3,000 cancer cases documented in large-format histological sections and worked up with detailed and systematic radiological–pathological correlation. Studying early breast carcinomas using this approach allowed us to formulate the most probable patterns of breast cancer development at the earliest phase of its natural history.

Because the malignant transformation may appear at any locus of the sick lobe, its timing will determine the focality of the disease. Many combinations may exist, but three patterns seem to be seen most often (Fig. 1.6). If most of the potentially malignant cells within the sick lobe are transformed into malignant clones simultaneously, the entire lobe of the breast (the entire ductal tree together with the lobules) will become cancerous. From a theoretical point of view, this pattern may be a result of the accumulation of further mutations in that subtype of mutant stem cells, which are capable of renewing an entire lobe. Because the size of the lobes vary from 2% to 23% of the breast volume (Going and Moffat 2004), this lobar scenario of cancer development may result in tumors that are several centimeters in size from the very beginning of their development. In this case, the tumor is large and extensive, involving a large volume of the breast tissue, and the tumor burden (the number of malignant cells present) is very high. A typical example is high-grade comedo-type or micropapillary in situ carcinomas (Fig. 1.7a), which are the cases in which the lobar nature of breast carcinoma is easiest to perceive upon radiological examination. On the other hand, these tumors are difficult to treat and may have an unfavorable prognosis (Tabár et al. 2004).

The second scenario is the malignant transformation involving a segment of the lobe, a branch of the ductal tree together with the lobules belonging to this branch (Fig. 1.7b). As in the case of the lobar pattern of cancer development within the sick lobe, the transformation is nearly continuous in this segmental pattern and involves most of the structures of the segment at the same time, or with a time difference. Theoretically, this pattern may be a result of a disturbed arborization process due to an accumulation of mutations in that type of mutant stem/progenitor cells that are capable of producing branching ducts. The tumor burden and extent of the disease is relatively limited, usually intermediate between that of the lobar and the peripheral pattern.

The peripheral pattern of malignant transformation within the sick lobe is characterized by the involvement

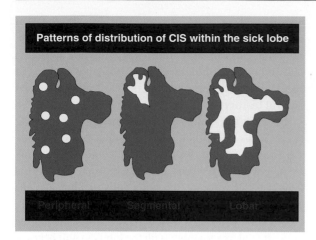

Fig. 1.6 Schematic illustrations of the three subgross morphological patterns of in situ breast carcinoma

capable of producing secretory lobules. The tumor burden is usually low, even if a large number of lobules are involved, but the disease may be extensive, because the involved lobules may be distant from each other in a large sick lobe. Consequently, this form of the disease is not easy to treat, but the prognosis is favorable. Typical examples of this pattern of cancer development within the breast are lobular carcinoma in situ and low-grade ductal carcinoma in situ.

The size of the sick lobe, the distribution of the mutant stem cells/committed progenitor cells within it, and the biological timing of their malignant transformation will determine the extent of the disease and the distribution of the tumor foci during the natural evolution of the breast carcinoma. In addition, the genetic construction (high-grade versus low-grade pathway of genetic changes) will influence the morphology, molecular characteristics, and speed of evolution; tumors with a high-grade genetic pathway will progress more rapidly than tumors with a low-grade pathway (Wiechmann and Kuerer 2008).

In the earliest phase of cancer development, the malignant cells are confined to the preexisting ducts and/or lobules, which may be distended and distorted

of the lobules, usually without involvement of segmental and lactiferous ducts (Fig. 1.7c). The lobules may be involved simultaneously or with a considerable time difference. This pattern may be a result of a disturbed lobularization process due to an accumulation of mutations in that type of mutant stem/progenitor cells that are

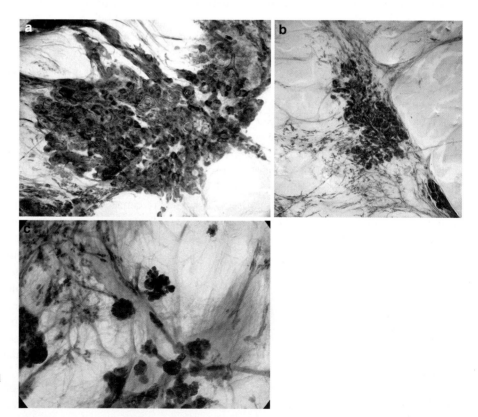

Fig. 1.7 Large-format thick (1 mm) section images demonstrating lobar (**a**), segmental (**b**), and peripheral (**c**) subgross patterns of in situ breast carcinoma

by the accumulation of malignant cells and their products. Low-grade lesions tend to be localized within the terminal ducts and lobules, whereas high-grade lesions often involve the larger ducts (Tot and Tabár 2005). The neoplastic process itself may maintain the lobular architecture and/or lead to the formation of new lobules and small ducts. Some high-grade in situ carcinomas are also able to form new larger ducts within the involved sick lobe, a pathological process termed neoductgenesis. These tumors may histologically exhibit not only a substantially higher number of ducts than anatomically expected within the breast tissue, but also early signs of epithelial–stromal interaction in the form of periductal tenascin C accumulation and lymphocytic infiltration, and they are regarded as being at an intermediate step between conventional in situ and conventional invasive lesions (Tabár et al. 2007).

Breast cancer cells are epithelial in character, but the myoepithelial cell layer and tissue environment of the tumor also participate in tumor development. Most breast tumor suppressor genes are expressed in the myoepithelial cells, which act to restrict tumoral growth to its in situ phase (Sager 1997). Further mutations in the malignant cells and the cells of the surrounding stroma may, however, lead to deregulation of the epithelial–stromal balance; consequently, the cancer cells lose their ability to maintain the myoepithelial layer and the basal membrane around the ducts and lobules and the normal periductal, intralobular, and interlobular stroma undergoes remodeling. Individual cancer cells and their groups come into direct contact with stromal elements and become entrapped in the remodeled stroma. They may change their phenotype and undergo epithelial–mesenchymal transition. The cancer cells may also come into contact with prelymphatic spaces and lymphatic vessels, invade them, and become transported via the lymphatic system within the breast, resulting in intramammary tumor spread (Asioli et al. 2008) and development of multiple invasive tumor foci. In this manner, the invasive tumor may spread beyond the area of the sick lobe. Thus, the invasive component of the tumor may grow by proliferation of the malignant cells, not only around the preexistent in situ process but also in distant places. New tumor foci may coalesce to form a larger tumor mass with more complex morphology. New cell clones may appear in the invasive foci by further mutations and dedifferentiation, leading to intratumoral and intertumoral heterogeneity within the same breast. The

cancer cells or the committed progenitor cells that spread from the breast to the lymph nodes and other organs may develop into a metastasis by cell proliferation and interaction with the components of the targeted tissue. By these mechanisms, the tumor gradually enters its advanced phase.

Mutant stem cells and committed progenitor cells share many characteristics with malignant stem cells. These mobile cells may, in some cases, enter the circulation and be transported to lymph nodes and other organs. Malignant transformation of the cell progeny may require several years or decades, like their counterparts within the breast. Transformation of these relocated mutant progenitor cells prior to the transformation of the intramammary compartment of these cells may give rise to a metastasis of "unknown origin." This concept may represent a possible explanation for, at least some cases of, the so-called CUP (cancer with unknown primary) syndrome. Such a transformation may also take place decades later than the intramammary transformation.

1.5.3 Early Breast Cancer is Not Necessarily "Small"

Using large-format two- and three-dimensional histological sections and the approach of detailed and systematic radiological–pathological correlation, we demonstrated that in situ carcinoma may be confined to lobules, ducts, or both and manifest as a unifocal, multifocal, or diffuse process as described above (Tot and Tabár 2005). We also analyzed a large number of early and more advanced invasive breast carcinomas and found that roughly one-third were unifocal, consisting of a single invasive focus (containing or not containing an in situ component), one-third were multifocal due to the multifocality of the in situ component, and one-third contained multiple invasive foci. A small proportion of advanced breast carcinomas grow diffusely, much like a spider web (Tot 2007c, 2009; Tot et al. 2009). Figure 1.8 illustrates our results regarding lesion distribution and disease extent in a series of 907 consecutively diagnosed breast carcinomas at our department during the period of 2005–2009. Only a minority of the cases were unifocal, regardless of the phase of development (in situ or invasive) or the size of the invasive component; roughly 40–50% of the

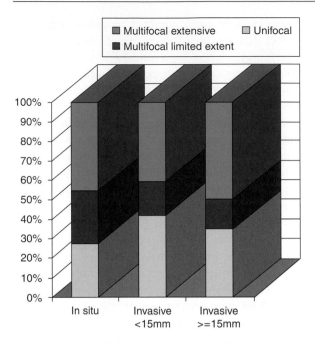

Fig. 1.8 Subgross distribution of cases in a series of 907 (Falun, 2005–2009) consecutively diagnosed new breast carcinomas by extent of the disease

cases were extensive and spread in a tissue volume of 40 mm or more in the largest dimension. Breast cancer is not necessarily small at the earliest stages of its development; on the contrary, it is widespread and multifocal in the majority of cases. These results are fully concordant with the results of similar studies using large-format histology (Andersen et al. 1987; Holland et al. 1990; Faverly et al. 2001; Foschini et al. 2007).

1.6 Practical Consequences, Future Perspectives

The theory of the sick lobe defines the risk tissue of malignant transformation that corresponds to a lobe with increased susceptibility to oncogenic effects compared to other lobes. The risk tissue is not a single TDLU but a field of genetic instability, which may be several centimeters large. Regardless of the size of the tumor (size of the largest invasive tumor focus), multiple in situ and invasive foci are often present in this field and may be located several centimeters from each other. Some of these lesions may be radiologically or

clinically undetectable. Early breast carcinomas are as often multifocal and extensive as are their more advanced counterparts.

An intervention that aims to remove only the detectable part of the already malignant component of the process and leaves the rest of the sick lobe in the breast is associated with a high risk of local recurrence. Nearly 40% of patients who undergo breast conserving surgery without additional irradiation and/or antihormonal therapy get ipsilateral local recurrences within 20 years (Fisher et al. 2002). The vast majority of local recurrences appear in the area adjacent to the surgical scar, indicating that they have developed in the rest of the partially removed sick lobe. According to our concept, an adequate surgical intervention has to remove not only the detected malignant tissue, but also the risk tissue, the entire sick lobe, around it. Although intravital marking of the sick lobe is not fully possible, the risk of local recurrence can be substantially lowered by sector resection (removing a lobe-like part of the breast) compared to lumpectomy (aiming to excise the malignant tissue). Cases resulting from extensive involvement of a large sick lobe, on the other hand, require mastectomy.

Removing or destructing the sick lobe prior to the development of malignant cells within it would eliminate the risk of getting breast carcinoma in the vast majority of cases. Efficient methods for the detection and intravital indication of the sick lobe are required to allow the wide application of the method in treating and preventing breast carcinoma.

1.7 Conclusions

The theory of the sick lobe and the theory of biological timing connect the process of carcinogenesis to an existing and well-defined anatomic structure, a breast lobe, and provide a possible explanation for the progressive character and morphological heterogeneity of breast carcinoma. These theories are more than a description of morphological patterns. They put these patterns into a unifying concept with genetic, developmental, and morphological perspectives of understanding breast carcinoma as a process that develops over time under endogenous and exogenous influences, not like a photo, but like a lifelong movie.

We are only at the beginning of exploring the advantages of this new concept, but we can already present promising research and important results. As knowledge is the most powerful weapon of mankind, the most important expected impact of this book will be a better understanding of the disease called breast cancer due to a critical rethinking of traditional paradigms. This understanding will allow us and future generations to alter the negative trend of increasing breast cancer incidence and relieve the women of the twenty-first century of the risk of getting breast carcinoma.

References

Agelopoulos K, Buerger H, Brandt B (2008) Allelic imbalance of the egfr gene as key event in breast cancer progression – the concept of committed progenitor cells. Curr Cancer Drug Targets 8:431–445

Al-Hajj M, Wicha MS, Benito-Hernandez A, Morrison SJ, Clarke MF (2003) Prospective identification of tumorigenic breast cancer cells. Proc Natl Acad Sci USA 100: 3983–3988

Andersen JA, Blichert-Toft M, Dyreborg U (1987) In situ carcinomas of the breast. Types, growth pattern, diagnosis and treatment. Eur J Surg Oncol 13:105–111

Asioli S, Eusebi V, Gaetano L, Losi L, Bussolati G (2008) The pre-lymphatic pathway, the roots of the lymphatic system in the breast tissue: a 3D study. Virchows Arch 453:401–406

Baik I, Becker PS, Devito WJ, Lagiou P, Ballen K, Quesenberry PJ, Hsiech CC (2004) Stem cells and prenatal origin of breast cancer. Cancer Causes Control 15:517–530

Boecker W, Burger H (2003) Evidence of progenitor cells of glandular and myoepithelial cell lineages in the human adult female breast epithelium: a new progenitor (adult stem cell) concept. Cell Prolif 36(Suppl 1):73–84

Boyle P, Ferlay J (2005) Cancer incidence and mortality in Europe 2004. Ann Oncol 16(3):481–488

Buell P (1973) Changing incidence in breast cancer in Japanese-American women. J Natl Cancer Inst 51:1479–1483

Buerger H, Otterbach F, Simon R, Poremba C, Diallo R, Decker T, Reithdorf L, Brinkschmidt C, Dockhorn-Deorniczak B, Boecker W (1999) Comparative genomic hybridization of ductal carcinoma in situ of the breast – evidence of multiple genetic pathways. J Pathol 187:396–402

Cardiff RD, Wellings SR (1999) The comparative pathology of human and mouse mammary glands. J Mammary Gland Biol Neoplasia 4:105–122

Cariati M, Purushotham AD (2008) Stem cells and breast cancer. Histopathology 52:99–107

Cerhan JR, Sellers TA, Janney CA, Pankratz VS, Brandt KR, Vachon CM (2005) Prenatal and perinatal correlates of adult mammographic breast densities. Cancer Epidemiol Biomarkers Prev 14:1502–1508

Cheatle GL (1921) Benign and malignant changes in duct epithelium of the breast. Br J Cancer 8:306

Clarke RB (2005) Isolation of characterization of human mammary stem cells. Cell Prolif 38:375–386

Clarke CA, Glaser SL, West DW, Ereman RR, Erdmann CA, Barlow JM, Wrensch MR (2002) Breast cancer incidence and mortality trends in an affluent population: Marin County, California, USA, 1990–1996. Breast Cancer Res 4:R13

Clarke CL, Sandle J, Jones AA, Sofronis A, Patani NR, Lakhani SR (2006a) Mapping loss of heterozygosity in normal human breast cells from BRCA1/2 carriers. Br J Cancer 95: 515–519

Clarke MF, Dick JE, Dirks PB, Eaves CJ, Jammison CH, Jones DL, Visvader J, Weissman IL, Wahl GM (2006b) Cancer stem cells – perspectives on current status and future directions. Cancer Res 66:9339–9344

Dawson FK (1933) Carcinoma in the mammary lobule and its origin. Edinb Med J 40:57–82

De Angelis R, Tavilla A, Verdechia A, Scoppa S, Hachey M, Feuer EJ, Mariotto AB (2009) Breast cancer survivors in the United States: geographic variability and time trends, 2005–2015. Cancer 115:1954–1966

Deng G, Lu Y, Zlotnikov G, Thor AD, Smith HS (1996) Loss of heterozygosity in normal tissue adjacent to breast carcinoma. Science 274:2057–2059

Deome KB, Faulkin IJ Jr, Bern HA, Blair PB (1959) Development of mammary tumors from hyperplastic alveolar nodules transplanted into gland-free mammary fat pads of female C3H mice. Cancer Res 19:515–520

Donnenberg VS, Donnenberg AD (2005) Multiple drug resistance in cancer revisited: the cancer stem cell hypothesis. J Clin Pharmacol 45:872–907

Dooley WC (2003) Routine operative breast endoscopy during lumpectomy. Ann Surg Oncol 10:38–42

Easton DF, Steele L, Fields P, Orminston W, Averill D, Daly PA, McManus R, Neuhausen ST, Ford D, Wooster R, Cannon-Albright LA, Stratton MR, Goldgar DE (1997) Cancer risk in two large breast cancer families linked to BRCA2 on chromosome 13q12-13. Am J Hum Genet 61:120–128

Ewing J (1940) Neoplastic diseases. A treatise of tumors, 4th edn. Saunders WB, Philadelphia, p 568

Faverly DRG, Henricks JHCL, Holland R (2001) Breast carcinoma of limited extent. Frequency, radiologic–pathologic characteristics, and surgical margin requirements. Cancer 91:647–659

Fisher B, Costantino JP, Wickerham DL, Redmond CK, Kavanah M, Cronin WM, Vogel V, Robidoux A, Dimitrov N, Atkins J, Daly M, Wieand S, Tan-Chiu E, Ford L, Wolmark N (1998) Tamoxifen for prevention of breast cancer: report of the National Surgical Adjuvant Breast and Bowel Project P-1 Study. J Natl Cancer Inst 90:1371–1388

Fisher B, Anderson S, Bryant J, Margolese RG, Deutsch M, Fisher ER, Jaong JH, Wolmark N (2002) Twenty-year follow-up of a randomized trial comparing total mastectomy, lumpectomy, and lumpectomy plus irradiation for the treatment of invasive breast cancer. N Engl J Med 347:1233–1241

Ford D, Easton DF, Bishop DT, Narod SA, Godgar DE (1994) Risk of cancer in BRCA1-mutation carriers. Breast Cancer Linkage Consortium. Lancet 343:692–695

Foschini MP, Flamminio F, Miglio R, Calo DG, Cucchi MC, Masetti R, Eusebi V (2007) The impact of large sections on the study of in situ and invasive duct carcinoma of the breast. Hum Pathol 38:1736–1743

Gallagher S, Martin JE (1969) Early phases in the development of breast cancer. Cancer 24:1170–1178

Going JJ, Moffat DF (2004) Escaping from flatland: clinical and biological aspects of human mammary duct anatomy in three dimensions. J Pathol 203:538–544

Going JJ, Mohun TJ (2006) Human breast duct anatomy, the 'sick lobe' hypothesis and intraductal approaches to breast cancer. Breast Cancer Res Treat 97:285–291

Goldstein NS, Kestin LJ, Vicini FA (2007) Monomorphic epithelial proliferations. Characterization and evidence suggesting they are the pool of partially transformed lesions from which some invasive carcinomas arise. Am J Clin Pathol 128:1023–1034

Gudjonsson T, Magnusson MK (2005) Stem cell biology and the pathways of carcinogenesis. APMIS 113:922–929

Harper S, Lynch J, Meersman SC, Breen N, Davis WW, Reichman MC (2009) Trends in area-socioeconomic and race-ethnic disparities in breast cancer incidence, stage at diagnosis, screening, mortality, and survival among women ages 50 years and over (1987–2005). Cancer Epidemiol Biomarkers Prev 18:121–131

Harris JR, Lippman ME, Veronesi U, Willet W (1992) Breast cancer. N Engl J Med 327:319–328

Heaphy CM, Griffith JK, Bisoffi M (2009) Mammary field cancerization: molecular evidence and clinical importance. Breast Cancer Res Treat 118:229–239

Hill AD, Doyle JM, McDermott EW, O'Higgins NJ (1997) Hereditary breast cancer. Br J Surg 84:1334–1339

Holland R, Hendricks JH, Vebeek AL, Mravunac M, Schuurmans Stekhoven JH (1990) Extent, distribution, and mammographic/histological correlation of breast ductal carcinoma in situ. Lancet 335:519–522

Honeth G, Bendahl PO, Ringnér M, Saal LH, Gruvbenger-Saal SK, Lövgren K, Grabau D, Fernö M, Borg A, Hegardt C (2008) The CD44+/CD24− phenotype is enriched in basal-like breast tumors. Breast Cancer Res 10:R53

Hortobagyi GN (2005) Trastuzumab in the treatment of breast cancer. N Engl J Med 353:1734–1736

Howard BA, Gustersson BA (2000) Human breast development. J Mammary Gland Biol Neoplasia 5:119–137

Jolicoeur F, Gaboury LA, Oligny LL (2003) Basal cells of second trimester fetal breasts: immunohistochemical study of myoepithelial precursors. Pediatr Dev Pathol 6:398–413

Jones C, Merrett S, Thomas VA, Barker TH, Lakhani SR (2003) Comparative genomic hybridization analysis of bilateral hyperplasia of usual type of the breast. J Pathol 199:152–156

Kawamura T, Sobue T (2005) Comparison of breast cancer mortality in five countries: France, Italy, Japan, the UK and the USA from the WHO mortality database (1960–2000). Jpn J Clin Oncol 35:758–759

Lakhani SR, Collins N, Sloane JP, Stratton MR (1995a) Loss of heterozygosity in lobular carcinoma in situ of the breast. Clin Mol Pathol 48:M74–M78

Lakhani SR, Collins N, Stratton MR, Sloane JP (1995b) Atypical ductal hyperplasia of the breast: clonal proliferation with loss of heterozygosity on chromosome 16q and 17p. J Clin Pathol 48:611–615

Lakhani SR, Slack DN, Hamoudi RA, Collins N, Stratton MR, Sloane JP (1996) Detection of allelic imbalance indicates that a proportion of mammary hyperplasia of usual type are clonal, neoplastic proliferations. Lab Invest 74:129–135

Lakhani SR, Chaggar R, Davies S, Jones C, Collins N, Odell C, Stratton MR, O'Hare M (1999) Genetic alterations in "normal" luminal and myoepithelial cells of the breast. J Pathol 189:496–503

Lányi M (1977) Differential diagnosis of microcalcifications, X-ray film analysis of 60 intraductal carcinoma, the triangle principle. Radiologe 17:213–216

Little P, Boice JD Jr (1999) Comparison of breast cancer incidence in the Massachusetts tuberculosis fluoroscopy cohort and in the Japanese atomic bomb survivors. Radiat Res 151:218–224

Liu S, Ginestier C, Charafe-Jauffret E, Foco H, Kleer CG, Merajver SD, Dontu G, Wisha MS (2008) BRCA1 regulates human mammary stem/progenitor cell fate. Proc Natl Acad Sci USA 105:1680–1685

Mai KT, Yazdi HM, Burns BF, Perkins DG (2000) Pattern of distribution of intraductal and infiltrating ductal carcinoma: Three-dimensional study using serial coronal giant sections of the breast. Hum Pathol 31:464–474

Meng ZH, Ben Y, Li Z, Chew K, Ljung BM, Lagios MD, Dairkee SH (2004) Aberrations of breast cancer susceptibility genes occur early in sporadic breast tumors and in acquisition of breast epithelial immortalization. Genes Chromosomes Cancer 41:214–222

Middleton LP, Vlastos G, Mirza NQ, Eva S, Sahin AA (2002) Multicentric mammary carcinoma, evidence of monoclonal proliferation. Cancer 94:1910–1916

Ohtake T, Abe R, Kimijima I, Fukushima T, Tsuchiya A, Hashi K, Wakasa H (1995) Intraductal extension of primary invasive breast carcinoma treated by breast-conservative surgery. Computer graphic three-dimensional reconstruction of the mammary duct-lobular systems. Cancer 76:32–45

Page DL, Rogers LW, Schuyler PA, Dupont WD, Jensen RA (2002) The natural history of ductal carcinoma in situ of the breast. In: Silverstein MJ (ed) Ductal carcinoma of the breast, 2nd edn. Lippincott Williams & Wilkins, Philadelphia, pp 17–21

Ramakrishnan R, Seema AK, Badve S (2002) Morphologic changes in breast tissue with menstrual cycle. Mod Pathol 15:1348–1356

Reya T, Morrison SJ, Clarke MF, Weissmann IL (2001) Stem cells, cancer, and cancer stem cells. Nature 414:105–111

Ruder EH, Dorgan JF, Kranz S, Kris-Etherton PM, Hartman TJ (2008) Examining breast cancer growth and lifetime risk factors: early life, childhood and adolescence. Clin Breast Cancer 8:334–342

Rudland PS (1991) Histochemical organization and cellular composition of ductal buds in developing human breast: evidence of cytochemical intermediates between epithelial and myoepithelial cells. J Histochem Cytochem 39:1471–1484

Russo J, Russo IH (2004) Molecular basis of breast cancer. Prevention and treatment. Springer, Berlin/Heidelberg/New York/Hong Kong/London/Milan/Paris/Tokio

Sager R (1997) Expression genetics in cancer: shifting the focus from DNA to RNA. Proc Natl Acad Sci USA 94:952–955

Sakakura T, Ishihara A, Yatani R (1991) Tenascin in mammary gland development: from embryogenesis to carcinogenesis. Cancer Treat Res 53:383–400

Simpson PT, Gale T, Reis-Filho JS, Jones C, Parry S, Sloane JP, Hanby A, Pinder SE, Lee AH, Humphreys S, Ellis IO, Lakhani SR (2005) Columnar cell lesions of the breast: the missing link in breast cancer progression? A morphological and molecular analysis. Am J Surg Pathol 29:734–736

Slaughter DP, Southwick HW, Smejkal W (1953) Field cancerization in oral stratified squamous epithelium: clinical implications of multicentric origin. Cancer 6:963–968

Smith GH, Boulanger CA (2003) Mammary epithelial stem cells transplantation and self-renewal analysis. Cell Prolif 36(Suppl 1):3–15

Smith RA, Duffy SW, Gabe R, Tabár L, Yen AM, Chen TH (2004) The randomized trials of breast cancer screening: what have we learned? Radiol Clin North Am 42:793–806

Smith BD, Smith GL, Hurria A, Hortobagyi GN, Buchholz TA (2009) Future of cancer incidence in the United States: burdens upon aging, changing nation. J Clin Oncol 27:1–10

Stratton MR, Collins N, Lakhani SR, Sloane JP (1995) Loss of heterozygosity in ductal carcinoma in situ of the breast. J Pathol 175:195–201

Tabár L, Chen HT, Yen MFA, Tot T, Tung TH, Chen LS, Chiu YH, Duffy SW, Smith RA (2004) Mammographic tumor features can predict long-term outcomes reliably in women with 1–14 mm invasive carcinoma. Cancer 101:1745–1759

Tabár L, Tot T, Dean PB (2007) Breast cancer. Early detection with mammography. Casting type calcifications: sign of a subtype with deceptive features. Thieme, Stuttgart/New York

Tabár L, Tot T, Dean PB (2008) Crushed stone-like calcifications: the most frequent malignant type. Thieme, Stuttgart/New York

Tavassoli FA, Devili P (eds) (2003) World Health Organization classification of tumors. Pathology & genetics. Tumors of the breast and female genital organs. IARC, Lyon, p 63

Teboul M, Halliwell M (1995) Atlas of ultrasound and ductal echography of the breast: the introduction of anatomic intelligence into breast imaging. Wiley-Blackwell, UK, p 380

The Swedish Organized Service Screening Evaluation Group (2006) Reduction in breast cancer mortality from organized service screening with mammography: 1. Further confirmation with expanded data. Cancer Epidemiol Biomarkers Prev 15:45–51

Tot T (2005a) Correlating the ground truth of mammographic histology with the success or failure of imaging. Technol Cancer Res Treat 4:23–28

Tot T (2005b) DCIS, cytokeratins, and the theory of the sick lobe. Virchows Arch 447:1–8

Tot T (2007a) The theory of the sick breast lobe and the possible consequences. Int J Surg Pathol 15:369–375

Tot T (2007b) How to eradicate breast carcinomas: a hypothetical way of breast cancer prevention based on the theory of the sick lobe. In: Litchfield JE (ed) New research in precancerous conditions. Nova, New York, pp 165–181

Tot T (2007c) The clinical relevance of the distribution of the lesions in 500 consecutive breast cancer cases documented in large-format histological sections. Cancer 110:2551–2560

Tot T (2009) The metastatic capacity of multifocal breast carcinomas: extensive tumors versus tumors of limited extent. Hum Pathol 40:199–205

Tot T, Tabár L (2005) Radiologic–pathologic correlation of ductal carcinoma in situ of the breast using two- and three-dimensional large histologic sections. Semin Breast Dis 8:144–151

Tot T, Tabár L, Dean PB (2000) The pressing need for better histologic–mammographic correlation of the many variations in normal breast anatomy. Virchows Arch 437:338–344

Tot T, Tabár L, Dean PB (2002) Practical breast pathology. Thieme, Stuttgart/New York

Tot T, Pekár G, Hofmeyer S, Sollie T, Gere M, Tarján M (2009) The distribution of lesions in 1–14-mm invasive breast carcinomas and its relation to metastatic potential. Virchows Arch 455:109–115

Trichopoulos D (1990) Hypothesis: does breast cancer originate in utero? Lancet 335:939–940

Tsai YC, Lu Y, Nichols PW, Zlotnikow G, Jones PA, Smith HS (1996) Contiguous patches of normal human mammary epithelium derived from a single stem cell: implications for breast carcinogenesis. Cancer Res 56:402–404

Villadsen R (2005) In search of stem cell hierarchy in the human breast and its relevance in breast cancer evolution. APMIS 113:903–921

Villadsen R, Fridriksdottir AJ, Ronnov-Jenssen L, Gudjunsson T, Rank F, LaBarge MA, Bissell MJ, Petersen OW (2007) Evidence for stem cell hierarchy in the adult human breast. J Cell Biol 177:87–101

Wang Y, Yang J, Zheng H, Tomasek GJ, Zhang P, McKeever PE, Lee EY, Zhu Y (2009) Expression of mutant p53 proteins implicates a lineage relationship between neural stem cells and malignant astrocytic glioma in a murine model. Cancer Cell 15:514–526

Wellings SR, Jensen HM, Marcum RG (1975) An atlas of subgross pathology of the human breast with special reference to possible precancerous lesions. J Natl Cancer Inst 55:231–273

Wiechmann L, Kuerer HM (2008) The molecular journey from ductal carcinoma in situ to invasive breast cancer. Cancer 112:2130–2142

Wolff MS, Collman GW, Barrett JC, Huff J (1996) Breast cancer and environmental risk factors: epidemiological and experimental findings. Annu Rev Pharmacol Toxicol 36:573–596

Xue F, Michels KB (2007) Intrauterine factors and risk of breast cancer: a systemic review and meta-analysis of current evidence. Lancet Oncol 8:1088–1100

Yan PS, Venkataramu C, Ibrahim A, Liu JC, Shen RZ, Diaz NM, Centeno B, Webel F, Leu UW, Shapiro CL, Eng C, Yeatman TJ, Huang TH (2006) Mapping geographic zones of cancer risk with epigenetic biomarkers in normal breast tissue. Clin Cancer Res 12:6626–6636

Lobar Anatomy of Human Breast and Its Importance for Breast Cancer

2

James J. Going

I have heard a good anatomist say, "the breast is so complicated I can make nothing clear of it."

Astley Paston Cooper, *On the Anatomy of the Breast* (Cooper 1840).

When a powerful new method emerges the study of those problems which can be dealt with by the new method advances rapidly and attracts the limelight, while the rest tends to be ignored or even forgotten, its study despised.

Imre Lakatos, Proofs and Refutations: The Logic of Mathematical Discovery (Lakatos 1976).

2.1 Introduction: Anatomy of Human Breast as a Subject of Scientific Study

Some believe that anatomy has experienced the fate described by Lakatos (Marušič 2008). But, while molecular explanations are more highly favored in biology, no single "thought-style" (Fleck 1979) can explain a process as complex as breast cancer, influenced by events at every scale from molecules to society and the environment, occurring over time scales from less than a second to a human lifetime. This chapter addresses a neglected order of breast organization which deserves closer attention: its partitioning into *lobes*.

Reasons for this neglect include a human tendency not to notice gaps in our knowledge. Anatomist and pioneer senologist Sir Astley Cooper may also be partly responsible: a serious commentator as recently as the mid-twentieth century could suggest that Cooper had said all that needed to be said about the large-scale anatomy of the breast (Brock 1952), including its lobar structure.

Cooper's own comment ("it was absolutely necessary to give an account of the natural structure of the breast, before its morbid changes could be properly explained or understood"; Cooper 1840) was true then, and is true today. But while *On the Anatomy of the Breast* still contains more original data about lobar organization of human breast tissue than almost any twentieth or twenty-first century primary source, Astley Cooper did not say the last word on the subject, and would, I think, have been surprised by such an idea; so it is satisfying that new work on morphology of human breast is being undertaken (Ramsay et al. 2005; Going 2006; Geddes 2007; Rusby et al. 2007).

Cooper was one of the last first-rate anatomists not also to be a microscopist, though he did see it in use (Cooper 1843). Joseph Jackson Lister had invented the achromatic microscope in the 1820s, but the rise of histology as a discipline (von Gerlach 1848) waited on theoretical and practical developments including cell theory (Schleiden and Schwann), Virchow's insight that all cells arise from preexisting cells ("omnis cellula e cellula"), development of the microtome by Wilhelm His, senior, and improved staining, all of which emphasized *the cell* as the fundamental unit of tissue organization.

The molecular revolution of the twentieth century may, then, seem to place large-scale aspects of anatomy at two removes from contemporary biological science, but the breast parenchyma and its stroma remain the theater of the cellular and molecular dramas of normal mammary development

J.J. Going
Institute of Cancer Sciences, Glasgow University and
Pathology Department, Glasgow Royal Infirmary,
Glasgow, UK
e-mail: going@udcf.gla.ac.uk

and breast disease during infancy, adulthood, and old age, and as these processes occur on multiple spatial scales, including that with which we are concerned (the lobe), its present relevance is greater than ever.

2.2 Limitations of Classical Microscopy

While microscopy is well adapted to the study of microscopic entities, including small portions of human breast tissue, and an entire murine mammary gland can be easily embedded in a single block of paraffin wax for histology, only a tiny portion of a complete human breast is easily handled like this. Giant histological sections do address this problem, with advantages recognized by breast pathologists from Cheatle (1920) to Eusebi (Foschini et al. 2006) and Tot (Tot et al. 2000), but their use is routine only in a few dedicated laboratories.

Also, histology is naturally two dimensional: 3D information can be extracted only with considerable effort, especially for larger objects. Virtuoso serial section studies of 3D anatomy and embryology have been performed from the time of His onwards, but the knotty problem of describing the lobar anatomy of the breast has received relatively little attention, being correctly perceived as difficult (Osteen 1995); incorrectly as having been done already (a perception suggested by its neglect), and perhaps also as lacking particular significance for breast cancer, which in recent years has been widely seen as a disease of the mammary lobules.

2.2.1 The "Lobular Origins" Hypothesis of Breast Cancer

It has never been obvious where breast cancers come from. Early investigators saw cells looking like cancer cells lining ducts and glandular acini of cancer-associated breast tissue (Cheatle 1906, 1920). It seemed plausible that these cells were progenitors of invasive breast carcinomas, and indeed, they could sometimes be observed apparently in the act of exiting ductal or glandular structures to invade the adjacent stroma.

Even before Foote and Stewart (1941) published their definitive description of lobular carcinoma in situ (LCIS), lesions recognizable as LCIS had also been illustrated (e.g., plate II in Cheatle and Cutler 1931:162). Ewing (1940:563) distinguished between "duct carcinoma arising from the lining cells of ducts" and "acinar carcinoma arising from the epithelium of the acini."

Given morphologically distinct ducts and lobules of the mammary parenchyma, and site-of-origin as a classifier for neoplasia, the formula of ductal and lobular carcinoma in situ, arising from epithelium of ducts and lobules respectively, as precursors of ductal and lobular invasive carcinoma is neat, tidy, and plausible, but seemed to have been dealt a severe blow by studies of subgross breast anatomy in the 1970s onward, which emphasized that many duct-like structures colonized by neoplastic cells were actually enlarged and distorted ("unfolded") lobules (Wellings et al. 1975). This has given rise to a frequently stated belief that breast cancer is of lobular origin, which appears to contradict the notion of a "sick lobe."

This "lobular origins" viewpoint was strongly endorsed by John Azzopardi in his discussion of work by Wellings and colleagues in his influential book *Problems in Breast Pathology* (Azzopardi 1979). He observed "the first fundamental conclusion that stems from this superb work is that the vast bulk of breast disease, much of which has been traditionally regarded as of ductal origin, is in fact of lobular and/or terminal duct origin." Other workers have published data interpreted to support the lobular hypothesis (Ohuchi et al. 1985; Faverly et al. 1992), and the degree to which it has been accepted by the senological community as a "scientific fact" can be confirmed by any student of the literature from how often it is asserted without citation of primary data to support it.

A key argument advanced by proponents of the lobular origins hypothesis is that structures considered to be ductal by workers advocating a ductal cancer origin were really expanded lobules which the pioneers had failed to recognize. It is difficult to assess the degree to which this is true, but insightful observers like Lenthal Cheatle were perfectly able to recognize even highly deformed lobules, and illustrate them in their works (e.g., Cheatle 1920:288, Fig. 204). Cheatle also recognizes that discriminating between abnormal ducts and lobules may be difficult, and notes the utility of serial sections in making this distinction. The same publication also illustrates a case (page 290, Fig. 208) in which, based on his study of giant histological sections, Sir Lenthal explicitly proposes a lobar distribution of epithelial proliferation leading to cancer.

2.2.2 A Critique of the "Lobular Origins" Theory

Subgross studies *do not* reveal the origins of breast cancer.

If we accept the proposition that neoplasia are monoclonal (Fialkow 1976), we accept that all neoplastic cells in a tumor (not counting stromal, inflammatory, and other nonneoplastic cells) are descendents of a somatic cell, which have acquired (epi)genetic changes sufficient to confer a neoplastic phenotype. (We may note that this point of view is not universally accepted (Parsons 2008), but shall not explore the arguments here.)

If tumor monoclonality is correct, to identify where breast cancers begin could be easily taken to mean this: to identify where in the mammary parenchyma that cell was located from which all the neoplastic cells of a particular cancer are descended, maybe years or decades even before that cancer became detectable clinically or by screening. It is safe to say that this has never been achieved for even one case of breast cancer, let alone often enough to allow anything to be said about the origins of breast cancer in general, and I intend to argue there is in reality *no such thing* as a "founder" cell to which all the cells in a cancer can be traced back in anything other than a trivial sense.

2.2.3 What Does It Mean to Speak of a Cancer's "Origin"?

Further reflection shows how elusive this idea is.

In the standard model, invasive breast cancer and most other cancers are usually thought to be clonally descended from proximate precursor lesions variously called severe dysplasia, high-grade intraepithelial neoplasia, or carcinoma in situ (essentially synonymous terms for lesions with which most invasive carcinomas are intimately associated) (Sinn 2009). If so, the origin of the in situ carcinoma is as legitimate a "beginning"

of the whole process as the moment a tumor cell first broke through a basement membrane.

But the same argument applies to in situ carcinomas: many of these arise on a background of atypical hyperplasia, itself likely to be clonally descended from still earlier ancestors, perhaps hyperplasias of usual type; columnar cell change; otherwise altered lobules; normal-looking but abnormal parenchyma; truly normal parenchyma; or even a remote ancestor cell in existence before the breast even began to form, early in fetal life; or the zygote itself, in which a germ line mutation in *TP53*, *BRCA1*, *BRCA2*, *CDH1*, *STK11*, or *PTEN* would already represent a major step on the long road to breast cancer (Campeau et al. 2008).

The common Icelandic *999del5 BRCA2* mutation has been causing breast cancer since the mid-sixteenth century (Thorlacius et al. 1996). Many women who have experienced breast cancer would never have done so had they not inherited this defective gene. In what sense, exactly, would it be incorrect to say these cancers began in the sixteenth century, or even earlier?

2.2.4 Cancers Have No "Beginning" in Time or Space

To sum up, cancers do not begin at a definable point in time or space. Even if a one-celled cancer was conceivable, which it isn't, it would only be apparent after many cellular generations that is what it was, when there is no prospect that unique individual cell can be identified. Even if the existence of such a cell could be inferred from indirect evidence, the chain of molecular causation extends over many cellular generations, into a remote past, and there is no reason to confer privileged status on the last to occur of the set of mutations driving the transformed phenotype, over all others: the first of them to occur may be as necessary as the last for the phenotype, and on that basis have a better claim to have begun the process of cancer formation.

To accept these arguments is to accept that "breast cancer *begins* in the terminal duct lobular units" is a *meaningless statement* which posits nothing with which one might agree or disagree. It will be obvious that the statement "breast cancer begins with a sick lobe" is equally meaningless: which is not to say "sick lobes" (and lobules) are not deeply and intimately connected with the evolution of breast cancer in an individual.

2.2.5 Another Reason for Doubting the "Lobular Hypothesis"

There are usually many abnormal lobules in both cancer-bearing and noncancerous breasts. Jensen, Rice, and Wellings (Jensen et al. 1976) found a median of 15 atypical lobules in cancer-containing breasts (3rd quartile 51, maximum 225) and a median of 5 in breasts without cancer (3rd quartile 11, maximum 91).

Each of these atypical lobules *must* have arisen independently, *if* their existence is to support a "lobular origin" theory of breast cancer, because, if they do share some common causation, their mere existence implies the involvement of a greater portion of breast parenchyma (necessarily including ducts as well as lobules) in that process.

At most, we may perhaps say that changes associated with breast cancer visibly affect lobules earlier than other parts of the mammary parenchyma.

A "lobular origins" theory *would* be supported by the existence of monolobular neoplasia, analogous to aberrant crypt foci or monocryptal adenomas in colon, which implicate the colonic crypt as a niche in which a founder cell was resident (Preston et al. 2003). Establishing the existence of isolated lobules colonized by recognizably neoplastic cells, but not involving any other lobules in the neighborhood of the abnormal one would require careful examination of all adjacent lobules not merely in the plane of a single histological section, but in other planes as well. This, subgross studies such as those of Wellings and others, including even the careful 3D studies of Ohuchi (Ohuchi et al. 1984a, b, 1985; Ohuchi, 1999) and Holland (Faverly et al. 1992) which found in almost every case multiple abnormal lobules, have not done. And even if they had, it would still not exclude the existence of a field in which a phenotypically silent mutation was present.

2.3 Evolution of Breast Cancer Precursors: Clonal Expansion

So, we should forget about where breast cancer or its putative precursors "begin" and ask instead, how do they evolve? The distribution in space of morphologically and genetically abnormal parenchymal cells in a cancer-containing breast is clearly informative about events in the evolution of a breast cancer.

The evolution of neoplasia in Barrett's esophagus, which is more accessible to direct observation over time than breast parenchyma, affords an instructive comparison. In Barrett's esophagus, a clone of cells with a mutation giving a selective advantage is capable of colonizing >10 cm of a long-segment Barrett esophagus, and of out-competing other clones (Maley 2007).

If this process is completed, the mutation is said to have "gone to fixation" by a "selective sweep" (Maley et al. 2004). If such events also occur in the breast, they would be expected to create a "sick lobe" if confined to one lobe, analogous to a "sick segment" of Barrett's esophagus. Cells with a markedly abnormal morphological phenotype, such as those of DCIS and LCIS, can be observed in the act of colonizing preexisting parenchymal structures including ducts and lobules, more or less extensively (Fig. 2.1), and DCIS does sometimes appear to colonize whole lobes.

This can occur in a continuous and possibly also a discontinuous fashion (Faverly et al. 1992), but in both cases, expansion is likely to be confined to parenchyma of the lobe in which the abnormal clone of cells is expanding, at least prior to the emergence of any invasive elements capable of transgressing basement membranes.

In the absence of an obviously abnormal morphological phenotype, such clonal expansion would be harder to observe. However, the expansion of a clone of cells at increased risk of completed neoplastic

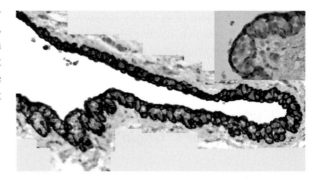

Fig. 2.1 Neoplastic epithelial cells can infiltrate widely within the epithelial bilayer of mammary ducts and lobules. In this immunostained duct, both basal and luminal cells express cytokeratin 5 strongly. Pale, moderately atypical, sometimes vacuolated cells individually and in clumps characteristically colonize the virtual space between basal and luminal cells. This example of so-called "Pagetoid spread" by atypical lobular hyperplasia was an incidental finding following surgical reduction of a breast contralateral to a previously treated cancer. Inset: Loss of E-cadherin expression is also characteristic of these cells

transformation could manifest itself indirectly by the emergence of in situ or invasive neoplasia throughout a field of genetically altered but morphologically normal or minimally abnormal cells.

Another possibility is that a mutation in a cell of the prepubertal breast or even the fetal breast anlage could give rise to a clone of cells from which a large part of the mature breast might be derived, and if that mutation was associated with increased risk of neoplastic transformation, it could manifest itself as a field of increased risk in which multifocal mammary neoplasia might develop.

A prescient, but little-noticed paper (Sharpe 1998) looking at breast cancer origins had received only five citations by October of 2009 (ideas which do not resonate with fashionable thought-styles are not attacked, but ignored). In it, Sharpe suggests that breast cancer multifocality could arise by intraductal spread of abnormal precursor cells or by a developmental mechanism in which anatomically connected branches of developing mammary duct trees might be populated by cells derived from a mutant precursor arising early in development. These first of these ideas would correspond to an initially healthy lobe becoming sick, and the second to a lobe "born sick" ab initio.

Both could be true. The maximal sensitivity of the human breast to radiation-induced carcinogenesis – before the age of five – is at least compatible with the latter concept. Females exposed to radiation in the atomic bombings at Hiroshima and Nagasaki experienced an increased incidence of breast cancer. This excess relative risk (ERR) was greatest (4.6) for women exposed as very young girls (0–4 years) (Tokunaga et al. 1994). Land (1995) found this surprising, given the much smaller mass of breast epithelium in this age-group, but women who were irradiated as infant girls for "thymic enlargement" have a comparable ERR (3.6) for breast cancer, so the susceptibility of the infant female breast to breast cancer initiation by ionizing radiation is well established, and the mutagen N-nitroso N-methylurea is likewise more carcinogenic to the mammary gland of sexually immature than of mature rats (Ariazi et al. 2005).

A radiation-induced mutation in a mammary precursor cell could be inherited by many descendents following thelarche, even perhaps to the extent of being disseminated throughout a complete lobe. The well-known ability of a single precursor cell to reconstitute an entire rodent mammary gland (Kordon and Smith

1998) highlights the potential for one cell to create an extensive glandular domain for itself.

While multifocal neoplasia might also occur following exposure of all the parenchyma of the breast to a common environment promoting neoplasia, e.g., an external carcinogen or an endocrine influence, one would expect such a process to be nonlobar.

2.4 The Need for Whole-Breast Parenchymal Visualization

To investigate fully the evolution of breast neoplasia up to cancer formation in its parenchymal context requires the ability to visualize morphology of parenchymal systems (lobes) in complete breasts, a scale much larger than is commonly attempted in 3D histological studies.

The need for this capability is imposed by the prediction that clonal expansion setting the scene for multifocal mammary carcinogenesis is likely to act over and within a lobe, as in the case of an abnormal clone spreading along ducts after the adult breast structure has been established following thelarche, or of a mutation disseminated in the descendents of a cell belonging to the prepubertal breast, in which early branching by the mammary anlage is established well before birth.

Growth (elongation and branching) of individual duct systems at thelarche could offer an opportunity for the expansion of mutation-bearing clones of cells possessing a growth advantage, which, while not necessarily having a morphologically abnormal phenotype, might be able to colonize more than their fair share of the developing breast and set the scene for future neoplastic development. It is known that breast lobe development is highly unequal (Going and Moffat 2004).

Because the emphasis over the last 30 years has been so strongly on the lobule as the relevant unit of organization of human mammary parenchyma, this larger scale, long-range structure of the breast has been neglected and techniques for its study are not mature. Nevertheless, possibilities for development in this area are attractive.

The rest of this chapter describes central and peripheral ductal/lobar anatomy of breast, as far as it is known; examines evidence for anastomoses within and between lobes, by which intraepithelial neoplasia might be able to spread from lobe to lobe; looks at whether precursors of breast cancer and cancer itself are distributed in a lobe-like manner, in keeping with the "sick lobe" hypothesis; and considers how gaps in our knowledge of lobar breast anatomy might be filled, and the scope for developing techniques allowing morphological and molecular data to be optimized in research and diagnostic settings.

2.5 Lobar Anatomy of the Breast

Many published illustrations of lobe anatomy in human breast are at best artist's impressions, attractive but without primary evidential value.

Cooper's original illustrations, in contrast, are primary research data. In these illustrations, the most noticeable features are the ducts, variable in caliber, radiating from the center, branching and rebranching, with the last branches terminating in glandular parenchyma. Note that glandular tissue is present in all parts of the breast, not just the periphery, although in the nipple itself lobules are said to be sparse (Stolier and Wang 2008). There is noticeable variation in the extent of different lobes (Fig. 2.2), and to some degree their branches intertwine, but not to the extent that their distributions overlap greatly.

The tracing of all ducts and their branches in an autopsy breast of a young woman by Moffat and Going (Moffat and Going 1996; Going and Moffat 2004) was a rare attempt to capture duct branching lobe-by-lobe in a complete human breast. Such studies are dauntingly laborious by manual methods (Osteen 1995), but the scope for developing more streamlined procedures has yet to be fully exploited (Going 2006).

Features of different ducts systems (lobes) revealed in these studies include great variability in total extent (Figs. 2.3 and 2.4): one lobe can account for as much as 25% of a whole breast, as little as 1%, or even less; variability in envelope profile (including predominantly convex, concavo-convex, and cuneiform or wedge-shaped); variability in the length of the central duct before first branching (short or long); and the existence of vestigial or abortive lobes with relatively long ducts penetrating deeply into the central breast, but little or no peripheral branching or associated glandular parenchyma. Minimal lobes with longish but unbranching ducts imply that duct elongation is allowed even when side branching is inhibited (Going and Moffat 2004),

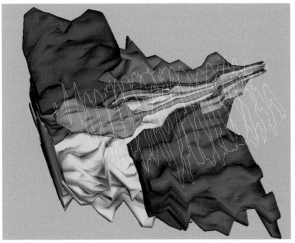

Fig. 2.3 Variation in mammary lobe morphology, I. Seven representative lobes of a single breast vary greatly in size and distribution. Each duct system was traced through serial subgross sections. In each slice, the area occupied by branches of any one duct system may have complex borders, but can be drawn around. Lobes are visualized in "Reconstruct" (Fiala 2005). Boissonnat surfaces are shown for six lobes; the seventh by wire-frame outlines, so as not to obscure the central part of the model behind this lobe. Obvious lobe-to-lobe differences include size; early branching close to the nipple and the breast surface (tan) versus late branching in the depths of the breast (orange, green), or none at all (sky blue). This last is a vestigial lobe in the form of a duct with no peripheral branching at all. This was the longest of several "failed lobes" in this breast, which was studied by Moffat and Going (1996, 2004)

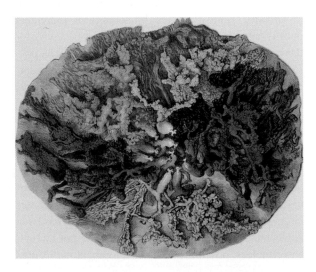

Fig. 2.2 On the Anatomy of the Breast, Plate VI, Fig. 3 (Cooper 1840). Individual lobes have been injected separately with different colored waxes. This figure is less often reproduced than Fig. 2 of the same plate, in which breast segmentation into lobes is more uniform. This may reflect an esthetic bias in favor of uniformity, which may account for the many published artists' impressions of lobes in human breast which emphasize a regularity of development and arrangement not sanctioned by any primary source

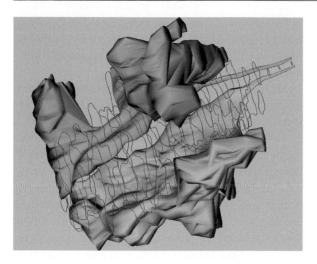

Fig. 2.4 Variation in mammary lobe morphology, II. Three other lobes belonging to the breast shown in Fig. 2.3. The turquoise lobe has two largely separate domains, one close to the surface, and a deep extension. Both lobes (represented by their Boissonnat surfaces) are wrapped around the blue system represented in wire-frame section profiles. One can speculate that the blue system developed in advance of the other two

perhaps implying a mechanism in humans akin to asymmetric (monopodial) branching characteristic of rodent mammary morphogenesis (Davies 2002).

The existence of a largely convex lobe with a concave lobe wrapped around it (Fig. 2.4) seems to suggest that growth of the convex lobe was dominant over growth of the concave lobe. Possibly the "convex" lobe began its growth earlier or grew more rapidly than the concave lobe, and hence growth of duct branches belonging to the concave lobe into virgin territory was inhibited by the fact that elongating branches of the convex lobe had got there first. This apparent competition between lobes in breast growth is of interest in the context of a possible role for the female human breast as a signifier of reproductive fitness (Møller et al. 1995), and the relationship between breast symmetry and cancer risk (Scutt et al. 2006).

2.5.1 Are There Anastomoses Between Lobes?

An abnormal clone of cells expanding within an epithelial domain bounded by a basement membrane must remain limited to that domain as long as the clone is confined by the basement membrane. In the case of a breast lobe, the expanding clone would remain monolobar,

provided the lobe was isolated from neighboring lobes. We ignore for the time being the theoretical possibility of cells of the clone escaping from the lobe into the epidermis of the nipple, and entering another lobe via its duct opening on the nipple surface.

If lobes are not isolated from each other, but are linked by epithelium-lined anastomotic ducts, then a clone might escape from its lobe of origin into an adjacent lobe to which it was connected; thence it might spread to any lobe that second lobe was also connected to; and so on, potentially putting any part of the entire breast parenchyma within reach of such an expanding clone. Such a process would be analogous to the dissemination of pneumococcal lobar pneumonia throughout a lung via the interalveolar pores of Kohn.

Anastomoses between lobes could also influence sampling of the mammary environment by techniques such as duct lavage and duct endoscopy (Tondre et al. 2008; Dooley 2009), and might have a physiological role in lactation, by providing alternate pathways for drainage of milk from parenchyma to nipple, by which a duct blockage might be bypassed. This could help to maximize effective lactating tissue mass, as impaired milk drainage inhibits milk secretion via feedback inhibitors of lactation (Wilde et al. 1995), one of which is thought to be serotonin acting on the 5HT7 receptor in both human breast and murine mammary glands (Stull et al. 2007). Whether anastomoses exist is therefore important, but an entirely satisfactory answer has not yet been given.

2.5.2 The Challenge of Lobar Anatomy

Lobes remain intractable objects of study. To define a lobe completely, all its "branches" (ducts) and "leaves" (lobules) must be visualized. Ducts are thin-walled, embedded in tough fibrous tissue, and can ramify extensively, branching again and again. One breast contains many lobes, and neither macroscopic nor microscopic examination of breast tissue gives any clues to lobe boundaries.

Practically, lobes can be defined by injection with a marker fluid (colored wax, resin, latex, urethane, mercury), or by tracing through serial thick ("subgross") sections, after they have been stained and cleared. Giant histological sections of conventional thickness may hint at the lobe architecture, but a sampling gap of 3–5 mm between sections does not allow confident duct tracing from slice to slice.

2.5.3 Duct Injection Studies

Cooper was a pioneer in this area (it is salutary to remember that he began to research normal breast when he was already 67 years old). Sir Astley's opinion is clear: physiological anastomoses do not connect separate duct systems (lobes): "The mammary ducts do not communicate with each other, as is easily shown by throwing injections of different colours into the ducts, or by injecting one duct only."

"If various colours are thrown into each duct, they proceed to the gland without any admixture of colour. If one duct be most minutely injected with quicksilver, it does not escape into any other. And this remark is also applicable to the mammary glands of other animals, where there are many, as in the hare, the bitch and the pig, the ducts are separate and distinct from those of the other gland."

"I have only seen one instance to the contrary of this position, in injecting a milk tube from the interior of the gland towards the nipple, two large branches of ducts crossing each other, where they laid in contact, the injection found its way by rupture, or by a deviation from the natural structure, from the one into the other duct, of which I have given a figure [Plate VIII, Fig. 7] (Fig. 2.5); and as this has only occurred once in more than two hundred times, it shows that it is not the result of a common structure." (Cooper 1840).

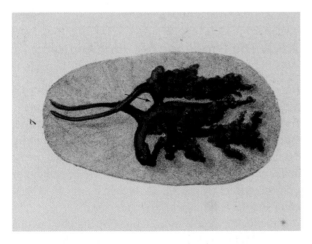

Fig. 2.5 On the Anatomy of the Breast, Plate VIII, Fig. 7. Rare anastomosis (arrow) between ducts of separate lobes. Cooper remarks this figure is "taken from a preparation which shows a rare deviation from a general law, viz., of two ducts communicating, of which this is the only instance I have seen. One of the ducts was injected from a branch near the circumference of the gland, and the injection was thrown towards the nipple, when either by laceration or unusual communication, two ducts became filled"

Cooper used a technique well adapted to the detection of anastomoses, in "more than two hundred" injection experiments, a breadth of experience unparalleled before or since.

Moffat and Going could find no anastomoses when tracing all identifiable branches of all ducts in subgross sections of an autopsy breast (Going and Mohun 2006).

Further evidence that anastomoses between lobes are rare is the absence of any reference in the galactography literature to retrograde filling of another central duct following injection of contrast medium down one central duct (Fig. 2.6). Love and Barsky detected no anastomoses in their studies (Love and Barsky 2004) which included a review of many galactograms performed by Otto Sartorius in Santa Barbara, California. Likewise, I am not aware of any published evidence of retrograde flow of fluid during nipple duct lavage, although such flow might not always be detected.

A theoretical consideration is that during mammary gland development, elongating mammary ducts mutually inhibit each others' continuing growth, and both rodent (Faulkin and DeOme 1960) and human (Going and Moffat 2004) mammary gland duct distributions show clear evidence of repulsion (Fig. 2.7), which would be calculated to interfere with the formation of anastomoses (Faulkin and DeOme 1960). TGFβ is likely to be a critical negative regulator of this mammary duct spacing (Lee and Davies 2007).

Ohtake et al., on the other hand, do describe interlobar and intralobar duct anastomoses in their subgross studies (Ohtake et al. 1995, 2001). This interesting and important question will be resolved only by further careful morphological studies. Experience of recording x, y, and z coordinates of all branch points and duct terminations of a complete mammary lobe (Going 2006) makes one aware of how fatally easy it is in such studies to confuse branches, and some of the apparent anastomoses identified by Ohtake et al. could have been a consequence of duct mistracing, however carefully they tried to avoid this.

2.5.4 Are Breast Cancer Precursors Lobar in Their Distribution?

There is only a distant relationship between breast quadrants and lobes, so studies of breast cancer and its precursors which look only at the distribution of disease between quadrants tell us little or nothing about the distribution of disease between lobes.

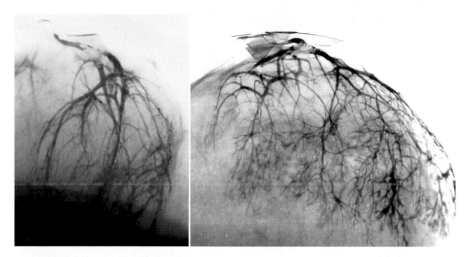

Fig. 2.6 Two views of the same lobe in a galactogram (oblique on left, cranial–caudal on right). This extensive system accounts for a significant fraction of breast volume. In the craniocaudal view glandular tissue is clearly visible. A filling defect (*) visible in both views is due to an intraductal papilloma. Note the single central duct and absence of retrograde filling of any other duct system. Galactograms, courtesy of Dr Jean Murray, South East Scotland Breast Screening Centre. Images have been contrast-reversed to maximize duct visibility

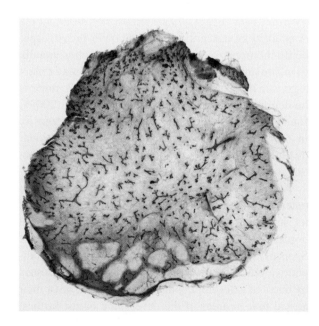

Fig. 2.7 Hematoxylin-stained subgross section cleared in methyl salicylate (oil of wintergreen). Section is in the coronal plane through a complete (autopsy) breast. Spacing of parenchymal elements maximizes the distance between adjacent units (implying repulsion during development)

Extensive intraductal carcinoma is a risk factor for local recurrence (Holland et al., 1990a, b), and finding a small or large, often wedge-shaped area of DCIS is common experience for the practicing breast pathologist. Other published studies support this segmental distribution of disease in breast cancer, in keeping with a lobar process (Johnson et al. 1995). The proposal that segmental treatment should be employed seems plausible, but the lobar hypothesis is not thereby proved, and the difficulty of doing this rigorously has been pointed out (Osteen 1995): "to prove the segmental anatomy of breast cancer would require serial sectioning of the breast in such a way as to establish the continuity of each duct and lobule. Such a monumental task is probably beyond the resources of any department and the patience of any individual." In the same editorial, Osteen reviewed findings by Holland et al. (1990b) of lobe-like regional DCIS in 81/82 mastectomies they subjected to subgross examination, but points out that while consistent with a segmental (lobar) distribution, such a distribution was not thereby established, because the lobe anatomy was unknown even in this thorough study. Indeed, few have attempted to extract such anatomy, and the small numbers of cases examined reflect the difficulty of the task.

In this same editorial, we also find another adumbration of the "sick lobe," in the remark that "some patients with breast cancer may have a segment that is, in some biologically definable terms, 'bad'... These cases raise the question of whether other markers, such as atypical lobular hyperplasia, microcalcifications in benign epithelium, or some genetic or molecular biologic markers, might identify 'bad segments' that require wide excision or mastectomy for treatment."

A recent review (Jain et al. 2009) usefully surveys the literature concerning multicentric and multifocal ipsilateral breast cancer.

In the case of lobular neoplasia (ALH/LCIS), the segmental distribution of the process is less obvious. Lobular neoplasia is often presented as a marker of risk rather than a lineal precursor of breast cancer. The relationship is not entirely clear, but a 2003 paper by David Page and colleagues indicating an approximately 3:1 ipsilateral:contralateral ratio for invasive cancers diagnosed subsequently to a diagnosis of ALH strongly implies more than a marker function for ALH (Page et al. 2003).

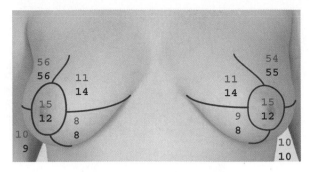

Fig. 2.8 Location of in situ and invasive carcinoma in human breast by side and quadrant. Data from Perkins et al. (2004). The percentages are based on the recorded locations of 223,053 invasive carcinomas (numbers in brown) and 36,280 in situ carcinomas (numbers in blue) in US cancer registries. The distributions of in situ and invasive carcinoma are closely matched. The upper outer quadrant is at greatest risk of cancer

2.5.5 Abnormalities of "Normal" Breast Tissue in the Vicinity of Cancers

There is now a considerable body of evidence that breast tissue which looks normal histologically may not be normal on genetic, epigenetic, or other molecular analysis (Ellsworth et al. 2004a, b; Meeker et al. 2004; Yan et al. 2006; Tripathi et al. 2008; Chen et al. 2009). These data are certainly in keeping with the idea of a sick lobe, but again, in the absence of anatomical data to anchor it in a lobar context, other possibilities are not excluded.

Chen et al. (2009) undertook global gene-expression microarray analysis of 143 histologically normal or non-atypical benign breast tissue samples from 90 patients with breast cancer. Eleven samples showed expression profile features in common with invasive carcinoma. Genes involved in cell proliferation and the cell cycle featured strongly in a "malignancy risk" expression signature derived by the authors from their data.

The finding of an increased frequency of molecular abnormalities in morphologically unremarkable tissue in the outer quadrants of the breast is of interest given the greater incidence of breast cancer in the outer and, especially, the upper outer quadrant of the breast (Ellsworth et al. 2004a). See also Fig. 2.8.

2.5.6 Inhomogeneity of Breast Cancer Risk by Quadrant

A majority of cancers occur in the outer breast, especially the upper outer quadrant. This applies equally to in situ and invasive cancers. While this may reflect a greater bulk of parenchymal tissue at risk, there is no definite evidence for this. Ellsworth et al. (2004a) found a greater prevalence of loss of heterozygosity in normal-looking breast tissue in outer than inner quadrants of cancer-bearing breasts, and thought that this might imply "field cancerization."

A unique feature of the parenchyma of the upper outer quadrant of the breast which may be relevant is its superolateral extension around the inferomedial border of pectoralis major to form the axillary tail (of Spence). If the growth of individual lobes is a competitive process, any competitive advantage possessed by ducts of a developing duct system might favor their arrival first in areas of the developing breast furthest from the nipple, which might therefore be most likely to harbor growth-promoting changes. Very marked variation in the depth of branching exists not only between lobes (Going and Moffat 2004) but also between divisions of individual lobes (Going 2006). This is a testable idea, in that it would be possible to look at molecular changes in normal-looking parenchyma in the axillary tail and other locations in the breast, and in relation to depth of duct branching associated with these different areas.

Apropos any relationship between depth of duct branching and breast cancer risk, many studies of breast size and cancer risk have yielded inconsistent results, but a large study (Kusano et al. 2006) of 89,268 participants in the Nurses' Health Study II did find a moderate excess risk in women with larger breasts, but only for those with body mass index <25 kg/m^2, in whom obesity is not a confounding factor.

2.6 The Nipple and Its Anatomy

The large number of ducts in the central duct bundle in the nipple has been mentioned already. These vary in size and open on the apex of the papilla. Similar ducts opening on the lateral aspects of the papilla and in the areola constitute the glands of Montgomery. Several ducts may apparently share a single ostium (Rusby et al. 2007); this could go some way toward explaining the apparent discrepancy between the large number of ducts in the nipple duct bundle and the substantially smaller duct numbers from which milk may be observed to issue during lactation, or which may be cannulated at the apex of the papilla. With hindsight, this feature of the human breast ducts in the nipple is hinted at in older publications; Cooper's atlas includes an illustration which hints strongly at ostium sharing, and Cheatle and Cutler (1931) include a photomicrograph of an ostium into which two separate ducts clearly discharge their secretions.

Figure 2.9 shows a cross section of the nipple duct bundle, illustrating the large number of ducts and their characteristically convoluted profile.

Figure 2.10 shows the squamocolumnar junction between the characteristic epithelial/luminal–myoepithelial/basal bilayer of the duct systems of the breast and the keratinizing squamous epithelium of the nipple epidermis. It is not uncommon to see a single nipple duct colonized by DCIS, but no evidence of Paget's disease; it appears that nipple epidermis usually resists colonization by DCIS, but in Paget's disease of the nipple, colonization of nipple epidermis does occur.

HER2 amplification and Her2 overexpression by about 85% of Paget's disease suggest an important role in its pathogenesis. Heregulin-α is a motility factor made and released by epidermal keratinocytes, and Paget cells express heregulin receptors Her3 and Her4 as well as their coreceptor Her2 (Schelfhout et al. 2000). Heregulin binding to the receptor complex on

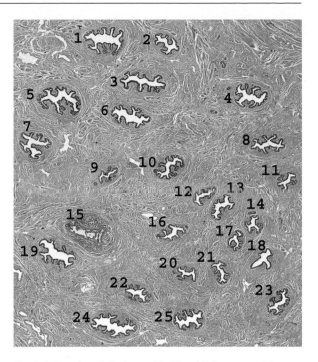

Fig. 2.9 Duct bundle in the papilla, H and E, low power. Twenty-five individual ducts are present, implying twenty-five individual lobes, not all of which would have developed to a significant degree. Only one system (15) is involved by DCIS

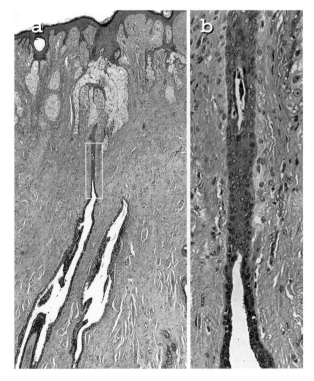

Fig. 2.10 Squamocolumnar junction in a duct approximately 0.5 mm deep to the epidermal surface of the papilla; Low (**a**) and high power views (**b**). Notice how small the duct is at this point

Paget cells is probably responsible for their migration into nipple epidermis. As normal mammary duct epithelium also expresses heregulins (de Fazio et al. 2000), this mechanism could equally promote expansion of Her2-positive DCIS in the breast itself.

Figure 2.11 shows a (previously unpublished) 3D reconstruction by the author of all the ducts in a mastectomy nipple as they approach the apex of the papilla, and a closer view of ducts sharing a single ostium. Clearly, it would be difficult to cannulate these ducts separately. This figure also reproduces a figure illustrating ostium sharing from Cooper's atlas (1840).

2.6.1 Clear Cells of Nipple Epidermis: Toker Cells

Finally, we take note of a population of cells to be found in many breasts, which have features which raise the possibility that they could act as vectors of risk in the creation of a "sick lobe" at increased risk of neoplastic transformation. These are the "clear cells of nipple epidermis" described by Cyril Toker (Toker 1970), and now known as Toker cells (Figs. 2.12 and 2.13).

Obviously, abnormal cells like those of high-grade DCIS can spread widely, to the extent of colonizing the ductal and glandular tissue of whole lobes. Less highly atypical cells of lobular neoplasia do the same. There is no a priori reason why other cells predisposed to neoplastic development should not do likewise, but if they did not have an obvious morphological phenotype, they would blend into the parenchymal background. Could Toker cells be representatives of such populations?

Toker cells are characteristically found in nipple epidermis in the vicinity of duct ostia. They express low molecular weight cytokeratins (cytokeratin 7, 19) in common with breast luminal epithelium and it has been plausibly suggested that they are of mammary origin (Marucci et al. 2002). Although inconspicuous in H and E sections (being observable in about 10% of cases), immunostaining with a marker such as cytokeratin 7 will reveal them in a much greater proportion of breasts (70–80%). They vary in numbers from scanty individual cells to so many, singly and in clumps there may be a possibility of mistaking them for Paget cells (which usually show much greater cytological atypia).

Their distribution implies an ability to migrate within nipple epidermis, and morphological features including the formation of lamellipodium- and filopodium-like cellular projections support this idea (unpublished observations by the author; Fig. 2.13). Despite apparently expressing steroid hormone receptors (although the literature is not entirely concordant on this point: Garijo et al. 2009), they can be just as numerous in breasts long postmenopausal as in breasts prior to the menopause. Also, their occasional presence in dead keratin suggests

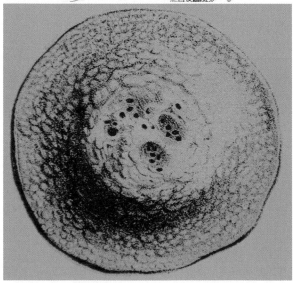

Fig. 2.11 Three dimensional reconstruction of ducts approaching the apex of the papilla in a mastectomy breast. Wire-frame views. Top view: all ducts shown. Middle: ostium sharing by four ducts. Below: ostium sharing depicted by Sir Astley Cooper (Cooper 1840)

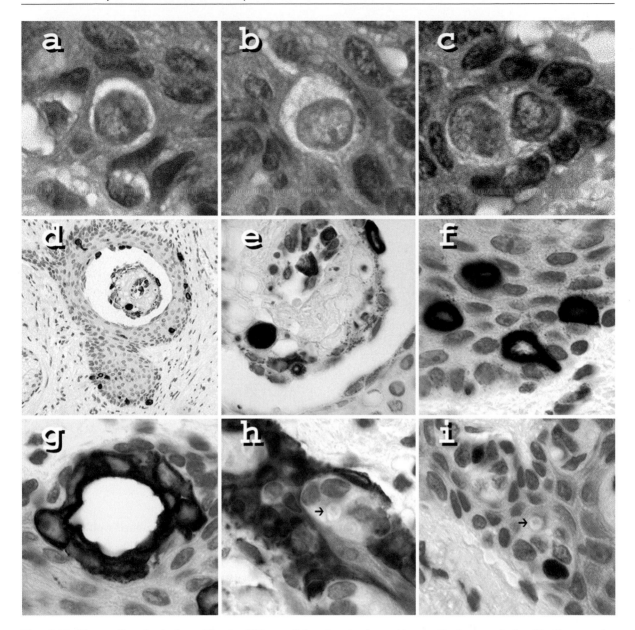

Fig. 2.12 Clear cells of nipple epidermis (Toker cells). (**a–c**) Hematoxylin and eosin. (**a, b**) Individual Toker cells resembling mammary small and large light cells. **c** Paired Toker cells; (**d–g**) CK7 immunostaining. (**d, e**) Numerous clear cells in the epidermis surrounding a duct ostium. CK7+ cells are also present in the keratin plug filling the lumen. (**f**) A suprabasal location is usual but a projection onto the basal lamina may give a gourd-like shape. (**g**) An acinus formed of CK7+ clear cells. (**h**) Clear cells negative for CK14 in contrast to surrounding keratinocytes. The arrow in this figure and in (i) indicates lumen formation. (**i**) Variable expression of estrogen receptor by Toker cells

an ability to survive in a situation in which they might have been expected to undergo anoikis (Fig. 2.12), suggesting apoptosis resistance. These hints at Toker cell autonomy and motility suggest a possible role not merely in relation to Paget's disease, with which a connection has been proposed, but more generally in breast cancer, especially as possible vectors of risk in the genesis of a "sick lobe."

Unfortunately, there are at present no specific markers allowing Toker cells to be recognized in mammary epithelium. Their expression profile for molecules related to cell motility, cell adhesion

Fig. 2.13 Clear cells of
nipple epidermis (Toker cells)
immunostained for cytokeratin 7, illustrating features
compatible with motility.
Top left: this cell has a broad
lamellipodium-like extension
from which a filopodium
("microspike") extends.
Top right: a long clavate
projection. *Bottom left* and
right: two cells with
wedge-shaped projections
with a flattened "contact
surface" on a neighboring
keratinocyte

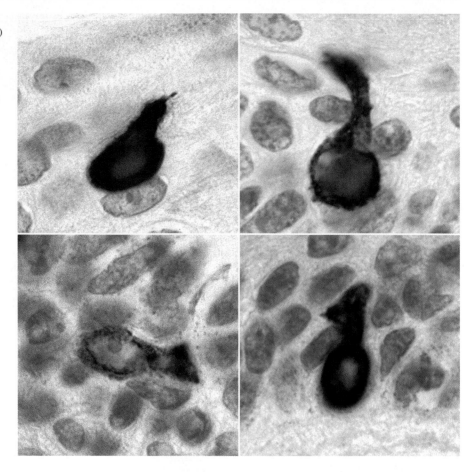

molecules, and receptors (e.g., Her3, Her4) for possible motogens (including heregulins) would be worth
investigating.

2.7 Cellular Supercompetition in the Making of a Sick Lobe

Clinically "early" neoplasia is nothing of the kind.
Waves of clonal expansion (at the expense of neighboring cells) over many years establish and consolidate
mutations in tissues and, by increasing after each new
event the number of cells in which the new mutation
and earlier mutations are present, pave the way to eventual malignancy.

Scope for competitive clonal expansion would be
increased by any reduction in the degree to which
stem cells remain tightly bound to a specific tissue
niche. (Any reduction in the ability of a cell and its

descendents to repair DNA damage would also favor
accumulation of further mutations, and several such
mechanisms are well known.) Recent research inter-
ests have focused on cell competition and supercom-
petition as a mechanism in carcinogenesis.

Cell competition is well attested in Drosophila
(Morata and Ripoll 1975). Cells heterozygous for
Minute ribosomal gene mutations grow into phenotypically normal flies, but in chimeric flies, M/wt
cells lose ground to wt/wt cells. The same occurs
with dmyc mutations (Johnston et al. 1999), and even
more strikingly, overexpression of dmyc creates
"supercompetitor" cells (Moreno and Basler 2004)
which outcompete wild-type cells. Supercompetitor
cells may also be created by aberrant Salvador/Warts
pathway signaling (Tyler et al. 2007). Particularly
important is that a population of "winner" cells can
expand at the expense of "loser" cells in a tissue without any visible histological alteration. Perhaps Toker
cells are supercompetitors.

2.8 Prospects for Improved Understanding of Breast Lobe Anatomy

2.8.1 Injection Studies

Injecting individual duct systems (lobes) with colored or radioopaque tracer fluids, gels, resins, polymers, liquid metals, and waxes (in vitro and in vivo) has a long history. These techniques have advantages but many disadvantages. Suitable fluids can define even fine duct branches, which certainly is an advantage, but human milk ducts are delicate and extraductal rupture and leakage are frequent; furthermore, few studies appear to record successful injection of anything approaching the number of ducts really present in a human breast. Primary sources for accurate ducts counts are hard to find in the literature but Going, who counted duct profiles in complete cross sections through the nipple duct bundle at the base of the papilla in cancer mastectomy breasts, found a median of 27 ducts (range 11–41; Q1 21, Q3 30) (Going and Moffat 2004), a number greater than the usual 10–20 or so quoted in secondary sources.

While many of these systems may be rudimentary or vestigial, in the absence of good data, this is speculative. At all events, many injection studies investigate far fewer systems. Khan et al. (2004) studied ducts yielding nipple aspirate fluid and were able to lavage and inject 39 systems in 28 breasts (1.4 per breast). On the other hand, Love and Barsky (2004) observed milk flow from a median of 5 nipple openings in lactating women and Ramsay et al. (2005) observed a mean of 9 ducts in right and left breasts of fully lactating women. Ultimately, these data are still difficult to explain fully. Some systems may be rudimentary, with little functional parenchyma; alternately, duct nonpatency could also be a factor, as a system disconnected from the nipple would not establish lactation, in that nondrainage inhibits lactation by the negative feedback mechanism mentioned earlier. Such nonpatency of main or branch ducts would also interfere with injection studies.

2.8.2 Duct Tracing

The other main technique for lobe studies has been tracing ducts as they ramify through serial thick stained and cleared (so-called subgross) sections.

Subgross techniques have a long history, going back at least to the studies of Werner Spalteholz (Spalteholz 1914). They were extensively applied by Adolf Dabelow (Dabelow 1957) and later workers including Wellings and colleagues (Wellings et al. 1975; Jensen et al. 1976), and remain widely used in developmental biology and experimental pathology most often in the form of wholemount preparations. Even in this venerable technique there are new developments: many fluorescent DNA-intercalating stains are incompatible with the classical hydrophobic clearing agents like benzyl alcohol/benzyl benzoate or methyl salicylate. Recently, thiodiethanol (refractive index = 1.52) was introduced into confocal microscopy as a watermiscible, low-toxicity (Reddy et al. 2005) high refractive index mounting medium compatible with many intercalating DNA dyes (Staudt et al. 2007; Appleton et al. 2009) and facilitating microscopy of substantially thicker specimens. The prospect of an improved, fluorescent subgross technique applicable to breast tissue is exciting.

Subgross techniques have the great advantage of allowing all parenchyma in a breast to be stained and visualized, but as a method of studying lobar breast anatomy, although all the data is present, the challenges remain great. Tissue distortions during sectioning and processing create a difficult registration problem, that is, points of correspondence between adjacent sections may be hard to identify, and duct tracing correspondingly difficult. (These difficulties were referred to above in the discussion of the work of Ohtake et al.)

Large sections certainly allow a greater appreciation of relationships over longer distances than conventional small histological sections in the size range 15–25 mm, but although 3D data can be inferred, great caution is required in the evaluation of duct connections. If a tissue block is 3 mm thick, a duct traversing that block at an angle of 10° to its surface will sustain more than 15 mm of lateral displacement. This makes inferring duct connections from histological sections of tissue blocks as little as 3 mm thick highly unreliable.

Conventional x-ray galactography is now little used with ready availability of other imaging modalities including ultrasound, but MRI galactography has potential in the area of defining lobe anatomy. However, it faces all the challenges of other duct injection techniques including contrast extravasation, the difficulty of injecting more than a few ducts, and (even if multiple ducts could be injected) it might be difficult to discriminate between systems.

Now, it would be a good time to bring together complementary techniques to advance the study of breast biology and pathology. Molecular and morphological analyses are powerful separately, but even more powerful together. Breast cancer is a disease of astonishing complexity. Neither approach on its own is optimal. The "sick lobe" hypothesis asks questions about the development of breast cancer in time and space, and observes that concentrating on events in a few cubic millimeters of tissue is not enough. To be able to analyze molecular events in different parts of duct trees, with a knowledge of how those ducts are physically connected, would allow for the testing of otherwise untestable hypotheses.

Almost all the necessary tools are available: fixatives less deleterious than formaldehyde to nucleic acids, proteins, and other important biological molecules; sensitive and specific fluorescent dyes to reveal structure; a new tissue clearing agent, thiodiethanol (Staudt et al. 2007), compatible with these dyes; data processing techniques for storage, extraction, processing, and visualization of that structure; and the whole gamut of molecular techniques.

Strangely, one of the challenges looks as if it ought to be easy, but isn't: making stacks of serial thick sections without distortion, essential for accurate duct tracing from section to section, and lobe reconstruction. Classically, investigators have used prolonged formaldehyde fixation, and deep-frozen the fixed tissue in agar for slicing. Egan introduced the slicing of deeply chilled tissue (Egan et al. 1969; Egan 1982). Neither is optimal, or free from artifacts.

The real challenge is to take unfixed breast tissue straight from the operating theater – be it a diagnostic biopsy, wide local excision, or mastectomy – and slice it within minutes into a stack of 2–3 mm thick slices, each collected on a dimensionally stable substrate for optimal fixation, staining, tissue clearing, visualization, and data collection for subsequent 3D analysis; followed by tissue processing for classical histology, immunohistochemistry, and any other including molecular analyses as indicated by clinical necessity. All to be done on a time scale no longer than we now accept for conventional histology. There are no grounds for thinking that this is not possible. Such a technique could allow us to be more accurate in our evaluation of diagnostic issues such as completeness of excision of in situ and invasive cancer, and achieving it is a highly desirable goal.

2.9 Conclusion

Astley Cooper's researches have been a theme in this chapter, and it is fitting to take final look at Sir Astley's work. His plate V, Fig. 1 (Fig. 2.14) illustrates different degrees of glandular development between areas of a lactating breast, to which Sir Astley draws particular attention. This may be the first published suggestion of significant variation in differentiation potential between human mammary gland lobes, and a very early hint at the possibility of a "sick lobe," given the possibility that failed attempts to establish lactation (in keeping with impaired glandular differentiation) may be associated with increased breast cancer risk (Yang et al. 1993).

Continuity in thought is interesting, and it is gratifying that such an "old" subject as the lobar organization of human breast tissue is, if anything, even more important in the postgenomic era than in 1840 when Cooper first laid the foundations for scientific senology.

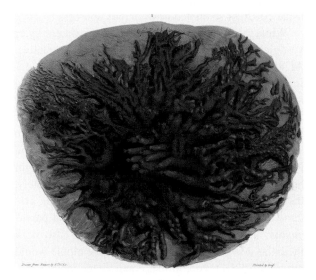

Fig. 2.14 On the Anatomy of the Breast, Plate V, Fig. 1. Cooper's caption reads "Lactiferous tubes, injected with red wax, in a woman who died during the period of lactation. Twelve ducts have been filled and ligatures are placed on their orifices. The ducts are seen forming large reservoirs at the roots of the mamillary tubes; these reservoirs are seen to be produced by the union of numerous branches from the ducts. The ducts are perceived to terminate at the margin of the gland in branches, but in some parts, in glandules." Glandular tissue is most obvious at 3–5 o'clock and 10–11 o'clock. This may be the first published suggestion of significant biological variation between human mammary gland lobes

Acknowledgement   Dr Going wishes to acknowledge grant support from the Dr Susan Love Research Foundation (Santa Monica).

References

Appleton PL, Quyn AJ, Swift S, Nathke I (2009) Preparation of wholemount mouse intestine for high-resolution three-dimensional imaging using two-photon microscopy. J Microsc 234:196–204

Ariazi JL, Haag JD, Lindstrom MJ, Gould MN (2005) Mammary glands of sexually immature rats are more susceptible than those of mature rats to the carcinogenic, lethal, and mutagenic effects of N-nitroso-N-methylurea. Mol Carcinog 43:155–164

Azzopardi JG (1979) Problems in breast pathology. W.B. Saunders, London

Brock RC (1952) The life and work of Astley Cooper. E. & S. Livingstone, Edinburgh

Campeau PM, Foulkes WD, Tischkowitz MD (2008) Hereditary breast cancer: new genetic developments, new therapeutic avenues. Hum Genet 124:31–42

Cheatle GL (1906) Clinical remarks on the early recognition of cancer of the breast. Br Med J 1:1205–1210

Cheatle GL (1920) Cysts, and primary cancer in cysts, of the breast. Br J Surg VIII:149–166

Cheatle GL, Cutler M (1931) Tumours of the breast: their pathology, symptoms, diagnosis and treatment. Edward Arnold, London

Chen DT, Nasir A, Culhane A, Venkataramu C, Fulp W, Rubio R, Wang T, Agrawal D, McCarthy SM, Gruidl M, Bloom G, Anderson T, White J, Quackenbush J, Yeatma T (2009) Proliferative genes dominate malignancy-risk gene signature in histologically-normal breast tissue. Breast Cancer Res Treat. doi:10.1007/s10549-009-0344-y

Cooper AP (1840) On the anatomy of the breast. Longman, Orme, Green, Brown and Longmans, London

Cooper BB (1843) The life of Sir Astley Cooper. John W. Parker, London

Dabelow A (1957) Die Milchdruse. Springer, Berlin/Gottingen/Heidelberg

Davies JA (2002) Do different branching epithelia use a conserved developmental mechanism? Bioessays 24:937–948

de Fazio A, Chiew YE, Sini RL, Janes PW, Sutherland RL (2000) Expression of c-erbB receptors, heregulin and oestrogen receptor in human breast cell lines. Int J Cancer 87: 487–498

Dooley WC (2009) Breast ductoscopy and the evolution of the intra-ductal approach to breast cancer. Breast J 15(Suppl 1):S90–S94

Egan RL (1982) Multicentric breast carcinomas: clinical-radiographic-pathologic whole organ studies and 10-year survival. Cancer 49:1123–1130

Egan RL, Ellis JT, Powell RW (1969) Team approach to the study of diseases of the breast. Cancer 23:847–854

Ellsworth DL, Ellsworth RE, Love B, Deyarmin B, Lubert SM, Mittal V, Hooke JA, Shriver CD (2004a) Outer breast quadrants demonstrate increased levels of genomic instability. Ann Surg Oncol 11:861–868

Ellsworth DL, Ellsworth RE, Love B, Deyarmin B, Lubert SM, Mittal V, Shriver CD (2004b) Genomic patterns of allelic imbalance in disease free tissue adjacent to primary breast carcinomas. Breast Cancer Res Treat 88:131–139

Ewing J (1940) Neoplastic diseases: a treatise on tumours. WB Saunders, Philadelphia/London

Faulkin LJ Jr, DeOme KB (1960) Regulation of growth and spacing of gland elements in the mammary fat pad of the C3H mouse. J Natl Cancer Inst 24:953–969

Faverly D, Holland R, Burgers L (1992) An original stereomicroscopic analysis of the mammary glandular tree. Virchows Arch A Pathol Anat Histopathol 421:115–119

Fiala JC (2005) Reconstruct: a free editor for serial section microscopy. J Microsc 218:52–61

Fialkow PJ (1976) Clonal origin of human tumors. Biochim Biophys Acta 458:283–321

Fleck L (1979) The genesis and development of a scientific fact. University of Chicago Press, Chicago

Foote FWJ, Stewart FW (1941) Lobular carcinoma in situ. A rare form of mammary cancer. Am J Pathol 17:491–496

Foschini MP, Flamminio F, Miglio R, Calo DG, Cucchi MC, Masetti R, Eusebi V (2006) The impact of large sections and 3D technique on the study of lobular in situ and invasive carcinoma of the breast. Virchows Arch 448:256–261

Garijo MF, Val D, Val-Bernal JF (2009) An overview of the pale and clear cells of the nipple epidermis. Histol Histopathol 24:367–376

Geddes DT (2007) Inside the lactating breast: the latest anatomy research. J Midwifery Womens Health 52:556–563

Going JJ (2006) Ductal-lobar organisation of human breast tissue, its relevance in disease and a research objective: vector mapping of parenchyma in complete breasts (the Astley Cooper project). Breast Cancer Res 8:107

Going JJ, Moffat DF (2004) Escaping from Flatland: clinical and biological aspects of human mammary duct anatomy in three dimensions. J Pathol 203:538–544

Going JJ, Mohun TJ (2006) Human breast duct anatomy, the 'sick lobe' hypothesis and intraductal approaches to breast cancer. Breast Cancer Res Treat 97:285–291

Holland R, Connolly JL, Gelman R, Mravunac M, Hendriks JH, Verbeek AL, Schnitt SJ, Silver B, Boyages J, Harris JR (1990a) The presence of an extensive intraductal component following a limited excision correlates with prominent residual disease in the remainder of the breast. J Clin Oncol 8:113–118

Holland R, Hendriks JH, Vebeek AL, Mravunac M, Schuurmans-Stekhoven JH (1990b) Extent, distribution, and mammographic/histological correlations of breast ductal carcinoma in situ. Lancet 335(8688):519–522

Jain S, Rezo A, Shadbolt B, Dahlstrom JE (2009) Synchronous multiple ipsilateral breast cancers: implications for patient management. Pathology 41:57–67

Jensen HM, Rice JR, Wellings SR (1976) Preneoplastic lesions in the human breast. Science 191(4224):295–297

Johnson JE, Page DL, Winfield AC, Reynolds VH, Sawyers JL (1995) Recurrent mammary carcinoma after local excision. A segmental problem. Cancer 75:1612–1618

Johnston LA, Prober DA, Edgar BA, Eisenman RN, Gallant P (1999) Drosophila myc regulates cellular growth during development. Cell 98:779–790

Khan SA, Wiley EL, Rodriguez N, Baird C, Ramakrishnan R, Nayar R, Bryk M, Bethke KB, Staradub VL, Wolfman J,

Rademaker A, Ljung BM, Morrow M (2004) Ductal lavage findings in women with known breast cancer undergoing mastectomy. J Natl Cancer Inst 96:1510–1517

Kordon EC, Smith GH (1998) An entire functional mammary gland may comprise the progeny from a single cell. Development 125:1921–1930

Kusano AS, Trichopoulos D, Terry KL, Chen WY, Willett WC, Michels KB (2006) A prospective study of breast size and premenopausal breast cancer incidence. Int J Cancer 118:2031–2034

Lakatos I (1976) Proofs and refutations. Cambridge University Press, Cambridge

Land CE (1995) Studies of cancer and radiation dose among atomic bomb survivors. The example of breast cancer. JAMA 274:402–407

Lee WC, Davies JA (2007) Epithelial branching: the power of self-loathing. Bioessays 29:205–207

Love SM, Barsky SH (2004) Anatomy of the nipple and breast ducts revisited. Cancer 101:1947–1957

Maley CC (2007) Multistage carcinogenesis in Barrett's esophagus. Cancer Lett 245:22–32

Maley CC, Galipeau PC, Li X, Sanchez CA, Paulson TG, Reid BJ (2004) Selectively advantageous mutations and hitchhikers in neoplasms: p16 lesions are selected in Barrett's esophagus. Cancer Res 64:3414–3427

Marucci G, Betts CM, Golouh R, Peterse JL, Foschini MP, Eusebi V (2002) Toker cells are probably precursors of Paget cell carcinoma: a morphological and ultrastructural description. Virchows Arch 441:117–123

Marusič A (2008) Jelena Krmpotic Namanic (1921–2008): conclusion of age of classical anatomy? Croat Med J 49:447–449

Meeker AK, Hicks JL, Gabrielson E, Strauss WM, De Marzo AM, Argani P (2004) Telomere shortening occurs in subsets of normal breast epithelium as well as in situ and invasive carcinoma. Am J Pathol 164:925–935

Moffat DF, Going JJ (1996) Three dimensional anatomy of complete duct systems in human breast: pathological and developmental implications. J Clin Pathol 49:48–52

Møller A, Soler M, Thornhill R (1995) Breast asymmetry, sexual selection, and human reproductive success. Ethol Sociobiol 16:207–219

Morata G, Ripoll P (1975) Minutes: mutants of drosophila autonomously affecting cell division rate. Dev Biol 42:211–221

Moreno E, Basler K (2004) dMyc transforms cells into super-competitors. Cell 117:117–129

Ohtake T, Abe R, Kimijima I, Fukushima T, Tsuchiya A, Hoshi K, Wakasa H (1995) Intraductal extension of primary invasive breast carcinoma treated by breast-conservative surgery. Computer graphic three-dimensional reconstruction of the mammary duct-lobular systems. Cancer 76:32–45

Ohtake T, Kimijima I, Fukushima T, Yasuda M, Sekikawa K, Takenoshita S, Abe R (2001) Computer-assisted complete three-dimensional reconstruction of the mammary ductal/lobular systems: implications of ductal anastomoses for breast-conserving surgery. Cancer 91:2263–2272

Ohuchi N (1999) Breast-conserving surgery for invasive cancer: a principle based on segmental anatomy. Tohoku J Exp Med 188:103–118

Ohuchi N, Abe R, Kasai M (1984a) Possible cancerous change of intraductal papillomas of the breast. A 3-D reconstruction study of 25 cases. Cancer 54:605–611

Ohuchi N, Abe R, Takahashi T, Tezuka F (1984b) Origin and extension of intraductal papillomas of the breast: a three-dimensional reconstruction study. Breast Cancer Res Treat 4:117–128

Ohuchi N, Abe R, Takahashi T, Tezuka F, Kyogoku M (1985) Three-dimensional atypical structure in intraductal carcinoma differentiating from papilloma and papillomatosis of the breast. Breast Cancer Res Treat 5:57–65

Osteen RT (1995) Strategies for breast-conserving surgery. An unresolved dilemma. Cancer 75:1563–1565, discussion 1566–1567

Page DL, Schuyler PA, Dupont WD, Jensen RA, Plummer WD Jr, Simpson JF (2003) Atypical lobular hyperplasia as a unilateral predictor of breast cancer risk: a retrospective cohort study. Lancet 361(9352):125–129

Parsons BL (2008) Many different tumor types have polyclonal tumor origin: evidence and implications. Mutat Res 659: 232–247

Perkins CI, Hotes J, Kohler BA, Howe HL (2004) Association between breast cancer laterality and tumor location, United States, 1994–1998. Cancer Causes Control 15:637–645

Preston SL, Wong WM, Chan AOO, Poulsom R, Jeffery R, Goodlad RA, Mandir N, Elia G, Novelli M, Bodmer WF, Tomlinson IP, Wright NA (2003) Bottom-up histogenesis of colorectal adenomas: origin in the monocryptal adenoma and initial expansion by crypt fission. Cancer Res 63: 3819–3825

Ramsay DT, Kent JC, Hartmann RA, Hartmann PE (2005) Anatomy of the lactating human breast redefined with ultrasound imaging. J Anat 206:525–534

Reddy G, Major MA, Leach GJ (2005) Toxicity assessment of thiodiglycol. Int J Toxicol 24:435–442

Rusby JE, Brachtel EF, Michaelson JS, Koerner FC, Smith BL (2007) Breast duct anatomy in the human nipple: three-dimensional patterns and clinical implications. Breast Cancer Res Treat 106:171–179

Schelfhout VR, Coene ED, Delaey B, Thys S, Page DL, De Potter CR (2000) Pathogenesis of Paget's disease: epidermal heregulin-alpha, motility factor, and the HER receptor family. J Natl Cancer Inst 92:622–628

Scutt D, Lancaster GA, Manning JT (2006) Breast asymmetry and predisposition to breast cancer. Breast Cancer Res 8:R14

Sharpe CR (1998) A developmental hypothesis to explain the multicentricity of breast cancer. CMAJ 159:55–59

Sinn HP (2009) Breast cancer precursors: lessons learned from molecular genetics. J Mol Med 87:113–115

Spalteholz KW (1914) Ueber das Durehsichtigmachen von Menschlichen und Tierischen Preparaten. S. Hirzel, Stuttgart

Staudt T, Lang MC, Medda R, Engelhardt J, Hell SW (2007) 2, 2'-thiodiethanol: a new water soluble mounting medium for high resolution optical microscopy. Microsc Res Tech 70:1–9

Stolier AJ, Wang J (2008) Terminal duct lobular units are scarce in the nipple: implications for prophylactic nipple-sparing mastectomy: terminal duct lobular units in the nipple. Ann Surg Oncol 15:438–442

Stull MA, Pai V, Vomachka AJ, Marshall AM, Jacob GA, Horseman ND (2007) Mammary gland homeostasis employs serotonergic regulation of epithelial tight junctions. Proc Natl Acad Sci USA 104:16708–16713

Thorlacius S, Thorlacius S, Olafsdottir G, Tryggvadottir L, Neuhausen S, Jonasson JG, Tavtigian SV, Tulinius H, Ogmundsdottir HM, Eyfjord JE (1996) A single BRCA2 mutation in male and female breast cancer families from Iceland with varied cancer phenotypes. Nat Genet 13:117–119

Toker C (1970) Clear cells of the nipple epidermis. Cancer 25:601–610

Tokunaga M, Land CE, Tokuoka S, Nishimori I, Soda M, Akiba S (1994) Incidence of female breast cancer among atomic bomb survivors, 1950–1985. Radiat Res 138:209–223

Tondre J, Nejad M, Casano A, Mills D, Love S (2008) Technical enhancements to breast ductal lavage. Ann Surg Oncol 15:2734–2738

Tot T, Tabar L, Dean PB (2000) The pressing need for better histologic–mammographic correlation of the many variations in normal breast anatomy. Virchows Arch 437:338–344

Tripathi A, King C, de la Morenas A, Perry VK, Burke B, Antoine GA, Hirsch EF, Kavanah M, Mendez J, Stone M, Gerry NP, Lenburg ME, Rosenberg CL (2008) Gene expression abnormalities in histologically normal breast epithelium of breast cancer patients. Int J Cancer 122:1557–1566

Tyler DM, Li W, Zhuo N, Pellock B, Baker NE (2007) Genes affecting cell competition in Drosophila. Genetics 175: 643–657

von Gerlach J (1848) Handbuch der allgemeinen und speciellen Gewebelehre des menschlichen Korpers fur Aerzte und Studirende. Janitsch, Mainz

Wellings SR, Jensen HM, Marcum RG (1975) An atlas of subgross pathology of the human breast with special reference to possible precancerous lesions. J Natl Cancer Inst 55: 231–273

Wilde CJ, Addey CV, Boddy LM, Peaker M (1995) Autocrine regulation of milk secretion by a protein in milk. Biochem J 305:51–58

Yan PS, Venkataramu C, Ibrahim A, Liu JC, Shen RZ, Diaz NM, Centeno B, Weber F, Leu YW, Shapiro CL, Eng C, Yeatman TJ, Huang TH (2006) Mapping geographic zones of cancer risk with epigenetic biomarkers in normal breast tissue. Clin Cancer Res 12:6626–6636

Yang CP, Weiss NS, Band PR, Gallagher RP, White E, Daling JR (1993) History of lactation and breast cancer risk. Am J Epidemiol 138:1050–1056

Breast Cancer May Originate In Utero: The Importance of the Intrauterine Environment for Breast Cancer Development

3

Fei Xue and Karin B. Michels

3.1 Introduction

Breast cancer is the most common female cancer worldwide and the second leading cause of cancer death (after lung cancer) (American Cancer Society 2009). The incidence of breast cancer varies four- to fivefold across countries, is the highest in Europe and North America, and the lowest in Asia (Ferlay et al. 2001). Breast cancer incidence has been on the rise since the 1930s, with more dramatic increase in the 1980s (White et al. 1990; Devesa et al. 1994). The incidence of breast cancer in the US stabilized from 2001 to 2003 and started to decline in 2003, possibly due, in part, to the reduced use of hormone replacement therapy (Howe et al. 2006). It was projected that in 2010, 207,090 women would develop invasive breast cancer and 39,840 women will die from the disease (American Cancer Society 2010).

Through decades of research, factors including family history of breast cancer in first-degree relatives, benign breast disease, mammographic density, endogenous hormone levels, younger age at menarche, low parity, older age at first birth, older age at menopause, postmenopausal hormone use, ionizing radiation exposure, height, high postmenopausal body mass index, and low premenopausal body mass index have been established as risk factors of breast cancer (Adami et al.

2002). Nonetheless, only a modest percentage of breast cancer cases are attributable to recognized risk factors (Madigan et al. 1995), and most epidemiologic investigations of the etiology of breast cancer have concentrated on events during women's reproductive years. To provide an alternative perspective on the etiology of breast cancer, this chapter reviews evidence supporting the effect of intrauterine exposures on breast cancer development and discusses potential underlying mechanisms including alterations in levels of pregnancy steroid hormones and growth factors and their impact on prenatal development of mammary stem cells.

3.2 Intrauterine Exposure and Breast Cancer Risk

In an early animal experiment, 19 out of 23 female pregnant rats (82.6%) injected with carcinogenic agents (dibenzanthracene in olive oil) through the uterine wall directly into amniotic fluid had offspring which developed primary carcinoma of the lung (Law 1940). Other animal studies have also suggested that when pregnant animals were exposed to any of at least 38 different chemical carcinogens, the offspring were more likely to develop tumors (Tomatis 1979). In parallel with findings from animals, descendants of women who were exposed to carcinogens such as diethylstilbestrol (DES) were reported to have increased risk of vaginal adenocarcinoma (Greenwald et al. 1971). Additionally, intrauterine exposure to ionizing radiation was found to be related to leukemia and other tumors in childhood (Macmahon 1962).

Based on evidence from early animal and human studies, Trichopoulos hypothesized that exposure to high levels of endogenous estrogens in utero might

F. Xue
Obstetrics and Gynecology Epidemiology Division,
Department of Obstetrics, Gynecology and Reproductive
Biology, Brigham and Women's Hospital, Harvard Medical
School, Boston, MA, USA and
Department of Epidemiology,
Harvard School of Public Health,
Boston, MA, USA
e-mail: n2fei@channing.harvard.edu

T. Tot (ed.), *Breast Cancer*, DOI: 10.1007/978-1-84996-314-5_3,
© Springer-Verlag London Limited 2011

initiate breast cancer development, and that perinatal factors might be used as surrogate measures of intra-uterine estrogen exposure (Trichopoulos 1990a, b). Subsequently, numerous epidemiologic studies have been conducted on various potential measures of intra-uterine exposure, including birth weight and other measures of birth size, parental age at delivery, gestational age, twin membership, radiation, and other pregnancy-related complications and maternal characteristics (Xue and Michels 2007a).

3.2.1 Birth Weight

As a potential marker of intrauterine exposure to insulin-like growth factor (IGF)-I (Bennett et al. 1983; Reece et al. 1994), IGF-II (Bennett et al. 1983; Reece et al. 1994; Baldwin et al. 1993; Hill 1990), and estrogen (Petridou et al. 1990; Liehr 2000), birth weight is the most studied intrauterine factor in the context of breast cancer. More than 30 publications have collectively suggested that higher birth weight is associated with around 15–25% increased risk of breast cancer relative to low birth weight (Michels and Xue 2006; Xue and Michels 2007a; Park et al. 2008; Xu et al. 2009). The thresholds usually identified were >4,000 g for high birth weight and <2,500 g for low birth weight. Results from a recent pooled analysis including 21,825 breast cancer cases from 29 studies on birth size and the risk of breast cancer also suggested that, relative to birth weight of 3,000–3,499 g, those weighing ≥4,000 g had a higher risk of breast cancer [Relative risk (RR) = 1.12, 95% CI 1.00–1.25] (Dos Silva et al. 2008). When breast cancer cases were separately assessed according to menopausal status, premenopausal cancer was more consistently associated with the risk of breast cancer than postmenopausal breast cancer (Michels and Xue 2006). The association persists across various study designs (case–control or cohort), method of birth weight assessment (birth records, self-reports, reports by the mother, etc.), and different countries. Furthermore, the association between birth weight and the risk of breast cancer does not seem to be confounded by other measured intrauterine factors, such as gestational age, birth length, maternal preeclampsia or eclampsia, parental age, birth order, parental smoking, or multifetal gestation, etc. (Michels and Xue 2006).

3.2.2 Maternal Age at Delivery

Women who give birth at older age have higher serum estrogen levels possibly exposing the fetus to elevated levels of this hormone (Petridou et al. 1990; Panagiotopoulou et al. 1990). At least 16 studies have evaluated the potential influence of maternal age at delivery on the risk of breast cancer among daughters (Xue et al. 2006; Park et al. 2008; Nichols et al. 2008). Results from the majority of studies which assessed this association regardless of the menopausal status at diagnosis suggest an increased risk of breast cancer associated with older maternal age at birth (Xue and Michels 2007a; Park et al. 2008). A meta-analysis has suggested a statistically significant 13% increase in breast cancer risk associated with older maternal age, and the association holds for both cohort and case–control studies. The cutoff point of high maternal age varied from late twenties to late thirties. Results did not differ materially between pre- and postmenopausal breast cancer (Xue and Michels 2007a). Several studies considered paternal age and birth order, both of which may be correlated with maternal age, as potential confounders. Adjustment for paternal age produced varying effects: the association was attenuated in several studies (Le Marchand et al. 1988; Zhang et al. 1995; Hemminki and Kyyronen 1999; Xue et al. 2006) but persisted in others (Janerich et al. 1989; Innes et al. 2000; Choi et al. 2005). Birth order was less influential and the maternal age-breast cancer association remained essentially the same in almost all studies that adjusted for it in the analysis (Xue and Michels 2007a).

3.2.3 Paternal Age at Delivery

Children born to older fathers have a higher incidence of autosomal dominant disorders, which have been related to increased base substitutions and structural chromosomal anomalies in spermatozoa (Jung et al. 2003; Glaser and Jabs 2004). Meiosis errors are also expected to be more prevalent in paternal than maternal germline with increased age, since sperm cells continued to divide after birth, unlike egg cells (Jung et al. 2003). Furthermore, DNA-repair activity and apoptosis of germ cells in response to mutagens were found to decline with paternal age (Wei et al. 1993;

Brinkworth 2000). At least 11 studies have examined older paternal age as a potential risk factor for breast cancer among daughters (Xue and Michels 2007a; Weiss-Salz et al. 2007), and findings from these studies have collectively suggested an approximate 10% increase in the risk of breast cancer associated with older paternal age at birth (the cutoff point ranged from early to late thirties). Studies that separately assessed premenopausal breast cancer collectively suggested a slightly stronger association with older paternal age (Xue and Michels 2007a; Weiss-Salz et al. 2007), though no study has separately evaluated postmenopausal breast cancer. After adjustment for maternal age as a potential confounding variable, the paternal age-breast cancer association persisted with statistical significance in two (Janerich et al. 1989; Choi et al. 2005) out of eight studies (Le Marchand et al. 1988; Janerich et al. 1989; Zhang et al. 1995; Hemminki and Kyyronen 1999; Innes et al. 2000; Hodgson et al. 2004; Choi et al. 2005; Xue et al. 2006), despite the potential collinearity between maternal and paternal age. Similar to studies on maternal age, most studies on paternal age adjusted for birth order as a potential confounding variable, and results remained essentially unchanged (Xue and Michels 2007a).

3.2.4 Birth Order

Pregnancy estrogen is higher for the first pregnancy than the second or later pregnancies (Panagiotopoulou et al. 1990). Levels of estradiol, estrone, and progesterone are also higher during the first pregnancy and decrease in subsequent pregnancies (Maccoby et al. 1979). Thus, in utero exposure to pregnancy hormones may be higher for a fetus of a primipara than a subsequent conception. A meta-analysis on the association between birth order and the risk of breast cancer included 17 published studies including 15 case–control and 2 cohort studies (Park et al. 2008). Among 14 studies which compared first births with 2nd or higher birth order, the risk of breast cancer in adulthood did not differ (summary RR = 0.97, 95% CI 0.91–1.04) across all studies or among case–control studies (OR = 0.99, 95% CI 0.94–1.04), though the one single cohort study reported a decreased risk for first birth (OR = 0.28, 95% CI 0.21–0.36). When higher birth orders were studied,

birth orders 2–4 did not differ in risk (OR = 0.97, 95% CI 0.91–1.03), but women with a birth order of 5+ were at a marginal reduced risk (OR = 0.88, 95% CI 0.75–1.01) relative to first birth. A recent case–control study suggested that breast-feeding status in infancy may modify the association between birth order and breast cancer as birth order was inversely associated with breast cancer only among breast-fed women (Nichols et al. 2008).

3.2.5 Gestational Age

Gestational age has also been suggested to be related to the risk of breast cancer, mainly because hypothalamic maturation in utero, which is closely related to the length of gestation, determines the level of postnatal gonadotropin. In fact, during the first 10 weeks after birth, daughters born with a shorter gestational age have substantially higher levels of gonadotropins (Tapanainen et al. 1981), which may lead to ovarian hyperstimulation and consequently elevated estradiol levels and breast cancer risk (Ekbom et al. 2000). Furthermore, girls who survive preterm birth are likely to experience an accelerated postnatal growth which has been suggested to be associated with a higher risk of breast cancer later in life (Forman et al. 2005). The effect of gestational age on the risk of breast cancer has been assessed in at least 12 studies to date (Xue and Michels 2007a; Park et al. 2008). Despite the biological plausibility, these studies generated fairly mixed results with regard to both the direction and the significance of the association. The cutoff point for shorter gestational age used in the reviewed studies ranged from ≤32 weeks to <39 weeks, and for longer gestational age ≥35 weeks to ≥42 weeks. Meta-analyses based on these studies suggested a lack of significant association between gestational age or preterm birth and breast cancer (Xue and Michels 2007a; Park et al. 2008). When premenopausal breast cancer and postmenopausal breast cancer were separately assessed, neither was significantly associated with breast cancer risk. The results were also consistent across cohort and case–control studies. Adjustment for birth weight, birth order, family history of breast cancer and other early-life factors had minimal influence on the effect estimates for gestational age (Xue and Michels 2007a).

3.2.6 Birth Length

As a strong correlate of birth weight, birth length may affect the risk of breast cancer through the same underlying mechanisms, e.g., increased intrauterine exposure to estrogen, IGF-1, and IGF-II. Indeed, birth length was found to be positively related to estrogen levels in maternal blood (Troisi et al. 2003a; Mucci et al. 2003). To date, the association between birth length and the risk of breast cancer has been evaluated in at least eight published studies. A meta-analysis of these studies has suggested an approximate 28% (95% CI 11–48%) increased risk comparing higher birth length (cutoff point ≥49 to ≥53 cm) to lower birth length (cutoff point ≤44 to <50 cm) (Xue and Michels 2007a). Additionally, a recent pooled analysis involving 3,612 cases from 11 published and unpublished studies reported a significant 17% (95% CI 2–35%) increase in the risk of breast cancer for women with birth length ≥51 cm relative to those with birth length <49 cm (dos Silva et al. 2008). In the two studies that separately evaluated premenopausal breast cancer and postmenopausal breast cancer, the association of birth length with premenopausal breast cancer was more consistent than that with postmenopausal breast cancer (McCormack et al. 2003; Vatten et al. 2005). Other birth size measures, e.g., birth weight and head circumference, are likely confounders for the birth-length breast cancer association. However, these factors did not completely account for the observed association between birth length and breast cancer risk (McCormack et al. 2003).

3.2.7 Diethylstilbestrol (DES)

From 1938 through 1971, DES, a synthetic estrogen, was used in the US to support pregnancies which were threatened by miscarriage or premature birth. Adolescents exposed to DES before birth were found to have an elevated risk of vaginal adenocarcinoma (Greenwald et al. 1971). This observation suggested that cancer may originate in utero. Trichopoulos later hypothesized that prenatal exposure to high levels of estrogen may increase breast cancer risk later in life (Trichopoulos 1990a, b). To date, the association

between DES and breast cancer risk has been examined in at least five studies (Weiss et al. 1997; Hatch et al. 1998; Sanderson et al. 1998; Palmer et al. 2002; Troisi et al. 2007), and two of these studies (Hatch et al. 1998; Palmer et al. 2002) were updated by more recent analyses. Only one of the remaining three studies assessed breast cancer overall (RR = 1.40, 95% CI 0.86–2.28) and premenopausal breast cancer (RR = 1.87, 95% CI 0.72–4.83) comparing women with prenatal exposure to DES to those without it (Palmer et al. 2002). A meta-analysis of the remaining three studies on postmenopausal breast cancer produced a summary RR of 1.37 (95% CI 0.86–2.18) for women with prenatal exposure to DES (Xue and Michels 2007a). When other early-life exposure variables including gestational age at first DES exposure were adjusted for as potential confounders, the association remained essentially unchanged (Hatch et al. 1998).

3.2.8 Twin Membership

Compared with singleton pregnancies, twins can elicit almost twice the level of pregnancy-related hormones, including estrogen (TambyRaja and Ratnam 1981; Gonzalez et al. 1989), gonadotropin, and lactogen (Thiery et al. 1977). Furthermore, dizygotic twins may elicit a higher level of pregnancy-related hormones than monozygotic twins because they have two placentas (Kappel et al. 1985). Conversely, because multiple pregnancy likely induces earlier termination of pregnancy due to pregnancy-related complications, twins may experience shorter intrauterine exposure to pregnancy hormones than singletons. Despite conflicting results on the association between gestational age and the risk of breast cancer from existing studies, it is biologically plausible that longer duration of intrauterine exposure to pregnancy hormones may increase the risk of breast cancer later in life. At least 14 studies have investigated the association between twin membership and the risk of breast cancer (Xue and Michels 2007a; Park et al. 2008). Regardless of the menopausal status of breast cancer cases, these studies suggest a decrease in risk of about 7% in twins (marginal statistical significance) compared with singletons. When premenopausal and postmenopausal breast cancer cases were separately examined, the direction of the association was similar to the combined analysis (Xue and Michels 2007a). Interestingly, when monozygotic twins and dizygotic twins were separately assessed, dizygotic twin membership was associated with a marginally increased risk of breast cancer, though results from the included studies were heterogeneous; monozygotic twin membership was associated with a decreased risk (Xue and Michels 2007a). These results suggest that the extra pregnancy hormone secretion due to the two placentas in dizygotic twins may overpower the reduced duration of exposure due to early termination of pregnancy. Dizygotic twins are also more often conceived by women who are taller or overweight, older, or non-Hispanic blacks, factors that may also differentiate their risk profile of breast cancer from that of monozygotic twins (Shipley et al. 1967; Oleszczuk et al. 2001; Hamilton et al. 2006). Nonetheless, more data are needed to confirm these hypotheses, particularly because studies that directly assessed the effect of zygosity of twin membership on breast cancer risk by comparing dizygotic twins to monozygotic twins (Swerdlow et al. 1997) or opposite-sex twins to same-sex twins (Swerdlow et al. 1996) did not suggest any significant difference.

3.2.9 Preeclampsia and Eclampsia

Preeclampsia and eclampsia are characterized by pregnancy-related hypertension and edema, with or without seizure, respectively. It has been suggested that pregnant women with preeclampsia or eclampsia have lower estrogen levels in blood (Zeisler et al. 2002) and urine (Long et al. 1979) than those without these disorders. Furthermore, preeclampsia and eclampsia may induce early termination of pregnancy because they are related to increased maternal and fetal morbidity and mortality, especially during the third trimester. Daughters born to mothers with preeclampsia or eclampsia are thus expected to have a decreased risk of breast cancer due to a reduced cumulative intrauterine exposure to estrogen and other pregnancy hormones than those born after normal pregnancy. To date, the effect of preeclampsia or eclampsia on the risk of breast cancer has been investigated in at least six studies, and a meta-analysis has suggested that preeclampsia or eclampsia is associated with a substantially

lower (52%) risk of breast cancer relative to normal pregnancy, though effect estimates from included studies were heterogeneous (Xue and Michels 2007a). Multiple pregnancy and maternal anthropometric factors prior to pregnancy may confound this association, but have not been considered in the studies available.

3.2.10 Other Intrauterine Exposures

Besides the aforementioned intrauterine factors or markers of intrauterine exposure that have been extensively studied, several other factors have also been suggested to be related to breast cancer risk, though the evidence is still sparse. Much has been learned from the bombing of Hiroshima and Nagasaki about the influence of intrauterine exposure to ionizing radiation on subsequent cancer risk. Children exposed to the atomic bombings in utero were at a higher risk of cancer overall, especially cancer in childhood, compared to children whose mothers were not exposed (Kato et al. 1989). Additionally, though intrauterine data were not reported, the relative risk associated with exposure to the atomic bomb blasts was the highest among the group who were youngest when exposed (0–5 years) (Land 1995).

Several perinatal conditions have also been studied in relation to subsequent risk of breast cancer, though the evidence is still insufficient to draw any conclusions. Neonatal jaundice is a potential marker for infection in utero or impaired fetal liver function, which increases endogenous estrogen levels (Lauritzen and Lehmann 1966; Robine et al. 1988). One study that assessed neonatal jaundice in relation to the risk of breast cancer later in life suggested a significant doubled risk among infants with neonatal jaundice compared to those without it (Ekbom et al. 1997). Maternal gestational diabetes has also been suggested to influence fetal growth through altering placental growth hormone levels, which may modify substrate availability and regulate paracrine actions in the placental bed (McIntyre et al. 2009). Maternal gestational diabetes was studied as a risk factor for breast cancer among daughters in one study, which found no association (Mogren et al. 1999). Maternal weight gain during pregnancy was positively associated with the risk of breast cancer in daughters in the one study considering this association [OR 1.5 (95%

CI 1.1–2.1) for a gain of 11–15 kg relative to a gain of <7 kg] (Sanderson et al. 1998). Maternal life style factors during pregnancy, e.g., coffee consumption and alcohol consumption, were not related to the daughter's breast cancer risk (Sanderson et al. 1998).

3.2.11 Summary of Evidence

A summary of the existing evidence regarding a range of intrauterine exposure variables in association with the risk of breast cancer is displayed in Table 3.1.

Table 3.1 Summary of evidence for intrauterine exposures and the risk of breast cancer

Intrauterine exposures	Direction of association	Strength of the evidence
Higher birth weight	↑	+++
Advanced maternal age at delivery	↑	++
Advanced paternal age at delivery	↑	++
Higher birth order	Ø	+
Longer gestational age	Ø	±
Higher birth length	↑	++
DES exposure	Ø	±
Twin membership overall	↓	+
Monozygotic	↓	+
Dizygotic	↑	+
Preeclampsia and eclampsia	↓	++
Other intrauterine factors		
Ionizing radiation	↑	++
Neonatal jaundice	↑	±
Maternal diabetes	Ø	±
Maternal weight gain during pregnancy	↑	±
Maternal coffee consumption	Ø	±
Maternal alcohol consumption	Ø	±

↑, increased risk of breast cancer; ↓, decreased risk of breast cancer; Ø, no association

+++, likely association; ++, probable association; +, possible association; ±, evidence is too sparse to draw any conclusion

3.3 Potential Mechanisms

As mentioned for each of the intrauterine exposures, the majority of the mechanisms underlying the association between these exposures and the risk of breast cancer likely involve alterations of maternal pregnancy hormones, growth hormones, and IGFs, as well as consequent mammary stem cell abnormalities.

3.3.1 Hormone Alterations

3.3.1.1 Estrogen

Intrauterine exposure to elevated endogenous estrogen levels was the basis of the initial hypothesis raised by Trichopoulos (1990a, b). Birth weight, maternal age, gestational age, birth length, twin membership, preeclampsia, and eclampsia all affect intrauterine estrogen levels and possibly subsequent breast cancer risk.

From the fourth week to the seventh week of gestation, the placenta supplants the maternal ovaries as the main source of estrogen in both the maternal and fetal circulation (Siiteri and MacDonald 1966; Csapo et al. 1973). By the end of gestation, maternal estriol production is 1,000 times the average daily level in normal ovulatory women, and it becomes the most important estrogen in pregnancy (Tulchinsky et al. 1971). Additionally, estradiol and estrone also increase in maternal blood and rise from 50–100 pg/ml to 30,000 pg/ml at term (Lindberg et al. 1974). On the fetus's side, by the end of the third trimester, around 90% of estriol is produced by placenta from 16a-hydroxydehydroepiandrosterone sulfate in fetal plasma, and 50% of estradiol is produced by placenta from fetal dehydroepiandrosterone sulfate (DHEAS). The majority of these steroid hormones (80–90%) from the placenta enter the maternal circulation (Casey and MacDonald 1992). Thus, the level of DHEAS production by fetal adrenal glands determines the level of circulating estrogens in both maternal and fetal blood. Fetal and maternal hormone levels were found to be correlated, with correlation coefficient of 0.26, 0.27, and 0.41 for estriol, estradiol, and estrone, respectively (Troisi et al. 2003b).

Estrogen has long been recognized as a promoter of cancer growth due to its growth-stimulating potential. It was believed that estrogen would stimulate cell proliferation and cell growth and promote cancer development by increasing the chances that a cell with potential cancer-causing mutations will multiply, while the initiation of the mutation was attributed to other internal or external carcinogens (Pike et al. 1993; Platet et al. 2004). Later studies based on cell culture suggested that estrogen metabolites can bind to DNA and trigger mutations; estrogen metabolites may also influence the levels of enzymes involved in the removal of active compounds such as 4-hydroxyestradiol that might initiate cancer (Zhu and Conney 1998). These data suggest that estrogen may also be a cancer initiator (Service 1998).

3.3.1.2 Insulin-Like Growth Factors (IGFs)

IGFs are 7-kDa polypeptides structurally homologous to proinsulin, synthesized by almost all tissues but mainly by liver in humans (Le Roith 1997; Zapf et al. 1984). They are important mediators in regulating cell growth, differentiation, and transformation (Le Roith 1997). Both *IGF1* and *IGF2* genes are expressed in fetal tissues throughout gestation and play important roles in the regulation of fetal–placental growth (Fowden 2003). IGF-I and IGF-II stimulate cell division and differentiation through autocrine, paracrine, and endocrine means during gestation (Ostlund et al. 2002). Fetal serum levels of IGF-I and IGF-II increase with gestational age (Giudice et al. 1995).

In humans, partial *IGF1* deletion has been linked to severe intrauterine growth failure (Morison et al. 1996). Studies have consistently shown that IGF-I levels in fetal blood are positively related to indicators of birth size, including birth weight (Gluckman et al. 1983; Osorio et al. 1996; Klauwer et al. 1997), birth weight independent of gestational age (Gluckman et al. 1983; Lassarre et al. 1991), birth length (Klauwer et al. 1997), ponderal index (Osorio et al. 1996), and placental weight (Osorio et al. 1996). Spencer et al. found that infants who were small for gestational age according to the first ultrasound measurement, with evidence of subsequent fetal growth restriction, had significantly lower cord blood IGF-I than did infants who were small for gestational age but with normal subsequent growth and infants appropriate for gestational age (Spencer et al. 1995).

The importance of IGF-II in determining intrauterine growth is less consistently supported by human studies that link fetal blood IGF-II level to birth size. In a study by Giudice et al., IGF-II in fetal cord serum was significantly lower in infants with intrauterine growth retardation (Giudice et al. 1995). Ong et al. found that fetal circulating IGF-II was weakly correlated to ponderal index at birth ($r = 0.18$) and placental weight ($r = 0.18$) (Ong et al. 2000). Bennett et al. also found a significant positive correlation between birth weight and cord IGF-II level (Bennett et al. 1983). However, other studies failed to confirm the association of fetal IGF-II level with measures of birth size, including birth weight (Gluckman et al. 1983; Lassarre et al. 1991; Osorio et al. 1996; Klauwer et al. 1997), birth weight independent of gestational age (Gluckman et al. 1983), birth length (Klauwer et al. 1997), ponderal index (Osorio et al. 1996), and placental weight (Osorio et al. 1996) possibly because IGF-II levels measured at birth do not reflect levels throughout pregnancy. The importance of IGF-II is greatest during intrauterine life, and it is thought to play a subsidiary role after birth.

Results of studies seeking to identify an association between circulating IGF-I and IGF-II levels in relation to breast cancer risk in human remain largely negative. Results from earlier studies on IGF-I suggested a positive though inconsistent association with premenopausal breast cancer (Hankinson and Schernhammer 2003); however, more recent studies based on larger prospective datasets did not support this association (Kaaks et al. 2002; Schernhammer et al. 2005, 2006). IGF-II was found to be associated with the risk of pre- or postmenopausal breast cancer in some (Grønbaek et al. 2004) but not all human studies (Holdaway et al. 1999; Li et al. 2001; Yu et al. 2002; Allen et al. 2005). Nonetheless, it is well-established that IGF-I and IGF-II can stimulate cell proliferation and inhibit cell death in many tissue types (Pollak 2000), including both normal and malignant breast tissue (Sachdev and Yee 2001). Although evidence for a link between circulating levels of IGF-I and IGF-II in adults and subsequent cancer risk is weak, it has not been explored whether any unique features of the fetal IGF system may affect the initiation or promotion of carcinogenesis in fetal mammary tissues. The fetal IGF system differs from the adult system in several ways. IGFs and insulin are the two factors that substantially regulate fetal growth, especially in the second and third trimesters, while growth hormone plays a minor role. Furthermore, in the second half of pregnancy, the IGF-II gene is more abundantly expressed than the IGF-I gene (Hill 1990), while IGF-I becomes predominant after birth as a result of the onset of growth hormone–stimulated IGF-I production by the liver. During late gestation, the fetal circulating level of IGF-II (150–400 ng/ml) can be three to four times higher than that of IGF-I (50–100 ng/ml) (Gluckman et al. 1983; Bennett et al. 1983; Reece et al. 1994). Therefore, IGF-II has been suggested to be primarily responsible for the regulation of fetal growth (Jones and Clemmons 1995; Allan et al. 2001).

3.3.1.3 Insulin

Insulin is known to have a significant mitogenic effect in normal mammary tissue as well as breast cancer cells (Belfiore et al. 1996; Papa and Belfiore 1996). The concentrations of insulin receptors were found to be higher in breast cancer tissues than in normal breast tissues (Papa et al. 1990), and directly related to tumor size (Papa et al. 1990), grade (Papa et al. 1990), and mortality (Mathieu et al. 1997). Epidemiologic studies have provided suggestive but conflicting results with regard to the effect of fasting insulin and the risk of breast cancer (Xue and Michels 2007b). However, more consistent results were generated suggesting that breast cancer is associated with levels of C-peptide (Xue and Michels 2007b), which is generally used as a marker to reflect insulin secretion (Clark 1999).

Because insulin receptor shares structural similarity with IGF-1 receptor, insulin can exert direct effect on fetal growth by binding to IGF-1 receptor (Grassi and Giuliano 2000). Further, insulin can also influence fetal growth by reversely controlling the expression of IGF binding proteins and thus regulating the bioavailability of IGF to high affinity receptors (Hill et al. 1998). Epidemiologic studies have suggested that the pattern of fetal growth can be influenced by maternal diet and metabolic function (Gluckman and Hanson 2004) and maternal insulin levels (Chiesa et al. 2008).

3.3.2 Hormone Alteration, Breast Stem Cells, and Carcinogenesis

3.3.2.1 Steroid Hormone and IGFs and Breast Development

Stem cells have the potential to perpetuate through self-renewal and generate mature cells of a particular tissue through differentiation (Reya et al. 2001). The differentiating potential of the human mammary gland is reflected by its development. The mammary gland is not fully developed at birth (Russo and Russo 1987) and in the human progresses through several stages, from in utero through the completion of the first full-term pregnancy. The development of the embryonic mammary gland culminates in a vesicle that contains colostrum at birth (Russo and Russo 2004). The stem cells further divide and become epithelial cells, alveolar cells, and myoepithelial cells. The mammary gland parenchyma consists of ducts terminating in end buds before puberty, undergoes proliferation and differentiation resulting in increased alveolar lobes during puberty (Rudland et al. 1996), and reaches maximal differentiation upon the first full-term pregnancy and lactation (Russo and Russo 1987).

Circulating hormone levels influence the growth of the mammary gland, with estrogen inducing ductal growth and progesterone promoting alveolar lobes (Rudland et al. 1996). Estrogen is the major steroid mitogen for the luminal epithelial cell population, which is often the target for carcinogenic transformation (Anderson et al. 1998). Estradiol has proliferative potential and affects DNA synthesis through binding to estrogen receptor in mammary epithelium. Steroid hormones modulate the synthesis of stimulatory and inhibitory growth factors, and growth factor receptors and binding proteins (Kenney and Dickson 1996).

Similarly, growth hormone, IGF-I and IGF-II also play a fundamental role in regulating the development of mammary gland by affecting proliferation, differentiation, and apoptosis of breast tissue (Laban et al. 2003). IGFs may also interact with estrogen in influencing mammary gland development by affecting the phosphorylation and function of steroid receptors and potentiating or reducing the mitogenic effect of steroid hormones (Kenney and Dickson 1996). Furthermore, IGF-I receptor gene expression was found to be upregulated in in vivo models, where normal human breast epithelial cells were treated with estradiol, and in in vitro models, where malignant cancer cells were treated with estradiol (Clarke et al. 1997).

3.3.2.2 Breast Stem Cells and Breast Cancer

It has been speculated that stem cells represent the cellular origin of cancer, as they exist quiescently over long periods of time, and therefore could accumulate mutations that eventually lead to cancer when stimulated to proliferate (Sell 2004). A relation between stem cells in the mammary gland and carcinogenesis was suggested by Rudland and Barraclough (Rudland and Barraclough 1988). At least a portion of breast cells have a long half-life, similar to stem cells, and play an important role in breast carcinogenesis, because a subset of breast cancers recur 10 years after initial diagnosis and excision of the primary tumor (Rosen et al. 1989).

The fetal mammary gland starts to develop at about 8–15 weeks of gestation, possibly as the progeny of a single embryonic stem cell (Kordon and Smith 1998). During the prenatal period, mammary gland cells are in a partially undifferentiated state and may be more susceptible to cancer initiation (Russo and Russo 1996), particularly considering intrauterine exposure to high levels of estrogen and growth factors that favor cell replication (Gluckman et al. 1983). Trichopoulos postulated that intrauterine exposure to high levels of estrogen and IGFs may favor the generation of breast stem cells, and the number of these cells is directly related to mammary mass, which provides increased opportunity for genetic mutations (Trichopoulos et al. 2005). Ekbom et al. reported that high-density mammographic parenchymal pattern (P2 or DY) was significantly associated with the weight of placenta, which is the main estrogen-generating organ during pregnancy (Ekbom et al. 1995). The observation suggests that altered intrauterine exposure to estrogen may be associated with breast cancer risk by increasing mammary density.

3.3.3 Current Pathologic Hypotheses About Breast Carcinogenesis

3.3.3.1 Multifocal Origin

Breast cancer is a complex disease with a wide range of morphology. Based on classic whole-organ studies, it has long been postulated that most in situ and invasive breast cancer cases are multifocal, multicentric, or diffuse (Gallager and Martin 1969; Holland et al. 1985). In 1975, Wellings et al. proposed that most lesions referred to as mammary dysplasia or fibrocystic disease arose in terminal ductal-lobular units (TDLU) or in the lobules themselves, based on the histological examination of whole human breasts. These lesions include apocrine cysts, sclerosing adenosis, fibroadenomas, various forms of lobules (sclerotic, dilated, hypersecretory, hyperplastic, atypical, or anaplastic), ductal carcinoma in situ, and lobular carcinoma in situ (Wellings et al. 1975). This postulation was later widely accepted as the classic theory of breast cancer development: most malignant tumors of the breast originate from the epithelial cells of the lobules, which are terminal ductal-lobular units and spread to the ducts and other lobules by migration of the malignant cells.

3.3.3.2 Single-Lobe Origin

Traditional whole-organ studies using routine histological techniques often do not allow repetition of results. Recently, the traditional theory of multifocal origin of breast cancer was challenged by findings from more modern diagnostic techniques that offer more thorough analysis of the extent and distribution of lesions in a breast carcinoma. Tot and colleagues have examined and analyzed more than 5,000 consecutive breast cancer cases over 20 years using advanced methods involving two- and three-dimensional large histological sections with detailed and systematic radiopathologic correlation (Tot 2005). They found that many cases of ductal carcinoma in situ demonstrate continuous distribution along the ducts over several centimeters. Such a distance is unlikely if the origin of the process was a few individual terminal units, which are typically millimeters in size. In addition, the migration of the malignant cells from the epithelial cells of the lobules to the ducts and other lobules is not supported by histological examinations. It was then postulated that ductal carcinoma in situ, and consequently breast carcinoma in general, is a lobar disease, i.e., that simultaneously or asynchronously occurring in situ (and invasive) tumor foci belong to a single lobe in one breast (Tot 2005). If this new hypothesis is proven true, it may suggest new approaches to reduce the incidence of breast carcinoma by selective visualization, excision, or destruction of the sick lobe before the malignant lesions develop (Tot 2007).

3.3.3.3 Intrauterine Risk Factors and Single-Lobe Origin of Breast Cancer

The mammary gland parenchyma develops from a single epithelial ectodermal bud. The prenatal development of the mammary gland has been suggested to include ten stages, including ridge, milk hill, mammary disk, lobule type, cone, budding, indention, branching, canalization, and end-vesicle. At birth, the mammary gland is composed of very primitive structures: ducts ending in short ductules, lined with one or two layers of epithelial and one of myoepithelial cells (Russo and Russo 2004). The structures in the newborn mammary gland grow and branch, producing terminal end buds, which develop into alveolar buds. The buds further develop into primitive lobules of alveolar buds, which consists of three to five lobes and continue to divide until reaching the greatest number in puberty (Rudland 1993).

As intrauterine exposures to potential carcinogens have been suggested to initiate and/or promote breast cancer development before birth, carcinogenesis is expected to affect breast stem cells, which are undergoing branching into the primitive structure of mammary lobes. Though the ramification and branching process is almost complete during intrauterine life, lobularization mainly occurs during the postpubertal period (Tot et al. 2002). Indeed, there are relatively few terminal ductal-lobular units before puberty (Vogel et al. 1981). Therefore, the genetic mutations or epigenetic abnormalities involved in breast cancer development are more likely to be perpetuated by cells undergoing continuous branching and ramification while the lobe is being formed, rather than

originating within the terminal ductal-lobular units, the majority of which are not developed before birth. These postulations are in accordance with the hypothesis of the "sick lobe" by Tot and colleagues (Tot 2005, 2007).

3.4 Conclusions

Findings from epidemiologic studies suggest that markers of intrauterine exposures, such as birth weight, parental age at delivery, birth length, DES exposure, twin membership, and preeclampsia and eclampsia are associated with the risk of breast cancer later in life. Thus breast cancer may originate in utero, possibly involving the exposure of mammary stem cells to alterations of estrogen and IGFs in utero. The human mammary gland undergoes prenatal development into the primitive structure of mammary lobes, but lobularization mainly occurs during the postpubertal period. Thus it is possible that the prenatal genetic and/or epigenetic events in breast cancer development occur among cells within the same lobe through continuous branching and ramification, rather than originating within the terminal ductal-lobular units, most of which are not yet formed before birth.

References

Adami H, Hunter D, Trichopoulos D (2002) Textbook of cancer epidemiology. Oxford University Press, New York, pp 301–373

Allan GJ, Flint DJ, Patel K (2001) Insulin-like growth factor axis during embryonic development. Reproduction 122:31–39

Allen NE, Roddam AW, Allen DS, Fentiman IS, Dos Santos Silva I, Peto J, Holly JM, Key TJ (2005) A prospective study of serum insulin-like growth factor-I (IGF-I), IGF-II, IGF-binding protein-3 and breast cancer risk. Br J Cancer 92:1283–1287

American Cancer Society (2010) Cancer facts & figures 2009. American Cancer Society, Atlanta, http://www.cancer.org/Cancer/BreastCancer/OverviewGuide/breast-cancer-overview-key-statistics. Last Accessed 12 Sep 2010

Anderson E, Clarke RB, Howell A (1998) Estrogen responsiveness and control of normal human breast proliferation. J Mammary Gland Biol Neoplasia 3:23–35

Baldwin S, Chung M, Chard T, Wang HS (1993) Insulin-like growth factor-binding protein-1, glucose tolerance and fetal growth in human pregnancy. J Endocrinol 136:319–325

Belfiore A, Frittitta L, Costantino A, Frasca F, Pandini G, Sciacca L, Goldfine ID, Vigneri R (1996) Insulin receptors in breast cancer. Ann NY Acad Sci 784:173–188

Bennett A, Wilson DM, Liu F, Nagashima R, Rosenfeld RG, Hintz RL (1983) Levels of insulin-like growth factors I and II in human cord blood. J Clin Endocrinol Metab 57:609–612

Brinkworth MH (2000) Paternal transmission of genetic damage: findings in animals and humans. Int J Androl 23:123–135

Casey ML, MacDonald PC (1992) Alterations in steroid production by the human placenta. In: Pasqualini JR, Scholler R (eds) Hormones and fetal pathophysiology. Marcel Dekker, New York, p 251

Chiesa C, Osborn JF, Haass C, Natale F, Spinelli M, Scapillati E, Spinelli A, Pacifico L (2008) Ghrelin, leptin, IGF-1, IGFBP-3, and insulin concentrations at birth: is there a relationship with fetal growth and neonatal anthropometry. Clin Chem 54:550–558

Choi JY, Lee KM, Park SK, Nah DY, Ahn SH, Yoo KY, Kang D (2005) Association of paternal age at birth and the risk of breast cancer in offspring: a case control study. BMC Cancer 5:143

Clark PM (1999) Assays for insulin, proinsulin(s) and C-peptide. Ann Clin Biochem 36:541–564

Clarke RB, Howell A, Anderson E (1997) Type I insulin-like growth factor receptor gene expression in normal human breast tissue treated with oestrogen and progesterone. Br J Cancer 75:251–257

Csapo AI, Pulkkinen MO, Wiest WG (1973) Effects of luteectomy and progesterone replacement therapy in early pregnant patients. Am J Obstet Gynecol 115:759–765

Devesa SS, Grauman DJ, Blot WJ (1994) Recent cancer patterns among men and women in the United States: clues for occupational research. J Occup Med 36:832–841

dos Silva IS, De Stavola B, McCormack V (2008) Collaborative Group on Pre-Natal Risk Factors and Subsequent Risk of Breast Cancer. Birth size and breast cancer risk: re-analysis of individual participant data from 32 studies. PLoS Med 5:e193

Ekbom A, Thurfjell E, Hsieh CC, Trichopoulos D, Adami HO (1995) Perinatal characteristics and adult mammographic patterns. Int J Cancer 61:177–180

Ekbom A, Hsieh CC, Lipworth L, Adami HO, Trichopoulos D (1997) Intrauterine environment and breast cancer risk in women: a population-based study. J Natl Cancer Inst 89:71–76

Ekbom A, Erlandsson G, Hsieh C, Trichopoulos D, Adami HO, Cnattingius S (2000) Risk of breast cancer in prematurely born women. J Natl Cancer Inst 92:840–841

Ferlay J, Bray F, Pisani P, Parkin DM (2001) GLOBOCAN 2000: cancer incidence, mortality and prevalence worldwide. International Agency for Research on Cancer, Lyon

Forman MR, Cantwell MM, Ronckers C, Zhang Y (2005) Through the looking glass at early-life exposures and breast cancer risk. Cancer Invest 23:609–624

Fowden AL (2003) The insulin-like growth factors and feto-placental growth. Placenta 24:803–812

Gallager HS, Martin JE (1969) The study of mammary carcinoma by mammography and whole organ sectioning. Cancer 23:855–873

Giudice LC, de Zegher F, Gargosky SE, Dsupin BA, de las Fuentes L, Fuentes L, Crystal RA, Hintz RL, Rosenfeld RG (1995) Insulin-like growth factors and their binding proteins in the term and preterm human fetus and neonate with normal and extremes of intrauterine growth. J Clin Endocrinol Metab 80:1548–1555

Glaser RL, Jabs EW (2004) Dear old dad. Sci Aging Knowledge Environ 2004:re1

Gluckman PD, Hanson MA (2004) Maternal constraint of fetal growth and its consequences. Semin Fetal Neonatal Med 9:419–425

Gluckman PD, Johnson-Barrett JJ, Butler JH, Edgar BW, Gunn TR (1983) Studies of insulin-like growth factor-I and -II by specific radioligand assays in umbilical cord blood. Clin Endocrinol (Oxf) 19:405–413

Gonzalez MC, Reyes H, Arrese M, Figueroa D, Lorca B, Andresen M, Segovia N, Molina C, Arce S (1989) Intrahepatic cholestasis of pregnancy in twin pregnancies. J Hepatol 9:84–90

Grassi AE, Giuliano MA (2000) The neonate with macrosomia. Clin Obstet Gynecol 43:340–348

Greenwald P, Barlow JJ, Nasca PC, Burnett WS (1971) Vaginal cancer after maternal treatment with synthetic estrogens. N Engl J Med 285:390–392

Grønbaek H, Flyvbjerg A, Mellemkjaer L, Tjønneland A, Christensen J, Sørensen HT, Overvad K (2004) Serum insulin-like growth factors, insulin-like growth factor binding proteins, and breast cancer risk in postmenopausal women. Cancer Epidemiol Biomarkers Prev 13:1759–1764

Hamilton BE, Ventura SJ, Martin JA, Sutton PD (2006) Final births for 2004. Health E-stats. National Center for Health Statistics, Hyattsville, Released 6 July 2006

Hankinson SE, Schernhammer ES (2003) Insulin-like growth factor and breast cancer risk: evidence from observational studies. Breast Dis 17:27–40

Hatch EE, Palmer JR, Titus-Ernstoff L, Noller KL, Kaufman HR, Mittendorf R, Robboy SJ, Hyer M, Cowan CN, Colton T, Hartge P, Hoover RN (1998) Cancer risk in women exposed to diethylstilbestrol in utero. JAMA 280:630–634

Hemminki K, Kyyronen P (1999) Parental age and risk of sporadic and familial cancer in offspring: implications for germ cell mutagenesis. Epidemiology 10:747–751

Hill DJ (1990) Relative abundance and molecular size of immunoreactive insulin-like growth factors I and II in human fetal tissues. Early Hum Dev 21:49–58

Hill DJ, Petrik J, Arany E (1998) Growth factors and the regulation of fetal growth. Diab Care 21(Suppl 2):B60–B69

Hodgson ME, Newman B, Millikan RC (2004) Birth weight, parental age, birth order and breast cancer risk in African-American and white women: a population-based case–control study. Breast Cancer Res 6:R656–R667

Holdaway IM, Mason BH, Lethaby AE, Singh V, Harman JE, MacCormick M, Civil ID (1999) Serum levels of insulin-like growth factor binding protein-3 in benign and malignant breast disease. Aust N Z J Surg 69:495–500

Holland R, Velling SH, Mravunac M, Hendricks JH (1985) Histologic multifocality of Tis, T1-2 breast carcinomas: implications for clinical trials of breast conserving surgery. Cancer 56:979–990

Howe HL, Wu X, Ries LA, Cokkinides V, Ahmed F, Jemal A, Miller B, Williams M, Ward E, Wingo PA, Ramirez A,

Edwards BK (2006) Annual report to the nation on the status of cancer, 1975–2003, featuring cancer among U.S. Hispanic/Latino populations. Cancer 107:1711–1742

Innes K, Byers T, Schymura M (2000) Birth characteristics and subsequent risk for breast cancer in very young women. Am J Epidemiol 152:1121–1128

Janerich DT, Hayden CL, Thompson WD, Selenskas SL, Mettlin C (1989) Epidemiologic evidence of perinatal influence in the etiology of adult cancers. J Clin Epidemiol 42:151–157

Jones JI, Clemmons DR (1995) Insulin-like growth factors and their binding proteins: biological actions. Endocr Rev 16:3–34

Jung A, Schuppe HC, Schill WB (2003) Are children of older fathers at risk for genetic disorders? Andrologia 35:191–199

Kaaks R, Lundin E, Rinaldi S, Manjer J, Biessy C, Söderberg S, Lenner P, Janzon L, Riboli E, Berglund F, Hallmans G (2002) Prospective study of IGF-I, IGF binding proteins, and breast cancer risk, in northern and southern Sweden. Cancer Causes Control 13:307–316

Kappel B, Hansen K, Moller J, Faaborg-Andersen J (1985) Human placental lactogen and dU-estrogen levels in normal twin pregnancies. Acta Genet Med Gemellol (Roma) 34:59–65

Kato H, Yoshimoto Y, Schull WJ (1989) Risk of cancer among children exposed to atomic bomb radiation in utero: a review. IARC Sci Publ 96:365–374

Kenney NJ, Dickson RB (1996) Growth factor and sex steroid interactions in breast cancer. J Mammary Gland Biol Neoplasia 1:189–198

Klauwer D, Blum WF, Hanitsch S, Rascher W, Lee PD, Kiess W (1997) IGF-I, IGF-II, free IGF-I and IGFBP-1, -2 and -3 levels in venous cord blood: relationship to birthweight, length and gestational age in healthy newborns. Acta Paediatr 86:826–833

Kordon EC, Smith GH (1998) An entire functional mammary gland may comprise the progeny from a single cell. Development 125:1921–1930

Laban C, Bustin SA, Jenkins PJ (2003) The GH-IGF-I axis and breast cancer. Trends Endocrinol Metab 14:28–34

Land CE (1995) Studies of cancer and radiation dose among atomic bomb survivors. The example of breast cancer. JAMA 274:402–407

Lassarre C, Hardouin S, Daffos F, Forestier F, Frankenne F, Binoux M (1991) Serum insulin-like growth factors and insulin-like growth factor binding proteins in the human fetus. Relationships with growth in normal subjects and in subjects with intrauterine growth retardation. Pediatr Res 29:219–225

Lauritzen C, Lehmann WD (1966) The importance of steroid hormones in the pathogenesis of hyperbilirubinemia and neonatal jaundice. Z Kinderheilkd 95:143–154

Law LW (1940) The production of tumors by injection of a carcinogen into the amniotic fluid of mice. Science 91:96–97

Le Marchand L, Kolonel LN, Myers BC, Mi MP (1988) Birth characteristics of premenopausal women with breast cancer. Br J Cancer 57:437–439

Le Roith D (1997) Seminars in medicine of the Beth Israel Deaconess Medical Center. Insulin-like growth factors. N Engl J Med 336:633–640

Li BD, Khosravi MJ, Berkel HJ, Diamandi A, Dayton MA, Smith M, Yu H (2001) Free insulin-like growth factor-I and breast cancer risk. Int J Cancer 91:736–739

Liehr JG (2000) Is estradiol a genotoxic mutagenic carcinogen? Endocr Rev 21:40–54

Lindberg BS, Johansson ED, Nilsson BA (1974) Plasma levels of nonconjugated oestrone, oestradiol-17b and oestriol during uncomplicated pregnancy. Acta Obstet Gynecol Scand Suppl 32:21–36

Long PA, Abell DA, Beischer NA (1979) Fetal growth and placental function assessed by urinary estriol excretion before the onset of pre-eclampsia. Am J Obstet Gynecol 135:344–347

Maccoby EE, Doering CH, Nagy Jacklin C, Kraemer H (1979) Concentrations of sex hormones in umbilical-cord blood: their relation to sex and birth order of infants. Child Dev 50:632–642

Macmahon B (1962) Prenatal x-ray exposure and childhood cancer. J Natl Cancer Inst 28:1173–1191

Madigan MP, Ziegler RG, Benichou J, Byrne C, Hoover RN (1995) Proportion of breast cancer cases in the United States explained by well-established risk factors. J Natl Cancer Inst 87:1681–1685

Mathieu MC, Clark GM, Allred DC, Goldfine ID, Vigneri R (1997) Insulin receptor expression and clinical outcome in node-negative breast cancer. Proc Assoc Am Physicians 109:565–571

McCormack VA, dos Santos Silva I, De Stavola BL, Mohsen R, Leon DA, Lithell HO (2003) Fetal growth and subsequent risk of breast cancer: results from long term follow up of Swedish cohort. BMJ 326:248

McIntyre HD, Zeck W, Russell A (2009) Placental growth hormone, fetal growth and the IGF axis in normal and diabetic pregnancy. Curr Diab Rev 5:185–189

Michels KB, Xue F (2006) Role of birthweight in the etiology of breast cancer. Int J Cancer 119:2007–2025

Mogren I, Damber L, Tavelin B, Hogberg U (1999) Characteristics of pregnancy and birth and malignancy in the offspring (Sweden). Cancer Causes Control 10:85–94

Morison IM, Becroft DM, Taniguchi T, Woods CG, Reeve AE (1996) Somatic overgrowth associated with overexpression of insulin-like growth factor II. Nat Med 2:311–316

Mucci LA, Lagiou P, Tamimi RM, Hsieh CC, Adami HO, Trichopoulos D (2003) Pregnancy estriol, estradiol, progesterone and prolactin in relation to birth weight and other birth size variables (United States). Cancer Causes Control 14:311–318

Nichols HB, Trentham-Dietz A, Sprague BL, Hampton JM, Titus-Ernstoff L, Newcomb PA (2008) Effects of birth order and maternal age on breast cancer risk: modification by whether women had been breast-fed. Epidemiology 19:417–423

Oleszczuk JJ, Cervantes A, Kiely JL, Keith DM, Keith LG (2001) Maternal race/ethnicity and twinning rates in the United States, 1989–1991. J Reprod Med 46:550–557

Ong K, Kratzsch J, Kiess W, Costello M, Scott C, Dunger D (2000) Size at birth and cord blood levels of insulin, insulin-like growth factor I (IGF-I), IGF-II, IGF-binding protein-1 (IGFBP-1), IGFBP-3, and the soluble IGF-II/mannose-6-phosphate receptor in term human infants. The ALSPAC Study Team. Avon Longitudinal Study of Pregnancy and Childhood. J Clin Endocrinol Metab 85:4266–4269

Osorio M, Torres J, Moya F, Pezzullo J, Salafia C, Baxter R, Schwander J, Fant M (1996) Insulin-like growth factors (IGFs) and IGF binding proteins-1, -2, and -3 in newborn serum: relationships to fetoplacental growth at term. Early Hum Dev 46:15–26

Ostlund E, Tally M, Fried G (2002) Transforming growth factor-beta1 in fetal serum correlates with insulin-like growth factor-I and fetal growth. Obstet Gynecol 100:567–573

Palmer JR, Hatch EE, Rosenberg CL, Hartge P, Kaufman RH, Titus-Ernstoff L, Noller KL, Herbst AL, Rao RS, Troisi R, Colton T, Hoover RN (2002) Risk of breast cancer in women exposed to diethylstilbestrol in utero: preliminary results (United States). Cancer Causes Control 13: 753–758

Panagiotopoulou K, Katsouyanni K, Petridou E, Garas Y, Tzonou A, Trichopoulos D (1990) Maternal age, parity, and pregnancy estrogens. Cancer Causes Control 1:119–124

Papa V, Belfiore A (1996) Insulin receptors in breast cancer: biological and clinical role. J Endocrinol Invest 19:324–333

Papa V, Pezzino V, Costantino A, Belfiore A, Giuffrida D, Frittitta L, Vannelli GB, Brand R, Goldfin ID, Vigneri R (1990) Elevated insulin receptor content in human breast cancer. J Clin Invest 86:1503–1510

Park SK, Kang D, McGlynn KA, Garcia-Closas M, Kim Y, Yoo KY, Brinton LA (2008) Intrauterine environments and breast cancer risk: meta-analysis and systematic review. Breast Cancer Res 10:R8

Petridou E, Panagiotopoulou K, Katsouyanni K, Spanos E, Trichopoulos D (1990) Tobacco smoking, pregnancy estrogens, and birth weight. Epidemiology 1:247–250

Pike MC, Spicer DV, Dahmoush L, Press MF (1993) Estrogens, progestogens, normal breast cell proliferation, and breast cancer risk. Epidemiol Rev 15:17–35

Platet N, Cathiard AM, Gleizes M, Garcia M (2004) Estrogens and their receptors in breast cancer progression: a dual role in cancer proliferation and invasion. Crit Rev Oncol Hematol 51:55–67

Pollak M (2000) Insulin-like growth factor physiology and cancer risk. Eur J Cancer 36:1224–1228

Reece EA, Wiznitzer A, Le E, Homko CJ, Behrman H, Spencer EM (1994) The relation between human fetal growth and fetal blood levels of insulin-like growth factors I and II, their binding proteins and receptors. Obstet Gynecol 84: 88–95

Reya T, Morrison SJ, Clarke MF, Weissman IL (2001) Stem cells, cancer, and cancer stem cells. Nature 414:105–111

Robine N, Relier JP, Le Bars S (1988) Urocytogram, an index of maturity in premature infants. Biol Neonate 54:93–99

Rosen PR, Groshen S, Saigo PE, Kinne DW, Hellman S (1989) A long-term follow-up study of survival in stage I (T1N0M0) and stage II (T1N1M0) breast carcinoma. J Clin Oncol 7:355–366

Rudland PS (1993) Epithelial stem cells and their possible role in the development of the normal and diseased human breast. Histol Histopathol 8:385–404

Rudland PS, Barraclough R (1988) Stem cells in mammary gland differentiation and cancer. J Cell Sci Suppl 10: 95–114

Rudland PS, Barraclough R, Fernig DG, Smith JA (1996) Growth and differentiation of the normal mammary gland and its tumors. Biochem Soc Symp 63:1–20

Russo J, Russo IH (1987) Development of the human mammary gland. In: Neville MC, Daniel CW (eds) The mammary gland. Plenum, New York, pp 67–93

Russo IH, Russo J (1996) Mammary gland neoplasia in long-term rodent studies. Environ Health Perspect 104: 938–967

Russo J, Russo IH (2004) Development of the human breast. Maturitas 49:2–15

Sachdev D, Yee D (2001) The IGF system and breast cancer. Endocr Relat Cancer 8:197–209

Sanderson M, Williams MA, Daling JR, Holt VL, Malone KE, Self SG, Moore DE (1998) Maternal factors and breast cancer risk among young women. Paediatr Perinat Epidemiol 12:397–407

Schernhammer ES, Holly JM, Pollak MN, Hankinson SE (2005) Circulating levels of insulin-like growth factors, their binding proteins, and breast cancer risk. Cancer Epidemiol Biomarkers Prev 14:699–704

Schernhammer ES, Holly JM, Hunter DJ, Pollak MN, Hankinson SE (2006) Insulin-like growth factor-I, its binding proteins (IGFBP-1 and IGFBP-3), and growth hormone and breast cancer risk in The Nurses Health Study II. Endocr Relat Cancer 13:583–592

Sell S (2004) Stem cell origin of cancer and differentiation therapy. Crit Rev Oncol Hematol 51:1–28

Service RE (1998) New role for estrogen in cancer? Science 279:1631–1633

Shipley PW, Wray JA, Hechter HH, Arellano MG, Borhant NO (1967) Frequency of twinning in California. Its relationship to maternal age, parity and race. Am J Epidemiol 85: 147–156

Siiteri PK, MacDonald PC (1966) Placental estrogen biosynthesis during human pregnancy. J Clin Endocrinol Metab 26: 751–761

Spencer JA, Chang TC, Jones J, Robson SC, Preece MA (1995) Third trimester fetal growth and umbilical venous blood concentrations of IGF-1, IGFBP-1, and growth hormone at term. Arch Dis Child Fetal Neonatal Ed 73:F87–F90

Swerdlow AJ, De Stavola B, MacOnochie N, Siskind V (1996) A population-based study of cancer risk in twins: relationships to birth order and sexes of the twin pair. Int J Cancer 67:472–478

Swerdlow AJ, De Stavola BL, Swanwick MA, MacOnochie NE (1997) Risks of breast and testicular cancers in young adult twins in England and Wales: evidence on prenatal and genetic aetiology. Lancet 350:1723–1728

TambyRaja RL, Ratnam SS (1981) Plasma steroid changes in twin pregnancies. Prog Clin Biol Res 69A:189–195

Tapanainen J, Koivisto M, Vihko R, Huhtaniemi I (1981) Enhanced activity of the pituitary–gonadal axis in premature human infants. J Clin Endocrinol Metab 52:235–238

Thiery M, Dhont M, Vandekerckhove D (1977) Serum HCG and HPL in twin pregnancies. Acta Obstet Gynecol Scand 56: 495–497

Tomatis L (1979) Prenatal exposure to chemical carcinogens and its effect on subsequent generations. Natl Cancer Inst Monogr 51:159–184

Tot T (2005) DCIS, cytokeratins and the theory of the sick lobe. Virchows Arch 447:1–8

Tot T (2007) The theory of the sick lobe and the possible consequences. Int J Surg Pathol 15:369–375

Tot T, Tabár L, Dean PB (2002) Practical breast pathology. Thieme, Stuttgart, pp 116–123

Trichopoulos D (1990a) Hypothesis: does breast cancer originate in utero? Lancet 335:939–940

Trichopoulos D (1990b) Is breast cancer initiated in utero? Epidemiology 1:95–96

Trichopoulos D, Lagiou P, Adami HO (2005) Towards an integrated model for breast cancer etiology: the crucial role of the number of mammary tissue-specific stem cells. Breast Cancer Res 7:13–17

Troisi R, Potischman N, Roberts J, Siiteri P, Daftary A, Sims C, Hoover RN (2003a) Associations of maternal and umbilical cord hormone concentrations with maternal, gestational and neonatal factors (United States). Cancer Causes Control 14:347–355

Troisi R, Potischman N, Roberts JM, Harger G, Markovic N, Cole B, Lykins D, Siiteri P, Hoover RN (2003b) Correlation of serum hormone concentrations in maternal and umbilical cord samples. Cancer Epidemiol Biomarkers Prev 12:452–456

Troisi R, Hatch EE, Titus-Ernstoff L, Hyer M, Palmer JR, Robboy SJ, Strohsnitter WC, Kaufman R, Herbst AL, Hoover RN (2007) Cancer risk in women prenatally exposed to diethylstilbestrol. Int J Cancer 121:356–360

Tulchinsky D, Hobel CJ, Korenman SG (1971) A radioligand assay for plasma unconjugated estriol in normal and abnormal pregnancies. Am J Obstet Gynecol 111:311–318

Vatten LJ, Nilsen TI, Tretli S, Trichopoulos D, Romundstad PR (2005) Size at birth and risk of breast cancer: prospective population-based study. Int J Cancer 114:461–464

Vogel PM, Georgiade NG, Fetter BF, Vogel FS, McCarty KS Jr (1981) The correlation of histologic changes in the human breast with the menstrual cycle. Am J Pathol 104:23–34

Wei Q, Matanoski GM, Farmer ER, Hedayati MA, Grossman L (1993) DNA repair and aging in basal cell carcinoma: a molecular epidemiology study. Proc Natl Acad Sci USA 90:1614–1618

Weiss HA, Potischman NA, Brinton LA, Brogan D, Coates RJ, Gammon MD, Malone KE, Schoenberg JB (1997) Prenatal and perinatal risk factors for breast cancer in young women. Epidemiology 8:181–187

Weiss-Salz I, Harlap S, Friedlander Y, Kaduri L, Levy-Lahad E, Yanetz R, Deutsch L, Hochner H, Paltiel O (2007) Ethnic ancestry and increased paternal age are risk factors for breast cancer before the age of 40 years. Eur J Cancer Prev 16:549–554

Wellings SR, Jensen HM, Marcum RG (1975) An atlas of subgross pathology of the human breast with special reference to possible precancerous lesions. J Natl Cancer Inst 55:231–273

White E, Lee CY, Kristal AR (1990) Evaluation of the increase in breast cancer incidence in relation to mammography use. J Natl Cancer Inst 82:1546–1552

Xu X, Dailey AB, Peoples-Sheps M, Talbott EO, Li N, Roth J (2009) Birth weight as a risk factor for breast cancer: a meta-analysis of 18 epidemiological studies. J Womens Health (Larchmt) 18:1169–1178

Xue F, Michels KB (2007a) Intrauterine factors and risk of breast cancer: a systematic review and meta-analysis of current evidence. Lancet Oncol 8:1088–1100

Xue F, Michels KB (2007b) Diabetes, metabolic syndrome, and breast cancer: a review of the current evidence. Am J Clin Nutr 86:s823–s835

Xue F, Colditz GA, Willett WC, Rosner BA, Michels KB (2006) Parental age at delivery and incidence of breast cancer: a prospective cohort study. Breast Cancer Res Treat 104:331–340

Yu H, Jin F, Shu XO, Li BD, Dai Q, Cheng JR, Berkel HJ, Zheng W (2002) Insulin-like growth factors and breast cancer risk in Chinese women. Cancer Epidemiol Biomarkers Prev 11:705–712

Zapf J, Schmid C, Froesch E (1984) Biological and immunological properties of insulin-like growth factors (IGF) I and II. Clin Endocrinol Metab 13:7–12

Zeisler H, Jirecek S, Hohlagschwandtner M, Knofler M, Tempfer C, Livingston JC (2002) Concentrations of estrogens in patients with preeclampsia. Wien Klin Wochenschr 114:458–461

Zhang Y, Cupples LA, Rosenberg L, Colton T, Kreger BE (1995) Parental ages at birth in relation to a daughter's risk of breast cancer among female participants in the Framingham Study (United States). Cancer Causes Control 6:23–29

Zhu BT, Conney AH (1998) Functional role of estrogen metabolism in target cells: review and perspectives. Carcinogenesis 19:1–27

Genetic Alterations in Normal and Malignant Breast Tissue

4

Chanel E. Smart, Peter T. Simpson, Ana Cristina Vargas, and Sunil R. Lakhani

Abbreviations

ADH	Atypical ductal hyperplasia
ALDH1	Aldehyde dehydrogenase 1
ALH	Atypical lobular hyperplasia
CAF	Cancer associated fibroblasts
CCL	Columnar cell lesion
CGH	Comparative genomic hybridization
DCIS	Ductal carcinoma in situ
ECM	Extracellular matrix
FEA	Flat epithelial atypia
FFPE	Formalin fixed paraffin embedded
G6PD	Glucose-6-phosphate dehydrogenase
HR	Homologous recombination
HUT	Hyperplasia usual type
ILC	Invasive lobular carcinoma
IDC	Invasive ductal carcinoma
LCIS	Lobular carcinoma in situ
LOH	Loss of heterozygosity
NS	Normal stroma
PLC	Pleomorphic lobular carcinoma
ROH	Retention of heterozygosity
SNP	Single nucleotide polymorphism
TDLU	Terminal ductal-lobular unit

4.1 Introduction

Breast cancer is a heterogeneous disease with a wide spectrum of morphological subtypes and a range of clinical behaviors. Over a long time period, pathologists have evolved a system of recording cancer-related data that reflects this heterogeneity as well as providing information relevant to prognosis and prediction of response to therapy. It is well established that subtype of breast cancer, grade, and stage (Ellis et al. 1992; Elston and Ellis 1991) provide prognostic information and the use of steroid receptor analysis as well as overexpression and amplification of HER2 provides prognostic and predictive data to manage patients (Oldenhuis et al. 2008). Nonetheless, there are limitations to these data and it is well known clinically that even within the same subtype (e.g., tubular carcinoma) or same stage of disease (e.g., lymph node positive), the behavior can be markedly different. Understanding the molecular abnormalities that drive the biology of each disease will assist our ability to specifically inhibit it.

4.2 The Genetic Basis of Cancer

We currently understand cancer to be a genetic disease: driven by changes in a cell's DNA. Some mutations can be inherited from the germline, thereby being present in every cell of the body and predisposing the individual to cancer development. Otherwise, mutations occur somatically and may be caused by environmental exposure such as chemical carcinogens or radiation or impaired DNA repair mechanisms that become compromised during tumor development. The type and scale of genetic/genomic changes that occur in cancer progression are also numerous and can have profound

S.R. Lakhani (✉)
University of Queensland Centre for Clinical Research,
School of Medicine, and Pathology Queensland,
The Royal Brisbane & Women's Hospital, Brisbane,
Queensland, Australia
e-mail: s.lakhani@uq.edu.au

T. Tot (ed.), *Breast Cancer*, DOI: 10.1007/978-1-84996-314-5_4,
© Springer-Verlag London Limited 2011

effects on driving the tumor phenotype. These can be (a) gross chromosomal gains and losses, which presumably affect the expression levels of numerous genes; (b) genomic amplifications whereby a specific genomic region is replicated numerous times and these are thought to harbor oncogenes whose expression probably drives tumor growth (e.g., amplification and subsequent overexpression of *ERBB2/HER2*); (c) inactivation of tumor or metastasis suppressor genes due to any combination of hemi/homozygous gene deletion, gene methylation, gene mutation, or transcription repression (e.g., E-cadherin inactivation in lobular breast cancers); (d) genomic rearrangements culminating in the formation of fusion genes (e.g., the *ETV6-NTRK3* fusion gene in secretory breast cancers, Tognon et al. 2002).

Over the last 2 decades, efforts to sequence the human genome and to study the molecular aspects of disease have led to significant advances in the technology now available for unraveling the genetic basis of diseases, such as cancer. The candidate gene/genomic loci approach of mutation detection or loss of heterozygosity (LOH) analysis are still valid applications for identifying specific alterations. To obtain more comprehensive characterization of somatic mutations (changes in DNA copy number) across the tumor genome, researchers have utilized the whole genome analyses called comparative genomic hybridization (CGH). Traditionally this was a low-resolution analysis providing only patterns of gross chromosomal abnormalities (Reis Fihlo et al. 2005), but nevertheless an important mechanism of identifying important events in tumor development and characterizing molecular relationships between entities. The introduction of microarray-based CGH (aCGH) has further revolutionized this technique, now providing resolution down to the 100 bp level and with the ability to characterize in detail the specific breakpoints of genomic alterations and to precisely map the genes involved. Furthermore, the drive to identify genetic variants associated with disease (genome wide association studies) has led to the development of high-density single nucleotide polymorphism (SNP) arrays that now enable genomic copy number alterations to be defined in an allele-specific manner. Of course, the explosion in genomic profiling has paralleled the boom in gene expression profiling studies that provide the next level of intricate control on the phenotype of the tumor cell. The gold standard in molecular analysis of tumor genomes is now driven by the massively high-throughput genomic and transcriptomic sequencing. This is not yet fully accessible to all researchers, but has the ability to define genomic rearrangements and gene mutations at nucleotide resolution, and obtain unbiased assessment of mRNA and microRNA expression levels (Stratton et al. 2009).

These methods have highlighted the genomic complexity of breast cancer and are fundamentally changing our understanding of the biology of breast disease. These efforts have identified important mutations in disease pathogenesis, led to the development of molecular targets for therapy (e.g., ER and HER2), supported the idea that certain preinvasive lesions are precursors for the development of invasive cancer, and are helping to refine the classification of the disease (Alizadeh et al. 2001; Buerger et al. 1999b; Lakhani 1997; Nishizaki et al. 1997; Pollack et al. 1999; Reis-Filho et al. 2005; Simpson et al. 2005b; Perou et al. 2000; Sorlie et al. 2001).

4.3 Molecular Analysis of Invasive Breast Cancer

Molecular genetic analyses of invasive breast cancers have defined common genomic alterations as gain of material on chromosome 1q, 8q, 17q, 20q, and losses of material affecting 4q, 5q, 8p, 11q, 13q and 16q. Some common high level genomic amplifications occur at 1q32, 8p12, 8q24, 11q13, 17q12 and 20q13. The pattern of genomic alterations has been shown to closely correlate with histological grade, molecular subtype, and, to a lesser extent, histological type. One of the most important molecular findings has provided fundamental evidence that low-grade breast cancers are different to high-grade breast cancers at the molecular level, and so presumably arise through different pathways of development (Buerger et al. 1999a, b, 2000; Roylance et al. 2006; Stratton et al. 1995). Overall, low-grade ductal carcinomas and tubular carcinomas show a low level of genomic instability with characteristic losses at chromosome 16q, gains on 1q, and few other recurrent alterations, whereas high-grade breast cancers show a greater degree of genetic instability with more complex genomic alterations and more high levels gains (amplifications) on regions such as 17q12, 8q24, and 20q13. These data, initially derived from loss of heterozygosity (LOH) and chromosomal CGH analysis, therefore suggested that the evolution of low-grade tumors from normal tissue was by a pathway independent to that of high-grade carcinomas. The loss of 16q for instance is frequent in low-grade tumors and involves the whole chromosomal arm, while in high-grade tumors, loss of 16q is less common, and when it does occur it is by a different mechanism (LOH with mitotic recombination) (Roylance et al. 2002, 2006; Cleton-Jansen et al. 2004; Natrajan et al. 2009a).

However, there may be some exceptions to this rule since around 20% of high-grade invasive ductal carcinomas (IDC) harbor loss of the whole of 16q. Grade III IDCs are a heterogeneous group of tumors, both morphologically and molecularly. Recent aCGH analysis of high-grade IDC revealed that the majority of tumors containing loss of the whole arm of 16q were estrogen receptor (ER) positive, suggesting that in these cases there maybe evidence to support progression from the low-grade/ER+ve pathway of tumor development to high-grade/ER+ve breast cancers (Natrajan et al. 2009a). Data in support of this come from the study of pleomorphic lobular carcinomas (PLC). PLC are a recently described variant of classic invasive lobular carcinoma (ILC) (Eusebi et al. 1992; Middleton et al. 2000; Weidner and Semple 1992; Palacios et al. 2003; Sneige et al. 2002; Simpson et al. 2003), with a reported aggressive biological behavior (Orvieto et al. 2008; Buchanan et al. 2008). Briefly, neoplastic cells in pleomorphic lobular carcinoma in situ (LCIS) and ILC show the typical discohesiveness of lobular neoplasms and lack E-cadherin expression; however, PLC are of high grade and show features of apocrine differentiation. Although molecular data on the PLC are scant, these tumors have overlapping genetic changes with both classic ILC and grade III invasive ductal breast carcinomas. Importantly, they harbor loss of 16q and overall a similar genomic profile to ILC. The data suggested that PLC arise from the same pathway as ILC. The sporadic accumulation of genetic alterations more common to high-grade cancers (*HER2, p53, MYC*) may then contribute to the more aggressive biology (Simpson et al. 2008).

CGH and conventional cytogenetic studies have demonstrated that there is a degree of variation in the pattern of genetic alterations between different histological subtypes of invasive breast cancer. Although differences between histological subtypes do exist, this association is not as strong as with histological grade (Buerger et al. 1999a; Reis-Filho and Lakhani 2003). Comparative analyses between IDCs and ILCs have

demonstrated that overall a lower number of genetic changes are found in ILCs relative to IDCs. Although some specific chromosomal abnormalities are found at a significantly different frequency in each histological type, this may only highlight the fact that most ILCs are of lower nuclear grade. Interestingly, several recurrent unbalanced changes, including physical loss of 16q, are common to both types, indicating that ILCs and low-grade IDCs may arise via common tumorigenic pathways.

As a result of this and other molecular data, some authors have questioned whether the boundary between ductal and lobular lesions should be removed and whether the designations "ductal" and "lobular" are appropriate. Since it is clear that the majority of neoplastic breast diseases arise from the terminal duct–lobular unit (TDLU), the terminology of "ductal" and "lobular" is not intended to reflect the micro-anatomical site of origin, but a difference in cell morphology and biology (Simpson et al. 2003). Hence, it is worth stressing that although loss of 16q is observed in both grade I IDC and ILC, the genes most affected by this deletion probably differ between these two lesions. The likeliest candidate tumor suppressor gene involved in loss of 16q in ILC is *CDH1* (E-cadherin), which maps to 16q22.1 (Cleton-Jansen et al. 2004; Palacios et al. 2003; Simpson et al. 2003). It is accepted that ILC harbor loss of 16q, followed by gene mutation, promoter methylation, or further loss of *CDH1*. Loss of E-cadherin, a critical cell adhesion molecule, is reflected at the morphological level by the characteristic discohesive nature of individual cells and overall growth pattern of lobular carcinomas. However, *CDH1* is almost certainly not the target gene in grade I IDCs as loss of E-cadherin expression and *CDH1* gene mutations are exceedingly rare in these tumors. The hunt for the tumor suppressor gene(s) involved in grade I ductal cancers continues (Cleton-Jansen 2002; Rakha et al. 2004b; Roylance et al. 2003).

4.4 Molecular Classification of Invasive Breast Cancer

Array-based techniques of CGH and gene expression profiling have led to the development of new molecular-based classification schemes for breast cancer.

These seem to be inter-related, whereby the genomic alterations and subsequent changes in gene expression are controlling tumor phenotype.

More recently, microarray-based expression profiling has added further insight into breast cancer heterogeneity and produced a new taxonomy of breast cancer, dividing tumors into five major molecular subclasses, namely luminal A, luminal B, HER2, basal-like, and normal-like (Perou et al. 2000; Sorlie et al. 2001, 2003). The major distinction is at the level of the ER. The ER positive cluster comprises tumors that have a gene expression signature similar to that seen for the normal luminal epithelial compartment of the breast with expression of low molecular weight keratins such as CK8/18 and ER and related genes. These "luminal" tumors are further divided into subclass A and B with luminal B being higher grade, having higher proliferation index and a poorer prognosis. It is worth noting that although the groups appear distinct on such an analysis, there is a continuum, and further there is at least data from lobular cancers (classic, luminal A; and pleomorphic variant, luminal B) that luminal A cancers can evolve into luminal B cancers through the stochastic acquisition of mutations in genes associated with worse prognosis such as *HER2* and *TP53*.

The ER negative group is more heterogeneous. The normal-like group is the least convincing and may be an artifact of the study, reflecting normal cell contamination in the samples. The HER2 and basal-like were shown to have the worst prognosis in the original studies although it is clear from many studies that the basal-like cancers are an extremely heterogeneous group with prognosis ranging from "good" to "bad." Basal-like cancers are so designated because these tumors express genes usually found in normal basal/myoepithelial cells of the breast, including high molecular weight cytokeratins (CK14, 5/6 and 17) as well as P-cadherin, P63, S100, and epidermal growth factor receptor (EGFR/HER1). The morphological features of these tumors are distinct with central acellular and necrotic zones, pushing borders, high degree of pleomorphism and mitotic index and areas of squamous and spindle cell differentiation (Fulford et al. 2006). These tumors are often but not invariably triple negative (ER, PR, and HER2 negative). HER2 tumors are also high grade and are characterized by overexpression of HER2 and genes associated with the HER2 pathway.

In clinical practice, some HER2 over-expressing tumors however fall into the luminal B category. The microarray studies have also identified further ER negative cancer subtypes including an "apocrine" subgroup (Farmer et al. 2005), an "interferon" subgroup, and a "claudin-low" subgroup (Hennessy et al. 2009). The clinical and biological significance of these subgroups remains to be elucidated.

The genomic architecture of invasive tumors, as characterized by array-based CGH analysis, can be classified as "simplex," "complex-firestorm" or "complex-sawtooth" (Hicks et al. 2006; Bergamaschi et al. 2006; Natrajan et al. 2009b), and these show correlation with the molecular subtypes classified by expression profiling. The "simplex" pattern is associated with a good outcome and is typical of low-grade luminal-like cancers, frequently displaying concurrent 1q gain and 16q loss. In contrast, the complex pattern is associated with poor outcome. The "firestorm" pattern involves a region of complex amplification affecting regions such as 11q13, 8p12, 8q, 17q12, and is typically seen in "HER2" and "luminal B" cancers. The "sawtooth" category has many narrow areas of duplication and deletion, affecting all chromosomes and the majority of the genome but with no/few amplifications and is typically seen in "basal-like" cancers. It is possible that the types of copy number profiles seen may be due to the different types of DNA repair defects/instability present in these tumors.

There is of course considerable excitement in the new molecular classification, but it is worth bearing in mind that the systems of classification are still likely to evolve as we get further insights into the biology of breast disease. For instance, the new taxonomy has led some to postulate a histogenetic classification of breast cancer with "luminal" subtypes arising from luminal epithelial cells and "basal-like" cancers arising from the basal/myoepithelial cells or even stem cell since they often express "luminal" and "myoepithelial" keratins. Data emerging from the study of normal cell populations and their progeny suggest that basal-like cancers may arise from luminal progenitors (Lim et al. 2009). There is much work to be done in understanding normal cell lineage differentiation and the plasticity of individual cell types, and we should be cautious in making too many leaps into histogenetic classification of disease.

4.5 Molecular Analysis of Preinvasive Breast Cancer

The frequent association and morphological similarities between invasive carcinomas and many forms of proliferative breast diseases have led pathologists to speculate that certain entities would be biologically related (e.g., LCIS and ILC, ductal carcinoma in situ (DCIS) and IDC) (Reis-Filho and Lakhani 2003). The complexity of these relationships has been thoroughly explored using the advancement in molecular pathology and has largely recapitulated the genotypic/phenotypic patterns observed in invasive ductal and lobular carcinomas in atypical ductal hyperplasia (ADH) DCIS and atypical lobular hyperplasia (ALH) LCIS (Buerger et al. 1999a, b; Lakhani et al. 1995; Lu et al. 1998; O'Connell et al. 1998). The distinct molecular genetic features found in different grades of invasive carcinomas are also mirrored in preinvasive lesions of comparable morphology (Buerger et al. 2000; Reis-Filho and Lakhani 2003).

In retrospect, it is clear that there are two major arms in the multi-pathway model of breast cancer progression: one comprising well-differentiated DCIS (low grade) that progress to grade I IDC, and the other encompassing poorly differentiated (high grade) DCIS that progress to grade III IDC. In the "low-grade arm," these in situ and invasive tumors are of low nuclear grade, usually ER and PR positive, negative for Her-2 and basal markers, and harbor low genetic instability and recurrent 16q loss, whereas in the "high-grade arm," the lesions show a higher degree of nuclear atypia, are more frequently hormone receptor–negative, frequently positive for either HER2 or basal markers, and are genetically advanced lesions, showing a combination of recurrent genomic changes including loss of 8p, 11q, 13q, 14q; gain of 1q, 5p, 8q, 17q; and amplifications on 6q22, 8q22, 11q13, 17q12, 17q22–24, and 20q13. Based on their pathological and genetic features, classic LCIS and ILC are remarkably similar to those tumors in the "low-grade arm" (Lu et al. 1998; Simpson et al. 2003). However, in contrast to well-differentiated DCIS/grade I IDC, the vast majority of these tumors lack E-cadherin expression owing to genetic and/or epigenetic changes in the *CDH1* gene (Rakha et al. 2004a; Roylance et al. 2003). On the other hand, the overlapping morphological features of PLCIS

and PLC with both classic lobular and grade III carcinomas, and the combination of E-cadherin (16q) loss with occasional HER2 positivity (Eusebi et al. 1992; Palacios et al. 2003; Sneige et al. 2002; Reis-Filho et al. 2005) add another level of complexity to these molecular pathways to breast cancer progression.

Apart from ADH and ALH, which bear stark morphological and molecular resemblance to low-grade DCIS and LCIS, respectively, the other non-obligate/premalignant lesions are more difficult to characterize and to establish their position along the multistep pathways (O'Connell et al. 1994, 1998; Reis-Filho and Lakhani 2003). Interestingly, ADH and low-grade DCIS show identical immunoprofiles with low numbers of chromosomal abnormalities, comprising recurrent loss of 16q. The similarities between ALH and LCIS are also at the morphological, immunohistochemical, and genetic level (Simpson et al. 2003). In fact, differentiating between ALH and LCIS is arbitrary and subjective, being based on subtle quantitative rather than qualitative morphological features. Hence, it is well accepted that both ADH and ALH are non-obligate precursors for the development of low-grade DCIS and LCIS, respectively. Alternatively, one could view them just as small DCIS or LCIS although this is not the view accepted by all.

Clonal diversity, evidenced by morphological and molecular intra-tumoral heterogeneity, adds further complexity to this model and probably accounts for some of the considerable diversity in the clinical nature of the disease. This diversity might be explained by ensuing genetic instability leading to the development of multiple neoplastic clones within the same tumor. Clonal diversity has been reported in DCIS, where up to 50% of cases studied showed heterogeneity in grade, with 9% of cases of low-grade DCIS also showing areas of intermediate and high-grade DCIS. Such cases exhibited heterogeneous expression of immunohistochemical biomarkers and, in particular this correlated with p53 positivity (Allred et al. 2008). The authors speculated that in some cases, ADH (the precursor to low-grade DCIS) could therefore be the precursor to high-grade DCIS and hence grade III IDC. The molecular data that low-grade disease is different to high-grade disease also raise the possibility of coexistence of independent clones of differing grades rather than one arising from the other.

For many years, hyperplasia of usual type (HUT) has been seen as the precursor of ADH and DCIS.

However, its role in the multistep model of breast carcinogenesis has been questioned (Aubele et al. 2000; Jones et al. 2003; Lakhani et al. 1996). The morphological features and immunoprofile of HUTs are different to those of the accepted precursors since they are composed of a mixed population of cell types with a variable proportion of ER, PR-positive luminal cells, and myoepithelial/basal marker-positive cells. At the molecular level, few fairly random chromosomal changes are observed (Aubele et al. 2000; Jones et al. 2003; Lakhani et al. 1996). Nonetheless, there is evidence to suggest that a small proportion of HUTs may be clonal, neoplastic proliferations (equivalent to colonic adenomas) that may putatively progress to ADH or DCIS, whereas the majority of them fail to show any evidence of a neoplastic/monoclonal nature using existing technology. Currently, most authors do not regard these lesions as playing any significant role in tumorigenesis and see these lesions as "dead-end."

A more likely candidate for precursor to ADH and low-grade DCIS is columnar cell lesion (CCL) (Fraser et al. 1998; Schnitt and Vincent-Salomon 2003; Simpson et al. 2005a). These comprise a spectrum of lesions with varying degrees of architectural and nuclear atypia. At the lower end of the spectrum are lesions referred to as columnar cell change and hyperplasia, and at the worst end, lesions that have atypia sufficient to be designated "flat epithelial atypia" (FEA) to fully developed ADH lesions. Throughout the spectrum, CCLs show an immunoprofile similar to that of ADH/low-grade DCIS (Schnitt and Vincent-Salomon 2003). However, the degree of proliferation, architectural, and cytological atypia are mirrored at the genetic level, with a stepwise increase in the number and complexity of chromosomal copy number changes as defined by CGH (Simpson et al. 2005a). Moreover, the hallmark genetic feature of "low-grade" lesions, loss of 16q, is the most frequently detected recurrent change and in addition, there is some degree of overlap in the molecular genetic profile of CCL and associated more advanced lesions (Moinfar et al. 2000b; Simpson et al. 2005a). Interestingly, it is not infrequent to observe ALH/LCIS in the context of multifocal CCLs. Hence CCLs may be the link between normal breast and ADH, as well as between "ductal" and "lobular" neoplasia (Abdel-Fatah et al. 2007, 2008). The precursor of poorly differentiated DCIS has been elusive. Based on morphological, immunohistochemical, and

molecular findings, CCL, ADH, and low-grade DCIS would be unlikely candidates.

Although apocrine change has long been considered a metaplastic process in breast tissues, usually associated with aging, this concept has come into question with the application of molecular findings (Jones et al. 2001; Selim et al. 2000, 2002). At least a subset of lesions with apocrine morphology show molecular changes, including LOH/allelic imbalance at 1p (*MYCL1*), 11q (*INT2*), 13q, 16q and 17q, and recurrent chromosomal changes as defined by CGH, including loss of 1p, 2p, 10q, 16q, 17q and 22q, and gain of 1p, 2q and 13q. These findings are more frequently observed in apocrine adenosis, and apocrine hyperplasia compared with apocrine cysts. For the large part, these observations have been ignored. Whether this prejudice is justified should be questioned. It may turn out to be wrong, but we would suggest that there is compelling molecular data that at least some of these lesions may be the precursors of high-grade DCIS and invasive cancer.

4.6 Molecular Alterations in Normal Breast

Since molecular alterations at genetic loci have been identified in many putative precursor lesions, the attention also shifted to whether "normal" tissues in the vicinity of preinvasive and invasive carcinomas may harbor mutations. With developments in microdissection in the early 1990s, Deng et al. (1996) reported that LOH identified in invasive carcinoma is indeed present in morphologically normal breast lobules adjacent to carcinomas, but not away from the tumor. Since their studies were carried out on microdissected tissues from paraffin-embedded sections, the possibility that the LOH was a result of tumor cells migrating to the lobular units via pagetoid spread could not be entirely excluded. Their findings could therefore be accounted for by one of three hypotheses: first, that the LOH identified is actually due to the presence of tumor cells, which have migrated into the normal lobule from the nearby invasive carcinoma; second, that the LOH is indeed present in the morphologically normal cells analyzed. The second hypothesis could imply that a "normal" area of the breast harbored genetic change preceding the development of the invasive carcinoma. Furthermore, that the carcinoma may arise as a result of additional changes to these "normal" cells. How this preliminary change arose is a major tenet of the sick lobe hypothesis (Tot 2005).

The sick lobe hypothesis suggests that changes to the breast epithelium occurring during its development can result in entire lobes or segments of the breast that are in someway predisposed to further changes (in adulthood) that result in the onset of cancer (see Fig. 4.1a, b). It is possible that this initial change in one cell, then passed on to all other cells derived from it to comprise a lobe of the breast, occurs at the genetic level by DNA mutation. This would suggest that the normal lobule is clonal, which would raise questions about the existence or otherwise of a common progenitor or stem cell from which all the epithelial cells

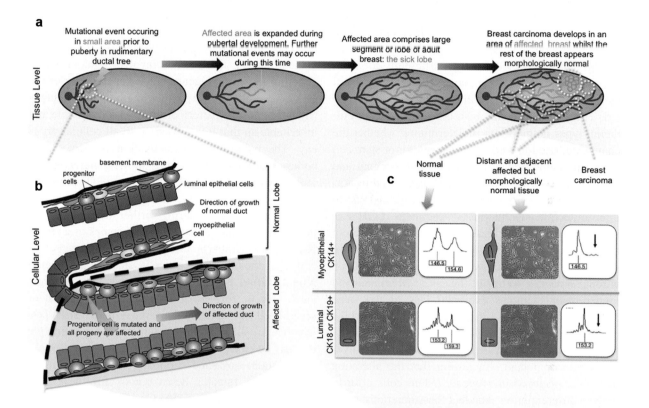

Fig. 4.1 Possible mechanisms of genetic alteration affecting the sick lobe. (**a**) Simplified diagram demonstrating how genetic change in the glandular epithelium of the developing breast may result in a "sick lobe" by passing this change onto progeny. Normal glandular epithelium is illustrated in red, while affected epithelium comprising the sick lobe is shown in blue. (**b**) Diagram illustrating possible cellular composition of bifurcating region of normal and sick lobes. Should a mutational event occur in a breast stem or progenitor cell, this change might be later observed in all cell types derived from it during expansion and differentiation of the ductal tree as it grows into the mammary fat pad, including both luminal and myoepithelial cells as well as other progenitors cells. It is also possible that the frequency of cell types, their function, and the molecular profiles of these affected areas may be altered (shown in blue), although it is possible that such change may not be detectable by traditional histomorphological examination. (**c**) The adult breast may therefore be comprised of normal lobes and sick lobes, the latter harboring genetic alteration that

may predispose to development of carcinoma. This model is supported by the findings of Clarke et al. Cell clones derived from fresh dissociated mastectomy samples from *BRCA1/BRCA2*-mutation carriers were identified as either luminal (CK18/19 positive) or myoepithelial (CK14 positive) features. While DNA derived from most clones demonstrated retention of heterozygosity (ROH) and were therefore considered normal, some rare clones of both luminal and myoepithelial phenotypes showed loss of heterozygosity (LOH) at *BRCA1* or *BRCA2* loci. Where these morphologically normal cells harbored the same mutation as the tumor residing in the breast, it could suggest that this change has predisposed to the development of the cancer. Indeed, LOH (particularly of tumor suppressor genes such as *BRCA1/2*) is considered one of the initial steps of tumor formation. Furthermore (not shown here), where both myoepithelial and luminal cell clones are shown to harbor the same genetic alteration, this could be interpreted to suggest that the initial change occurred in a progenitor cell, which is common to both cell types comprising the lobe were derived, there are several studies whose findings suggest this to be true.

Using an in vitro cell cloning technique, Lakhani et al. (1999) addressed these issues by looking for LOH in breast samples free of contamination from tumor cells and examined LOH independently in both the luminal and myoepithelial cells of the breast. Chromosomal loci exhibiting LOH at high-frequency in invasive breast cancer were investigated in "normal" breast tissue from patients with carcinoma and from reduction mammoplasty specimens. Ductal-lobular units dissected from paraffin-embedded tissues and 485 "normal" luminal and myoepithelial cell clones cultured from a fresh dissociation were studied. The ability to distinguish between different epithelial types is important in determining whether the change occurred in a common progenitor or stem cell whose progeny then differentiated into luminal and myoepithelial cells. Overall, LOH was found in normal cells in five of ten breast cancer cases and one of three reduction mammoplasty specimens. LOH was identified in normal cells adjacent to and distant from the tumor. One of 93 clones from three reduction mammoplasties also showed allele loss at a locus on chromosome 13q. In one of the cases, all luminal and myoepithelial samples exhibited loss of the same allele on chromosome 13q. These data confirmed the presence of LOH in normal tissues as well as demonstrated an independent loss in the luminal and myoepithelial component, suggesting that the alteration may have occurred in progenitor/stem cells prior to lineage differentiation. The fact that alterations are in both cell types and can also be identified using microdissection also provided evidence that the clonal patch derived from stem cells was likely to be large within the breast.

The ability to identify clonal patches is difficult in human samples but important, not just for normal biology but because there has been a huge body of literature suggesting clonal nature of lesions in the breast using X-linked inactivation methodologies. Many authors failed to realize that without knowledge of clonal patch size, these data were not meaningful. If the patch size is large, it is possible to get a proliferation from multiple cells but yet would appear clonal using X-linked methods. In order to examine the clonal architecture of normal tissue, it is necessary to have a cellular marker that can be used to identify a subset of germ-line cells.

Experimentally using chimeric or mosaic animals can achieve this.

As a result of the process of X inactivation, females heterozygous for X-linked polymorphisms are functionally mosaic at the mRNA and protein levels. Previous studies have used X-linked genes such as glucose-6-phosphate dehydrogenase (*G6PD*) (Fialkow 1976) or restriction fragment length polymorphisms (Vogelstein et al. 1985) without reference to patch size. In female mammals, the process of X inactivation occurs early during embryogenesis (day 16 in the human female). This process involves random inactivation of most of the genes on one or the other of the two X chromosomes by methylation of CpG islands (Lyon 1972). The pattern of methylation is stable and inheritable so that it is passed on to all cellular progeny. The pattern of X inactivation is also widely believed to be stable during tumorigenesis (Jones 1996). As X inactivation occurs at a relatively early stage of embryogenesis, although there is inevitably some mixing of cells during further development, in the adult mammal, many of the progenies of a single X-inactivated embryonic cell are arranged together. In epithelia, these groups of cells sharing a common X-inactivation pattern are termed patches. A single patch may be formed of the progeny of one cell or several cells all showing the same X-inactivation pattern. Thus, cells in a single patch are monophenotypic but may be clonal or polyclonal in derivation. Novelli et al. (2003) collected surgical resection specimens of Sardinian females heterozygous for the *G6PD* Mediterranean mutation (563 C → T). All patients had been previously shown to have reduced G6PD enzyme activity, and heterozygosity for the *G6PD* Mediterranean mutation was confirmed by PCR analysis of genomic DNA followed by *Mbo*II restriction endonuclease digestion. Using histochemical method on tissue sections, they confirmed that the clonal patch within the female breast was large, involving whole ducts and lobular units, providing further evidence to support the hypothesis generated from the LOH data.

In their original paper, Lakhani et al. (1999) had one case in which the patient had a germ-line truncating mutation in the *BRCA1* gene and they found LOH on 17q in 3 of 33 normal clones. One of these clones showed loss of wild-type allele, indicating gene inactivation. This sample also had LOH at markers on chromosomes 11p and 13q, suggesting that further alterations may have occurred as a result of genomic instability due to loss of homologous recombination (HR). This work was followed by further analysis of cases with germ-line *BRCA1/2* mutations. Clarke et al. (2006) studied LOH at the *BRCA1* and *BRCA2* loci in 992 normal cell clones derived from topographically defined areas of normal tissue in 4 samples from *BRCA1/BRCA2* mutation carriers. The frequency of LOH in the clones was low (1.01%), but it was found in all 4 samples, whether or not a tumor was present. Again, LOH could be detected in both luminal and myoepithelial clones, which indicates not only that both cell types can harbor such genetic changes (see Fig. 4.1c), but where those changes are identical it suggests they have been derived from a common progenitor cell. It is also possible the cell clones are themselves derived from committed progenitors by virtue of the fact that they can grow in in vitro culture. Interestingly, topographical mapping revealed that the genetic changes were clustered in a segmental distribution in some of the breast samples. The study provided further evidence that a field of genetic instability can exist around a tumor and that this size was greater than one TDLU. Although there are little additional data to confirm these findings, at face value, it does suggest that sufficient tissue must be removed at surgery to avoid local recurrence and raises questions about whether such alterations could account for some cases of local recurrence after apparent "complete excision" of the tumor.

Two other more recent studies provide further evidence that the normal breast of *BRCA*-mutation carriers is altered and shows early changes similar to those found in the subsequent carcinoma. Max Wicha's group not only reproduced the observation of *BRCA1* LOH in morphologically normal areas of the breast in *BRCA1*-mutation carriers (Liu et al. 2008), they also discovered that ALDH1 – a putative stem cell marker – could be used to identify those lobules which contained this genetic alteration. While ALDH1 positive cells appear to be extremely rare in the normal breast of healthy donors, *BRCA1*-mutation carriers have a higher frequency of ALDH1 positive cells that appear to comprise entire acini in breast lobules of these patients. This is significant because it provides evidence that entire areas of the *BRCA1*-breast can show both genetic and molecular (in this cases protein) differences despite appearing morphologically normal. In this way it is possible that the color used to delineate the sick lobe in Fig. 4.1a could be representing ALDH1 positivity in the breast of *BRCA1*-carriers, depending on how early these changes occur. Furthermore, as a putative stem cell marker, the expression of ALDH1 at high frequency in the lobules of *BRCA1*-mutation carriers may suggest that the initial genetic change that occurs in a breast stem cell, which although has then expanded to form the acini, may in someway be defective, unable to lose expression of this marker, and somehow blocked in its ability to differentiate. Another study that revealed an expanded and abnormal luminal progenitor population in mastectomy samples of *BRCA1*-mutation carriers adds weight to this hypothesis (Lim et al. 2009) although they did not investigate the presence of genetic differences in this population.

4.7 The Sick Stroma

LOH in the mammary stroma of patients with breast cancer has also been demonstrated by Moinfar et al. (2000a). By using 11 DNA markers on FFPE tissue, LOH was reported in the morphologically normal stroma in 11–57% of cases. A comparison of LOH frequency in the epithelial/stromal cells revealed that 73% of cases were associated with at least one identical LOH in both the epithelial and stromal components. This intriguing observation suggests that there may be common precursors for epithelial and stromal cells; however, these data need validation and are certainly contrary to other more recent analysis. Kurose et al. (2001) identified that genetic alterations occurred in the epithelial compartment, followed by LOH in the stromal compartments, indicating that genetic alterations in the epithelia precede the ones in the stroma.

Most of studies based on cDNA microarrays have focused mainly on the neoplastic transformation of the breast epithelial compartment. Recently attention has focused on the role of breast tumor stroma in breast cancer progression demonstrated by gene expression profile. In a series of 14 patients with matched DCIS, IDC, normal epithelium, IDC-associated stroma (IDC-S), DCIS-associated stroma (DCIS-S), and normal stroma (NS), Ma et al. (2003) provided evidence that gene expression changes occurred in the stroma during breast cancer progression, suggesting that tumor stroma may co-evolve along with the malignant epithelium even before epithelial transformation occurs. Genetic alterations mainly involved components of the extra cellular matrix (ECM) and ECM-remodeling matrix metalloproteases (MMP). While cytoplasmic ribosomal proteins were decreased in both compartments, mitochondrial ribosomal protein genes were increased. Differentially expressed genes between IDC-S and NS included antagonists of the WNT receptor signaling which were downregulated and upregulation of TGFb family members. The stroma showed genes enriched for extracellular matrix, MMP, and cell cycle–associated genes, indicating that increased proliferation is a feature of stroma. Particularly, the stroma showed significant expression of MMP11, MMP2, MMP14, and MMP13 in IDC-S compared to DCIS-S, suggesting that MMPs may play a role in the transition from in situ to invasive carcinoma (Fleming et al. 2008; Ma et al. 2009).

Allinen et al. (2004) developed a purification procedure that allows the isolation of pure cell populations from breast tissue. This method is based on cell type–specific cell surface markers and magnetic beads. BerEP4 sorted epithelial cells, CD45 was used for leukocytes, P1H12 for endothelial cells, and CD10 for sequential isolation of myoepithelial cells and myofibroblasts. The unbound fraction following the removal of all other cell types was regarded as the fibroblast-enriched stromal fraction. However, further differentiation between myoepithelial cells and myofibroblasts was not possible. As a result, these cell types were regarded as a single group. By aCGH analysis, no genetic changes were detected in myoepithelial cells/myofibroblasts isolated from DCIS/IDC. By contrast, numerous genetic changes were observed in tumor epithelial cells. Normal tissue adjacent to tumors did not express any genetic alterations. SNP arrays and LOH methodology were also applied to the same purified cell types and showed no evidence of LOH in any stromal cell from DCIS/IDC samples. Therefore, unlike the studies of Lakhani et al. and Clarke et al., genetic changes using these methodologies were only detected in luminal epithelial cells (Allinen et al. 2004).

Genomic alterations of breast cancer–associated fibroblasts/myofibroblasts are not consistent among the studies. Qiu et al. (2008) by using SNP array–based technologies studied cancer-associated fibroblasts

(CAFs) microdissected from fresh frozen primary human ovarian and breast cancers as well as some specimens derived from primary culture. None of the 10 CAFs from breast tumors harbored any evidence of copy number alteration or LOH on any chromosome. However, one fibroblast culture showed gains on chromosomes 7 and 10. Interestingly, when CAF cultures without any detectable somatic changes were injected in xenografts, tumor growth occurred more efficiently compared to normal breast stromal fibroblasts.

Although genomic alterations could not be demonstrated, epigenetic alterations cannot be ruled out. Qiu et al. (2008) showed in the same study that CAFs from primary cultures showed different methylation and expression patterns compared to normal counterparts, implying an abnormal phenotype of CAF cultures in the absence of somatic genetic changes (Qiu et al. 2008). Furthermore, genomic methylation profiling, bisulfite sequencing, and anti-5-methyl-C immunohistochemistry have been used to show global hypomethylation in myofibroblasts. Studies in a transgenic mouse model from gastric carcinoma indicate its early occurrence in cancer progression; however, the cause of genomic demethylation in cancer cells remains unknown (Jiang et al. 2008).

Hence overall, there is little doubt that normal tissue harbors molecular alterations and that epithelial cells do show genetic mutations; but whether stromal cells show mutations or whether they show changes in expression without DNA alterations remains to be clarified. What is clear is that changes in the normal cell compartments play an important and interesting role in breast cancer development.

4.8 Hypothesis

Taking together the totality of evidence relating to molecular alterations involved in the multistep model of breast cancer and the finding of changes with normal luminal and myoepithelial cells of the breast, it is plausible that the first alterations giving rise to tumorigenesis may occur in stem/progenitor cell populations. Since most mutations occur during the process of cell division when DNA replication occurs, it is also likely that mutations in these progenitor populations are occurring at a time of greatest cell division, i.e., at puberty when there is prolific cell division to produce the adult breast. Alterations in the stem/ progenitor cells at that time could conceivably give rise to large clonal patches with genetic alterations, which subsequently predispose the tissues to further changes and hence begin the journey toward tumor formation. Such a hypothesis would certainly explain the segmental distribution of many forms of breast diseases, e.g., DCIS, although it would not by itself explain multifocal disease such as seen with LCIS. Presumably, in these cases, there is a combination of germ-line predisposition and a somatic predisposition coming together to produce the risk and disease distribution seen in clinical practice. Current data on molecular alterations within the stroma and the increasing recognition of the importance of stromal–epithelial interactions raise the possibility that the stromal component as well as the epithelial component may be abnormal within the "sick lobe."

4.9 Conclusion: Is There Any Relevance to Clinical Practice?

This is a difficult question to answer other than that if the hypotheses are correct, it would suggest that recurrences may be new tumors arising from the already unstable clonal patch that has been left behind since the excision is currently done to excise the cancer without knowledge of the topography of the abnormal patch. It is not possible at present to excise in such an anatomically precise manner. Perhaps in the future, if these abnormal patches could be identified *in vivo*, intraductal or external methods to ablate the ductal tree may be feasible. This of course does not take into account the role that the stroma may play and hence in reality, the management could be a lot more complicated than we envisage.

The next decade will be critical as new technology combined with traditional pathology comes together to unravel the biology of breast tumorigenesis and hence provide insights into how we should manage our patients with breast disease.

Acknowledgments Ana Cristina Vargas is a clinical fellow funded by the Ludwig Institute for Cancer Research. We acknowledge Prof Michael O'Hare and Dr Catherine Clarke who made a significant contribution to our studies and understanding of normal breast epithelial cell biology.

References

Abdel-Fatah TM, Powe DG, Hodi Z, Lee AH, Reis-Filho JS, Ellis IO (2007) High frequency of coexistence of columnar cell lesions, lobular neoplasia, and low grade ductal carcinoma in situ with invasive tubular carcinoma and invasive lobular carcinoma. Am J Surg Pathol 31:417–426

Abdel-Fatah TM, Powe DG, Hodi Z, Reis-Filho JS, Lee AH, Ellis IO (2008) Morphologic and molecular evolutionary pathways of low nuclear grade invasive breast cancers and their putative precursor lesions: further evidence to support the concept of low nuclear grade breast neoplasia family. Am J Surg Pathol 32:513–523

Alizadeh AA, Ross DT, Perou CM, van de Rijn M (2001) Towards a novel classification of human malignancies based on gene expression patterns. J Pathol 195:41–52

Allinen M, Beroukhim R, Cai L, Brennan C, Lahti-Domenici J, Huang H, Porter D, Hu M, Chin L, Richardson A, Schnitt S, Sellers WR, Polyak K (2004) Molecular characterization of the tumor microenvironment in breast cancer. Cancer Cell 6:17–32

Allred DC, Wu Y, Mao S, Nagtegaal ID, Lee S, Perou CM, Mohsin SK, Ó'Connell P, Tsimelzon A, Medina D (2008) Ductal carcinoma in situ and the emergence of diversity during breast cancer evolution. Clin Cancer Res 14:370–378

Aubele MM, Cummings MC, Mattis AE, Zitzelsberger HF, Walch AK, Kremer M, Hofler H, Werner M (2000) Accumulation of chromosomal imbalances from intraductal proliferative lesions to adjacent in situ and invasive ductal breast cancer. Diagn Mol Pathol 9:14–19

Bergamaschi A, Kim YH, Wang P, Sørlie T, Hernandez-Boussard T, Lonning PE, Tibshirani R, Børresen-Dale AL, Pollack JR (2006) Distinct patterns of DNA copy number alteration are associated with different clinicopathological features and gene-expression subtypes of breast cancer. Genes Chromosomes Cancer 45:1033–1040

Buchanan CL, Flynn LW, Murray MP, Darvishian F, Cranor ML, Fey JV, King TA, Tan LK, Sclafani LM (2008) Is pleomorphic lobular carcinoma really a distinct clinical entity? J Surg Oncol 98:314–317

Buerger H, Otterbach F, Simon R, Poremba C, Raihanatou D, Decker T, Riethdorf L, Brinkschmidt C, Dockhorn-Dworniczak B, Boecker W (1999a) Comparative genomic hybridization of ductal carcinoma in situ of the breast – evidence of multiple genetic pathways. J Pathol 187:396–402

Buerger H, Otterbach F, Simon R, Schafer KL, Poremba C, Diallo R, Brinkschmidt C, Dockhorn-Dworniczak B, Boecker W (1999b) Different genetic pathways in the evolution of invasive breast cancer are associated with distinct morphological subtypes. J Pathol 189:521–526

Buerger H, Simon R, Schafer KL, Diallo R, Littmann R, Poremba C, van Diest PJ, Dockhorn-Dworniczak B, Bocker W (2000) Genetic relation of lobular carcinoma in situ, ductal carcinoma in situ, and associated invasive carcinoma of the breast. Mol Pathol 53:118–121

Clarke CL, Sandle J, Jones AA, Sofronis A, Patani NR, Lakhani SR (2006) Mapping loss of heterozygosity in normal human breast cells from BRCA1/2 carriers. Br J Cancer 95:515–519

Cleton-Jansen AM (2002) E-cadherin and loss of heterozygosity at chromosome 16 in breast carcinogenesis: different genetic pathways in ductal and lobular breast cancer? Breast Cancer Res 4:5–8

Cleton-Jansen AM, Buerger H, Haar N, Philippo K, van de Vijver MJ, Boecker W, Smith VT, Cornelisse CJ (2004) Different mechanisms of chromosome 16 loss of heterozygosity in well- versus poorly differentiated ductal breast cancer. Genes Chromosomes Cancer 41:109–116

Deng G, Lu Y, Zlotnikov G, Thor AD, Smith HS (1996) Loss of heterozygosity in normal tissue adjacent to breast carcinomas. Science 274:2057–2059

Ellis IO, Galea M, Broughton N, Locker A, Blamey RW, Elston CW (1992) Pathological prognostic factors in breast cancer. II. Histological type. Relationship with survival in a large study with long-term follow-up. Histopathology 20:479–489

Elston CW, Ellis IO (1991) Pathological prognostic factors in breast cancer. I. The value of histological grade in breast cancer: experience from a large study with long-term follow-up. Histopathology 19:403–410

Eusebi V, Magalhaes F, Azzopardi JG (1992) Pleomorphic lobular carcinoma of the breast: an aggressive tumor showing apocrine differentiation. Hum Pathol 23:655–662

Farmer H, McCabe N, Lord CJ, Tutt AN, Johnson DA, Richardson TB, Santarosa M, Dillon KJ, Hickson I, Knights C, Martin NM, Jackson SP, Smith GC, Ashworth A (2005) Targeting the DNA repair defect in BRCA mutant cells as a therapeutic strategy. Nature 434:917–921

Fialkow PJ (1976) Clonal origin of human tumors. Biochim Biophys Acta 458:283–321

Fleming JM, Long EL, Ginsburg E, Gerscovich D, Meltzer PS, Vonderhaar BK (2008) Interlobular and intralobular mammary stroma: genotype may not reflect phenotype. BMC Cell Biol 9:46

Fraser JL, Raza S, Chorny K, Connolly JL, Schnitt SJ (1998) Columnar alteration with prominent apical snouts and secretions: a spectrum of changes frequently present in breast biopsies performed for microcalcifications. Am J Surg Pathol 22:1521–1527

Fulford LG, Easton DF, Reis-Filho JS, Sofronis A, Gillett CE, Lakhani SR, Hanby A (2006) Specific morphological features predictive for the basal phenotype in grade 3 invasive ductal carcinoma of breast. Histopathology Jul;49(1):22–34

Hennessy BT, Gonzalez-Angulo AM, Stemke-Hale K, Gilcrease MZ, Krishnamurthy S, Lee JS, Fridlyand J, Sahin A, Agarwal R, Joy C, Liu W, Stivers D, Baggerly K, Carey M, Lluch A, Monteagudo C, He X, Weigman V, Fan C, Palazzo J, Hortobagyi GN, Nolden LK, Wang NJ, Valero V, Gray JW, Perou CM, Mills GB (2009) Characterization of a naturally occurring breast cancer subset enriched in epithelial-to-mesenchymal transition and stem cell characteristics. Cancer Res 69:4116–4124

Hicks J, Krasnitz A, Lakshmi B, Navin NE, Riggs M, Leibu E, Esposito D, Alexander J, Troge J, Grubor V, Yoon S, Wigler M, Ye K, Borresen-Dale AL, Naume B, Schlicting E, Norton L, Hagerstrom T, Skoog L, Auer G, Maner S, Lundin P, Zetterberg A (2006) Novel patterns of genome rearrangement and their association with survival in breast cancer. Genome Res 16:1465–1479

Jiang Y, Tong D, Lou G, Zhang Y, Geng J (2008) Expression of RUNX3 gene, methylation status and clinicopathological significance in breast cancer and breast cancer cell lines. Pathobiology 75:244–251

Jones PA (1996) DNA methylation errors and cancer. Cancer Res 56:2463–2467

Jones C, Damiani S, Wells D, Chaggar R, Lakhani SR, Eusebi V (2001) Molecular cytogenetic comparison of apocrine hyperplasia and apocrine carcinoma of the breast. Am J Pathol 158:207–214

Jones C, Merrett S, Thomas VA, Barker TH, Lakhani SR (2003) Comparative genomic hybridization analysis of bilateral hyperplasia of usual type of the breast. J Pathol 199:152–156

Kurose K, Hoshaw-Woodard S, Adeyinka A, Lemeshow S, Watson PH, Eng C (2001) Genetic model of multi-step breast carcinogenesis involving the epithelium and stroma: clues to tumour–microenvironment interactions. Hum Mol Genet 10:1907–1913

Lakhani SR (1997) Is there a benign to malignant progression? Endocr Relat Cancer 4:93–104

Lakhani SR, Collins N, Stratton MR, Sloane JP (1995) Atypical ductal hyperplasia of the breast: clonal proliferation with loss of heterozygosity on chromosomes 16q and 17p. J Clin Pathol 48:611–615

Lakhani SR, Slack DN, Hamoudi RA, Collins N, Stratton MR, Sloane JP (1996) Detection of allelic imbalance indicates that a proportion of mammary hyperplasia of usual type are clonal, neoplastic proliferations. Lab Invest 74:129–135

Lakhani SR, Chaggar R, Davies S, Jones C, Collins N, Odel C, Stratton MR, O'Hare MJ (1999) Genetic alterations in 'normal' luminal and myoepithelial cells of the breast. J Pathol 189:496–503

Lim E, Vaillant F, Wu D, Forrest NC, Pal B, Hart AH, Asselin-Labat ML, Gyorki DE, Ward T, Partanen A, Feleppa F, Huschtscha LI, Thorne HJ, Fox SB, Yan M, French JD, Brown MA, Smyth GK, Visvader JE, Lindeman GJ (2009) Aberrant luminal progenitors as the candidate target population for basal tumor development in BRCA1 mutation carriers. Nat Med 15:907–913

Liu S, Ginestier C, Charafe-Jauffret E, Foco H, Kleer CG, Merajver SD, Dontu G, Wicha MS (2008) BRCA1 regulates human mammary stem/progenitor cell fate. Proc Natl Acad Sci USA 105:1680–1685

Lu YJ, Osin P, Lakhani SR, Di Palma S, Gusterson BA, Shipley JM (1998) Comparative genomic hybridization analysis of lobular carcinoma in situ and atypical lobular hyperplasia and potential roles for gains and losses of genetic material in breast neoplasia. Cancer Res 58:4721–4727

Lyon MF (1972) X-chromosome inactivation and developmental patterns in mammals. Biol Rev Camb Philos Soc 47:1–35

Ma XJ, Salunga R, Tuggle JT, Gaudet J, Enright E, McQuary P, Payette T, Pistone M, Stecker K, Zhang BM, Zhou YX, Varnholt H, Smith B, Gadd M, Chatfield E, Kessler J, Baer TM, Erlander MG, Sgroi DC (2003) Gene expression profiles of human breast cancer progression. Proc Natl Acad Sci USA 100:5974–5979

Ma XJ, Dahiya S, Richardson E, Erlander M, Sgroi DC (2009) Gene expression profiling of the tumor microenvironment during breast cancer progression. Breast Cancer Res 11:R7

Middleton LP, Palacios DM, Bryant BR, Krebs P, Otis CN, Merino MJ (2000) Pleomorphic lobular carcinoma: morphology, immunohistochemistry, and molecular analysis. Am J Surg Pathol 24:1650–1656

Moinfar F, Man YG, Arnould L, Bratthauer GL, Ratschek M, Tavassoli FA (2000a) Concurrent and independent genetic alterations in the stromal and epithelial cells of mammary carcinoma: implications for tumorigenesis. Cancer Res 60:2562–2566

Moinfar F, Man YG, Bratthauer GL, Ratschek M, Tavassoli FA (2000b) Genetic abnormalities in mammary ductal intraepithelial neoplasia-flat type ("clinging ductal carcinoma in situ"): a simulator of normal mammary epithelium. Cancer 88:2072–2081

Natrajan R, Lambros MB, Geyer FC, Marchio C, Tan DS, Vatcheva R, Shiu KK, Hungermann D, Rodriguez-Pinilla SM, Palacios J, Ashworth A, Buerger H, Reis-Filho JS (2009a) Loss of 16q in high grade breast cancer is associated with estrogen receptor status: evidence for progression in tumors with a luminal phenotype? Genes Chromosomes Cancer 48:351–365

Natrajan R, Lambros MB, Rodríguez-Pinilla SM, Moreno-Bueno G, Tan DS, Marchió C, Vatcheva R, Rayter S, Mahler-Araujo B, Fulford LG, Hungermann D, Mackay A, Grigoriadis A, Fenwick K, Tamber N, Hardisson D, Tutt A, Palacios J, Lord CJ, Buerger H, Ashworth A, Reis-Filho JS (2009b) Tiling path genomic profiling of grade 3 invasive ductal breast cancers. Clin Cancer Res 15:2711–2722

Nishizaki T, Chew K, Chu L, Isola J, Kallioniemi A, Weidner N, Waldman FM (1997) Genetic alterations in lobular breast cancer by comparative genomic hybridization. Int J Cancer 74:513–517

Novelli M, Cossu A, Oukrif D, Quaglia A, Lakhani S, Poulsom R, Sasieni P, Carta P, Contini M, Pasca A, Palmieri G, Bodmer W, Tanda F, Wright N (2003) X-inactivation patch size in human female tissue confounds the assessment of tumor clonality. Proc Natl Acad Sci USA 100:3311–3314

O'Connell P, Pekkel V, Fuqua S, Osborne CK, Allred DC (1994) Molecular genetic studies of early breast cancer evolution. Breast Cancer Res Treat 32:5–12

O'Connell P, Pekkel V, Fuqua SA, Osborne CK, Clark GM, Allred DC (1998) Analysis of loss of heterozygosity in 399 premalignant breast lesions at 15 genetic loci. J Natl Cancer Inst 90:697–703

Oldenhuis CN, Oosting SF, Gietema JA, de Vries EG (2008) Prognostic versus predictive value of biomarkers in oncology. Eur J Cancer 44:946–953

Orvieto E, Maiorano E, Bottiglieri L, Maisonneuve P, Rotmensz N, Galimberti V, Luini A, Brenelli F, Gatti G, Viale G (2008) Clinicopathologic characteristics of invasive lobular carcinoma of the breast: results of an analysis of 530 cases from a single institution. Cancer 113:1511–1520

Palacios J, Sarrio D, Garcia-Macias MC, Bryant B, Sobel ME, Merino MJ (2003) Frequent E-cadherin gene inactivation by loss of heterozygosity in pleomorphic lobular carcinoma of the breast. Mod Pathol 16:674–678

Perou CM, Sorlie T, Eisen MB, van de Rijn M, Jeffrey SS, Rees CA, Pollack JR, Ross DT, Johnsen H, Akslen LA, Fluge O, Pergamenschikov A, Williams C, Zhu SX, Lonning PE, Borresen-Dale AL, Brown PO, Botstein D (2000) Molecular portraits of human breast tumours. Nature 406:747–752

Pollack JR, Perou CM, Alizadeh AA, Eisen MB, Pergamenschikov A, Williams CF, Jeffrey SS, Botstein D, Brown PO (1999) Genome-wide analysis of DNA copy-number changes using cDNA microarrays. Nat Genet 23:41–56

Qiu W, Hu M, Sridhar A, Opeskin K, Fox S, Shipitsin M, Trivett M, Thompson ER, Ramakrishna M, Gorringe KL, Polyak K, Haviv I, Campbell IG (2008) No evidence of clonal somatic genetic alterations in cancer-associated fibroblasts from human breast and ovarian carcinomas. Nat Genet 40:650–655

Rakha EA, Pinder SE, Paish CE, Ellis IO (2004a) Expression of the transcription factor CTCF in invasive breast cancer: a candidate gene located at 16q22.1. Br J Cancer 91: 1591–1596

Rakha EA, Pinder SE, Paish EC, Robertson JF, Ellis IO (2004b) Expression of E2F-4 in invasive breast carcinomas is associated with poor prognosis. J Pathol 203:754–761

Reis-Filho JS, Lakhani SR (2003) The diagnosis and management of pre-invasive breast disease: genetic alterations in pre-invasive lesions. Breast Cancer Res 5:313–319

Reis-Filho JS, Simpson PT, Jones C, Steele D, Mackay A, Iravani M, Fenwick K, Valgeirsson H, Lambros M, Ashworth A, Palacios J, Schmitt F, Lakhani SR (2005) Pleomorphic lobular carcinoma of the breast: role of comprehensive molecular pathology in characterization of an entity. J Pathol 207(1):1–13

Reis-Filho JS, Simpson PT, Gale T, Lakhani SR (2005) The molecular genetics of breast cancer: the contribution of comparative genomic hybridization. Pathol Res Pract 201: 713–725

Roylance R, Gorman P, Hanby A, Tomlinson I (2002) Allelic imbalance analysis of chromosome 16q shows that grade I and grade III invasive ductal breast cancers follow different genetic pathways. J Pathol 196(1):32–6

Roylance R, Droufakou S, Gorman P, Gillett C, Hart IR, Hanby A, Tomlinson I (2003) The role of E-cadherin in low-grade ductal breast tumourigenesis. J Pathol 200:53–58

Roylance R, Gorman P, Papior T, Wan YL, Ives M, Watson JE, Collins C, Wortham N, Langford C, Fiegler H, Carter N, Gillett C, Sasieni P, Pinder S, Hanby A, Tomlinson I (2006) A comprehensive study of chromosome 16q in invasive ductal and lobular breast carcinoma using array CGH. Oncogene 25:6544–6553

Schnitt SJ, Vincent-Salomon A (2003) Columnar cell lesions of the breast. Adv Anat Pathol 10:113–124

Selim AG, El-Ayat G, Wells CA (2000) c-erbB2 oncoprotein expression, gene amplification, and chromosome 17 aneusomy in apocrine adenosis of the breast. J Pathol 191:138–142

Selim AG, El-Ayat G, Wells CA (2002) Expression of c-erbB2, p53, Bcl-2, Bax, c-myc and Ki-67 in apocrine metaplasia and apocrine change within sclerosing adenosis of the breast. Virchows Arch 441:449–455

Simpson PT, Gale T, Fulford LG, Reis-Filho JS, Lakhani SR (2003) The diagnosis and management of pre-invasive breast disease: pathology of atypical lobular hyperplasia and lobular carcinoma in situ. Breast Cancer Res 5:258–262

Simpson PT, Gale T, Reis-Filho JS, Jones C, Parry S, Sloane JP, Hanby A, Pinder SE, Lee AH, Humphreys S, Ellis IO, Lakhani SR (2005a) Columnar cell lesions of the breast: the missing link in breast cancer progression? A morphological and molecular analysis. Am J Surg Pathol 29:734–746

Simpson PT, Reis-Filho JS, Gale T, Lakhani SR (2005b) Molecular evolution of breast cancer. J Pathol 205:248–254

Simpson P, Reis-Filho J, Lambros M, Jones C, Steele D, Mackay A, Iravani M, Fenwick K, Dexter T, Jones A, Reid L, Da

Silva L, Shin S, Hardisson D, Ashworth A, Schmitt F, Palacios J, Lakhani S (2008) Molecular profiling pleomorphic lobular carcinomas of the breast: evidence for a common molecular genetic pathway with classic lobular carcinomas. J Pathol 215:231–244

Sneige N, Wang J, Baker BA, Krishnamurthy S, Middleton LP (2002) Clinical, histopathologic, and biologic features of pleomorphic lobular (ductal-lobular) carcinoma in situ of the breast: a report of 24 cases. Mod Pathol 15:1044–1050

Sorlie T, Perou CM, Tibshirani R, Aas T, Geisler S, Johnsen H, Hastie T, Eisen MB, van de Rijn M, Jeffrey SS, Thorsen T, Quist H, Matese JC, Brown PO, Botstein D, Eystein Lonning P, Borresen-Dale AL (2001) Gene expression patterns of breast carcinomas distinguish tumor subclasses with clinical implications. Proc Natl Acad Sci USA 98:10869–10874

Sorlie T, Tibshirani R, Parker J, Hastie T, Marron JS, Nobel A, Deng S, Johnsen H, Pesich R, Geisler S, Demeter J, Perou CM, Lonning PE, Brown PO, Borresen-Dale AL, Botstein D (2003) Repeated observation of breast tumor subtypes in independent gene expression data sets. Proc Natl Acad Sci USA 100:8418–8423

Stratton MR, Collins N, Lakhani SR, Sloane JP (1995) Loss of heterozygosity in ductal carcinoma in situ of the breast. J Pathol 175:195–201

Stratton MR, Campbell PJ, Futreal PA (2009) The cancer genome. Nature 458:719–724

Tognon C, Knezevich SR, Huntsman D, Roskelley CD, Melnyk N, Mathers JA, Becker L, Carneiro F, MacPherson N, Horsman D, Poremba C, Sorensen PH (2002) Expression of the ETV6-NTRK3 gene fusion as a primary event in human secretory breast carcinoma. Cancer Cell 2:367–376

Tot T (2005) DCIS, cytokeratins, and the theory of the sick lobe. Virchows Arch 447:1–8

Vogelstein B, Fearon ER, Hamilton SR, Feinberg AP (1985) Use of restriction fragment length polymorphisms to determine the clonal origin of human tumors. Science 227: 642–645

Weidner N, Semple JP (1992) Pleomorphic variant of invasive lobular carcinoma of the breast. Hum Pathol 23:1167–1171

The Role of Ductal Lavage: A Cautionary Tale

5

Susan M. Love and Dixie J. Mills

5.1 Introduction

Nearly one hundred years ago, the English surgeon and author, Sir Geoffrey Keynes, wrote "the breast is a gland which throughout life is exhibiting some secretory activity, the difference between a lactating and a non-lactating breast being one partly of degree and partly of the chemical constitution of the secretion" (Keynes 1923). While knowledge about the histopathology of breast cancer has progressed significantly in the subsequent years, the intraluminal cells and secretions of the ductal system in the non-lactating or resting breast have received little attention. Most pathologists have considered these cells and secretions to be sloughed off degenerating epithelium and proteinaceous material and of little biological interest (Petrakis 1986). However, there has been isolated interest in looking more carefully at this fluid and determining its physiology and its clinical significance.

5.2 Nipple Aspirate Fluid (NAF)

Papanicolaou in 1958 (Papanicolaou et al. 1958) described applying suction to the nipple using a maternal bulb type breast pump to obtain small drops of fluid from the milk ducts (NAF). There was hope that this fluid could be used for early detection much like the Pap smear. However, due to poor cellularity and few positive results, the technique was not widely adopted.

In the 1970s, several researchers reevaluated and revived Papanicolaou's approach (Buehring 1979; Sartorius 1973; Sartorius et al. 1977). They were able to obtain fluid from a greater percentage of women by using a suction cup over the nipple that was attached to a 10cc syringe by a short plastic tube. They also found it useful to cleanse the nipple to remove any keratin plugs that could be sealing the pores. This breast pump was found to generate higher negative pressures and with repeated visits, they were able to elicit NAF from nearly 70% of women. Fluid yielders tended to be premenopausal, white and with a wet-type cerumen. Asian-Americans and post-menopausal women were the least likely group to be fluid yielders. NAF was also found to contain lipids, cholesterol, hormones, and diverse substances such as barbiturates, caffeine, nicotine, and pesticides (Petrakis 1986). Cytopathological examination of NAF shows ductal epithelial cells, apocrine cells, and foam cells now usually referred to as macrophages (King et al. 1975). Research has focused on epithelial cells in NAF as the progression from normal epithelium through hyperplasia, atypical hyperplasia, carcinoma in situ to cancer became well understood in breast pathology.

Wrensch and Petrakis demonstrated epithelial cells found in NAF correlate with a 21% increased risk for developing breast cancer over 30 years. Furthermore, cytological atypia in NAF results in an increased relative risk of 2.8 compared to women with no fluid (Wrensch et al. 2001). However, atypia in NAF is not an obligate precursor of breast cancer since only 11% of women with atypia in NAF went on to develop breast cancer. Three large clinical studies with 20-year follow-up have now confirmed that fluid yielders and especially those with atypical cytology in their fluid are at higher subsequent risk of breast cancer development (Wrensch et al. 2001; Buehring et al. 2006; Baltzell

S.M. Love
Dr. Susan Love Research Foundation, Santa Monica, CA, USA
e-mail: susan.love@dslrf.org

T. Tot (ed.), *Breast Cancer*, DOI: 10.1007/978-1-84996-314-5_5,
© Springer-Verlag London Limited 2011

Table 5.1 Major prospective NAF studies demonstrating relative risk of cancer

Study	N	Follow up (years)	No fluid	Fluid	Cells	Atypia
Wrensch et al. (2001)	3,627	21	1.0 (3.7%)	1.2 (7.5%)	1.3 (6.6%)	2.1 (11%)
Buehring et al. (2006)	972/1,744	25	1.0		2.27	
Baltzell et al. (2008)	946/1,706	20	1.0	1.4	1.7	2.0

et al. 2008) (see Table 5.1). However, use of NAF as a risk factor for screening was limited by the technique and the number of non-yielders and, perhaps more significantly, by the relatively poor epithelial cell count obtained and the need for a trained cytopathologist to read the sample.

5.3 Ductal Lavage (DL)

The idea of studying the ducts and ductal fluid through cannulating orifices in the nipple was actually first mentioned over 60 years ago by Leborgne, a Uruguayan doctor (Leborgne 1946). He described a way to pass a small catheter into a breast duct through the nipple and instill saline, remove the catheter, massage the breast manually and express and collect the fluid that returned. He termed this procedure "ductal rinse." With the advent of radiological imaging in this country, contrast mammography was pursued as a preoperative evaluation for nipple discharge (Love and Barsky 1996). While impressive X-rays of the ductal trees were obtained (Fig. 5.1) difficulty with the procedure and contrast reactions in women limited its use. Interest surged again however with the results from cytology stains of the cervix. Otto Sartorius, a surgeon and colleagues combined contrast ductography and ductal rinsing to collect fluid after imaging. Positive yields were higher with this technique (Sartorius et al. 1977). However, it was not until the development of a unique microcatheter by Love with a double lumen to maintain patency of the duct while lavaging that the procedure received widespread use (Love and Barsky 1996) (see Fig. 5.2). DL and the Cytyc catheter were developed and commercialized as a method and tool to sample a specific duct, based on the observation that DCIS and invasive ductal cancer are limited to one ductal system (Holland et al. 1985; Mai et al. 2000).

Evidence suggests that lavage procedures are capable of delivering fluid (dye or saline) to, and harvesting cells from, the junctions of the terminal

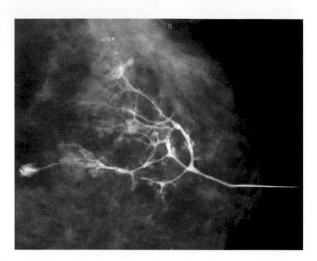

Fig. 5.1 Radiogram with dye (contrast medium) in one ductal system showing extent to lobules

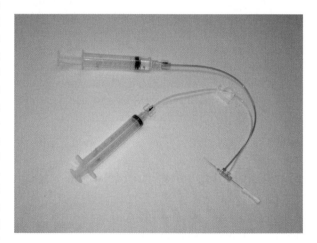

Fig. 5.2 Ductal lavage microcatheter

ductal lobular units of the mammary tree. Several studies involving the intraductal delivery of dyes to demarcate the path of lavage fluids have demonstrated permeation of the lobular-alveolar portion of the ductal systems (Love and Barsky 1996; Brogi et al. 2003; Khan et al. 2004). Moreover, the procedure has collected exfoliated cells exhibiting cytological features of lobular carcinoma in situ (LCIS) from a patient with pathology-confirmed LCIS (Brogi et al. 2003). In addition, lavage study participants have reported feeling the cooler (room) temperature of the lavage saline circulating within chest wall and axial regions (King and Love 2005). Collectively, these data suggest that epithelial cells can be collected from the terminal reaches of the mammary trees. The first multicenter study with 507 high risk women reported that large numbers of ductal cells could be collected by DL and that the procedure was safe and well-tolerated and found to be a more sensitive method of detecting cellular atypia than nipple aspiration (Dooley et al. 2001).

5.3.1 Superficial Nipple Anatomy

The fact that fluid, breast milk comes out of the nipple through several orifices like a watering can and not a hose is quite obvious to anyone who has observed a lactating woman. The nipple orifices however do not allow any substances naturally back into the breast and are thus seen as a one-way conduit. Gross examination of the surface of the nipple shows multiple clefts but the openings to the ducts are not always evident. In fact, the number of these openings is debated. Sir Astley Cooper (Cooper 1845) injected wax through the nipple at autopsies of women who had died from childbirth sepsis. He described being able to inject at most 12 lactiferous ducts and more commonly 7–10 per nipple. Love and Barsky (2004) observed over 200 lactating women in order to map milk duct orifices and indentified an average of 5–9 openings. There appeared to be consistently a central group of 4–5 orifices and a peripheral ring of 4–5 also. Teboul and Halliwell (1995) reported on over 6,000 ultrasound studies of the breast ducts and described 5–8 "milk pores" in the nipple. Ramsay et al. (2005) studied 21 lactating women with ultrasound and described 6–12 main ducts. The often-quoted finding of 15–20 ducts appears on pathological sectioning of the nipple and counting of the lumens (Rusby et al. 2007). The exact anatomy of the nipple is still being investigated as to whether some of these lumens are rudimentary or straight ducts or whether several lumens join at the nipple surface. Also, as the cross sections were not traced distally into the breast parenchyma, it is unclear what they represent. Whether each ductal tree is clonally unique is discussed elsewhere in this textbook.

5.3.2 The DL Technique

Because of the difficulty in identifying ductal orifices, lavage was initially performed only after the demonstration of fluid from one or multiple discharging pores with the use of a nipple aspiration suction device (Dooley et al. 2001). The nipple is first de-keratinized using a mild abrasive gel; the breast is then massaged by the subject or the physician for at least 1 min. A suction cup fitted with a 10–20 ml syringe is placed over the nipple and a small amount of suction (approximately 7–15 ml) is applied. If no fluid appears on the nipple, the lactiferous sinus at the base of the nipple is manually compressed. Repeated efforts at breast massage and suction are attempted until fluid is elicited or until the investigator determines the breast to be non-fluid yielding.

The first large study of DL (Dooley et al. 2001) used local or topical anesthesia (EMLA cream: 2.5% lidocaine and 2.5% prilocaine; Astra USA) to the nipple in the majority of cases. Twenty-eight percent of subjects underwent the procedure in an operating room while under general anesthesia or sedation.

Subcutaneous periareolar injections or nipple blocks, using a 30-gauge needle, of 1% lidocaine were attempted but were subsequently abandoned because of subject discomfort. DL is then usually attempted immediately after nipple aspiration on all ducts that yield fluid. The woman is placed in the supine position, the skin and nipple area are cleansed with 70% alcohol. After nipple anesthesia, ductal orifices are gently enlarged with microdilators to facilitate cannulation. To facilitate insertion 2% zylocaine jelly is used on the dilator tip . A separate microcatheter is used for each duct cannulation to prevent cellular cross-contamination between individual ductal systems. The microcatheter has been primed with 1% lidocaine or saline before insertion to eliminate air infusion. The catheter is inserted to a maximum depth of 1.5 cm and then 2 ml of normal saline, Plasmalyte or lactated ringers is infused. Then the breast is compressed or massaged to facilitate recovery of ductal fluid into the collection chamber. The lavage procedure (infusion, compression, and effluent collection) is repeated multiple times instilling a total volume of approximately 10–20 ml of normal saline and recovering approximately 5–10 ml of ductal effluent per duct. The effluent is then centrifuged at 2,500 rpm for 10 min and the cell pellet resuspended in 20 ml of Preservcyt (Hologic, MA) for cytological examination and the supernatant frozen for other biomarker analysis.

5.3.3 Modifications

More recently, Tondre et al. (2008) have used direct nipple injections with a 30-gauge needle of 1% lidocaine buffered with sodium bicarbonate (Fig. 5.3). Additional lidocaine and or marcaine can be injected depending on the subject's level of discomfort and the length of the procedure. Pain scores were low with this technique. This procedure also allows the nipple to become engorged and the ductal orifices are then more prominent. The dilators and stiffeners can also be used to identify non-discharging ducts. Pulling up on the nipple also permits the dilator and catheter to fall more easily into position. The use of a magnifying light also facilitates cannulation. With minimal instruction and practice, up to 6–8 non-fluid-yielding ducts can be cannulated in a short amount of time (Love et al. 2009).

Several investigators (Visvanathan et al. 2007; Loud et al. 2009) have reported poor tolerability for the procedure and a relatively high attrition rate (25%) when follow-ups were due. These procedures were done as part of high risk screening in *BRCA1* and *BRCA2* mutation carriers or other high risk women and it was seen that women with greater pre-existing emotional distress experience more DL-related discomfort than they anticipated (Loud et al. 2009). Others (Tondre et al. 2008) had a much higher (near 90%) 6-month return rate with healthy volunteers and with a 95% return rate in high risk women (Twelves and Gui 2008). Naturally, there is some contribution from subject involvement and understanding and clinician input and enthusiasm for DL. With some subjects finding DL to be more tolerable than a mammogram while others

experiencing it to be more uncomfortable, it's utility as a routine screening tool is again questioned.

The DL technique can be used with ultrasound to identify ductal structures or perforations. It can also be used after ductoscopy again to identify and confirm that the structure cannulated is a duct not a perforation (Tondre et al. 2008) (see Figs. 5.4 and 5.5). Danforth et al. present a feasibility study where they followed DL with breast endoscopy and in 11 subjects performed endoscopic sampling with a brush, coil, or aspiration device (Danforth et al. 2006). The later

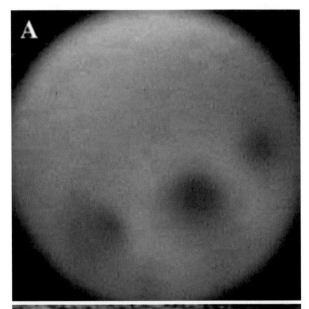

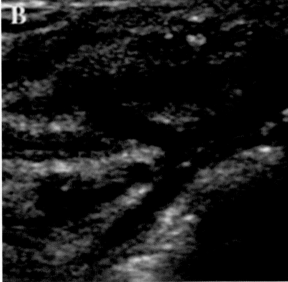

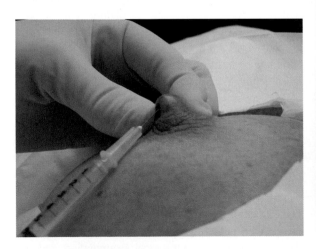

Fig. 5.3 Nipple block utilizing 30-gauge needle, note upward direction and site of injection

Fig. 5.4 A ductal trifurcaction visualized by ductoscopy (**a**) and its distention during lavage on ultrasound (**b**)

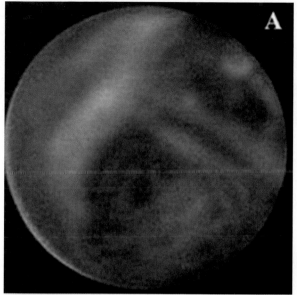

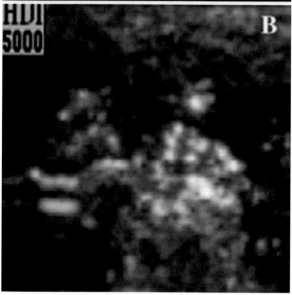

Fig. 5.5 A perforation appears as irregularity and increased light on the scope (**a**) and pooling on the ultrasound (**b**)

techniques obtained increased cells/sample with minimal trauma to the duct. This study was done under intravenous sedation.

5.4 Studies and Lessons Learned

Initial reports of the success of DL led multiple centers to undertake studies investigating its utility for risk assessment. Most centers involved subjects from their

breast cancer high risk centers. Management recommendations for DL were published in early 2003 (Danforth et al. 2006). The interpretation of lavage cytology as benign was seen as a basis for repeat lavage in 1–3 years. Mildly atypical cytology would warrant repeat lavage within a year or raise consideration of prevention therapy (see Fig. 5.6). Markedly atypical or "malignant" cytology would be the basis of additional studies to confirm the results, such as magnetic resonance imaging (MRI), ductoscopy, or performance of a ductograms. These procedures might lead to a tissue biopsy if a lesion were found or the lavage results could lead to the use of prevention therapy. It was not recommended that major surgical intervention be based on DL results. However, the initial enthusiasm with DL has waned as a number of the early hypotheses on which DL was based were found not to be completely accurate.

5.4.1 The Significance of Fluid Yielding Ducts

Initially the presumption was made that the duct that secreted most actively and therefore would be the most readily accessible would be the sentinel duct and represent the status of the whole breast (Dooley et al. 2001). In fact, if NAF represents a field defect within the whole breast, one would expect that sampling any duct with NAF in a breast with cancer would demonstrate atypical cells. Studies by Khan et al. (2004) and Brogi et al. (2003) demonstrated that this is not the case. Another assumption made was that the fluid yielding ducts would be the ones most likely to harbor atypical and malignant cells and that NAF and DL fluid would therefore be similar. Based on the previous NAF studies mentioned above, an assumption was made that ducts yielding NAF would be the duct most likely to be abnormal. However, several investigators have recently demonstrated that dry ducts are as likely to contain atypical cells as fluid yielding ones (Kurian et al. 2005; Bhandare et al. 2005; Maddux et al. 2004) have shown atypical cells in non-discharging ducts at a rate similar to their incidence in discharging ducts and Khan et al. (2005) showed that most ducts with ductal carcinoma in situ (DCIS) did not produce NAF. These findings are not surprising since spontaneous serosanguinous or watery discharge represents in situ or invasive cancer only about 5% of the time (Cabioglu et al. 2003).

Fig. 5.6 Ductal lavage cellular cytologies. (**a**) Benign. (**b**) Mild atypia. (**c**) Marked atypia. (**d**) Malignant

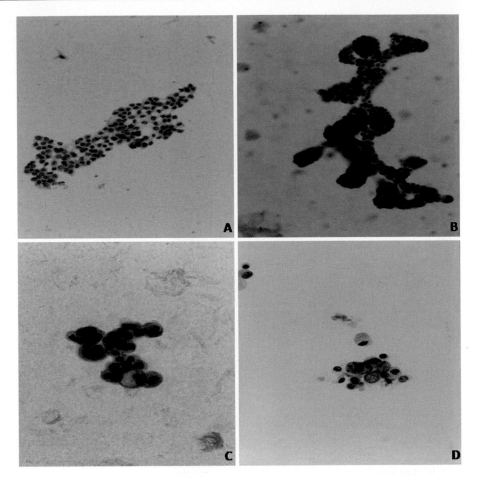

5.4.2 The Meaning and Clinical Utility of the Presence of Cytological Atypia

While atypical ductal hyperplasia from breast tissue biopsies has been shown to be a known risk factor by Dupont and Page in 1985 (Dupont and Page 1985) and cytological atypia in NAF has also shown an increased risk, although lower than histological in several studies by Wrensch, Buehring and Baltzell (Wrensch et al. 2001; Buehring et al. 2006; Baltzell et al. 2008), the risk of atypia in DL had only been presumed. While it may be intuitively reasonable and biologically plausible that atypia detected in DL specimens would be associated with a comparable measure of association, documentation of this assumption still awaits maturation of prospectively accumulated data. The one multicenter study, the "Serial Evaluation of Ductal Epithelium"

(SEDE) trial looking at this risk and designed to answer many of the questions surrounding DL was prematurely closed (Linder 2004). DL samples had been collected from women at high risk at 6-month intervals and assessed for both cytological features and supernatant fluid was frozen for future biomarker analysis. Attempts at follow-up of these subjects and their specimens are underway.

Cytological atypia in a DL sample was initially felt to merit clinical management. However, the reproducibility of atypia on DL over time has not held up so that its usefulness in risk assessment has been questioned. A study by Johnson–Maddox found that less than half of women producing atypical DL samples on the first attempt were found to have atypical samples on a subsequent attempt (Johnson-Maddox et al. 2005). In the Patil study (Patil et al. 2008), 58% of women showed a change to benign cytology at 6-months after being diagnosed with benign atypia at baseline, while 20% of women with benign cytology at baseline went on to mild atypia over 6-months. In a smaller study by Hartman et al. (2004), only one repeat DL in four women with mild atypia was persistent. Visvanathan et al. (2007), evaluated the reliability of NAF versus DL at two time points 6-months apart in women at increased risk for breast cancer where 24 ducts in 14 women were lavaged twice. Among these ducts, cellular yield for the two time points was inconsistent, and only fair cytologic agreement was observed. In our study of 100 community women of unspecified risk who underwent lavage of 3 ducts which were repeated in 6 months, only one of the initial 17 ducts with atypia remained atypical. The absence of reproducibility was seen in women at all risk levels.

One theory emerging from these and other studies is that the ductal epithelium requires more than 6 months to fully regenerate – a contradiction to the notion that atypia on exfoliative cytology represents a proliferative process. Euhus et al. (2007) recently reported on a series of 514 ductal fluid samples in 150 women where both atypia and DNA methylation were evaluated and found that both methylation and marked atypia were independently associated with risk. These observations led us to question whether all cytological atypia is in fact representative of a proliferative premalignant state or whether it is alternatively more indicative of another process that may also be related to subsequent cancer development such as a low grade state of chronic inflammation exiting in the breast. Thus, we would now propose that DL mild atypia be interpreted more as similar to an ASCUS cervical Pap smear and viewed as an interpretation of uncertainty.

5.4.3 Cytology and Other Biomarkers for Use as Indicators for Screening for Risk or Chemoprevention

While the reproducibility of atypia is being questioned, there are few mature studies of DL to answer the question if cytological atypia does indeed suggest increase risk. Only one study of 116 high risk women has followed their patients for 1–4 years. While 25 women had atypia on DL, none had atypical pathology on further examination or developed breast cancer. Two women did develop breast cancer but both had benign lavages. This group no longer utilizes DL as part of their screening of high risk patients (Carruthers et al. 2007).

As the field of biomarker discovery has mushroomed over the last 10-years, several groups have explored both NAF and DL as a means to identify a panel of breast markers for detection of risk, disease, response to therapy, and/or reoccurrence (Dua et al. 2006). Cytology, genomic changes, and protein profiling techniques have been analyzed; however, the results have been discouragingly variable and not reproducible, perhaps due to lack of precise measurement technology and reagents. A few studies have examined and compared cytology and biomarkers in paired DL studies (Table 5.2). Again, cytological evaluation consistently demonstrated low sensitivity while some biomarkers, particularly FISH had higher sensitivities and specificities. Other markers such as DNA methylation have been examined in DL samples. Euhus found that atypia and methylation were independently associated with Gail risk and independent risk factors (Euhus et al. 2007). Fackler et al. (2006) reported that quantitative multiplexed methylation-specific PCR

Table 5.2 Comparison of cytology and biomarkers in paired studies of ductal lavage

Fluid Collection	Cytology		Biomarker			Ref.
	Sensitivity (%)	Specificity (%)	Assay	Sensitivity (%)	Specificity (%)	
Lavage	33	89	FISH	100	100	Yamamoto et al. (2003)
Lavage	47	79	FISH	71	89	King et al. (2003)
Lavage	31	100	SELDI-TOF MS	75	NA	Mendrinos et al. (2005)

Comparison of cytology and biomarkers in paired studies in which breast fluids were collected presurgically from women scheduled for excisional breast biopsies or mastectomies. Sensitivities reflect the detection of invasive and/or ductal carcinoma in situ (DCIS), except when noted. FISH, fluorescence in situ hybridization; NA, not available; SELDI-TOF MS, surface-enhanced laser desorption and ionization-time of flight mass spectrometry when used to detect tumor suppressor gene silencing in DL samples doubles the sensitivity for cancer identification compared with cytomorphology alone.

Reproductive hormones have been studied in NAF and DL and found that the concentrations of estrogens in breast fluids are significantly higher than in serum with little variation with the menstrual cycle or menopause (Petrakis et al. 1993; Chatterton 2005). The use of a hormone as a biomarker of risk or response has not yet been established.

Khan et al. (2009) has looked at biomarkers in DL as part of a study of high risk women who had been offered Tamoxifen. They found over the study period that cytology was not an adequate marker of response to Tamoxifen. They also found that a 53% attrition rate, the expense of the catheter, the time required for the procedure, and the analysis of multiple samples per woman rendered DL an extremely expensive method of breast epithelial sampling. The variability of findings over time about put into question the utility of this procedure for biomarker assessment over time in high risk women.

The quest is still ongoing for a reliable marker or markers of success of a chemoprevention and how to best sample tissue. That DL will have a niche in risk stratification is not clear and the information to date would appear not to support it use in that arena (Fabian 2007). However, in the research field, it would seem that there is still a role for DL and the collection of cells, be they epithelial or histiocytes, and or other markers, such as endogenous hormones, proteins or exogenous carcinogens in the supernatant.

5.4.4 All Ducts Are the Same or Are They Unique

The breast has been looked upon as one organ with a right and a left side. Recent textbooks identify the ducts laid out radially in equal distributions of a pie. This is in direct opposition to anatomical studies by Cooper (Cooper 1845) and Going (Going and Moffat 2004) who showed variation in the size of the lobes and that the six largest ductal systems constituted 75% of the volume of the breast.

One area not analyzed in many studies is the inter-class coefficient of cytology, hormones, and other markers between ducts and between women. We have found that ducts from the same breast were no more similar than ducts from different breasts (Tondre et al. 2006). More data is currently still being analyzed. Moreover, this would support the hypothesis of unique ducts within the breast, rather than a field defect. However, if every duct is indeed unique and breast cancer a lobar disease (Tot 2005) this makes epithelial sampling difficult without a standardized anatomical map of the breast and nipple. It would seem imperative for imaging or other methods to be recognized as accurately directing and identifying which duct is abnormal.

5.4.5 Patient Selection

Candidates for DL were originally thought to be those who were at increased epidemiological risk of breast cancer, by the Gail model, women who have had contralateral breast cancer or have genetic risk such as BRCA1 or BRCA2 mutations. DL was not seen as a screening test but a method to more precisely quantify breast cancer risk. It was hoped that women could be advised by their DL result to choose a risk-reduction drug or other strategy. It was also hoped that DL could serve as an effective method of serial epithelial sampling to measure specific biomarkers to aid in the intermediate assessment of new preventive interventions (Fabian 2007).

While initially only high risk women were deemed candidates for DL, and primarily those with fluid yielding ducts, it has become evident that the value of DL may lie in understanding the basic anatomy and physiology of the breast and in future noninvasive treatment of the breast with ductoscopy and intraductal therapy.

5.5 The Future

The unsatisfying experience with cytological atypia has led us to pursue other facets and utility of DL. The Dr. Susan Love Research Foundation (DSLRF) is currently looking at macrophages and cytokine production in ductal fluid to see if we can identify a more promising risk factor. As the breast oncology field is looking at the tumor microenvironment, we are also looking more carefully at the ductal microenvironment. Our initial investigation of reproductive hormones in the ductal fluid is showing little correlation between ducts thus, suggesting that each ductal tree is its own system.

We are also reexamining the physiology and secretory activity of the non-lactating breast or resting breast. Bonser et al. (1961) found that mature non-lactating breasts contained secretion in the alveoli, tubules, ductules, and ducts and injected suspensions of India ink into the breast ducts of rabbits and found that the injected material moved out of lumen through the walls and eventually into the lymphatics. They felt that this supported their hypothesis that secretion and reabsorption were constantly taking place. Few studies in the last 50 years have been reported on the physiology of the resting breast. Our foundation is currently studying membrane transport mechanisms in the resting breast using several agents, including caffeine, cimetidine, aspirin, and mannitol. We are looking at the absorption of these ingested substances into parous and nulliparous women's breast over a 12-h period using DL and then comparing the curves to those of lactating women's breast milk.

Preliminary results showed significant and intriguing differences (Mills et al. 2009). In lactating women, caffeine passively diffuses into milk rapidly within 1 h and reflects serum levels. In resting breasts, caffeine levels generally peak at 6 h or later after injection. Cimetidine, on the other hand, is known to be concentrated in milk in the lactating woman but was not detected in ductal fluid from the resting breast. Since cimetidine is known to be actively transported in the lactating woman, this pattern is consistent with a transporter protein that is transcribed only during lactation. The concentrations and time course of drugs in NAF and DL also seem to differ suggesting some physiological difference other than dilution. There was a significant difference between parous and nulliparous women in terms of caffeine concentrations and uptake. Finally, preliminary analyses of injected mannitol into breast ducts are still undergoing investigation to better understand the bidirectional transfer of drugs as well as the study of other safe drugs that can be used with volunteers.

The experience with DL and the ability to cannulate non-discharging ducts has opened up the field to the possibility of intraductal therapy. While once assumed that the breast was impenetrable through the nipple, we have now been successful in instilling saline, lactated ringers, and mannitol through the orifices of the nipple in non-discharging ducts without sequelae. Success in the intraductal field starting with the animal model is discussed elsewhere in this textbook. Two human safety trials have been conducted with women undergoing mastectomies. The DSLRF is supervising the first clinical trial in a rural area looking at intraductal therapy of DCIS with liposomal doxorubicin (PLD). This study is testing the safety and feasibility of this neo adjuvant approach in women with ductal carcinoma in situ prior to definitive surgery. To date, with nine patients, we have been able to demonstrate our ability to correctly identify the orifice of the affected duct, and safely deliver 20 mg of PLD demonstrating histological changes. Further evaluation of markers, MRI changes, and pathology will be performed once accrual (30 women) has been completed (Mahoney 2009).

While the initial enthusiasm about DL for risk assessment has not been sustained, its use has led to an important reinvestigation into the field of the resting breast's anatomy and physiology. Every other year since 1999, the DSLRF has held an international symposium on the intraductal approach to breast cancer. Symposium highlights, abstracts and a listing of pilot grants given out are available on line at www.dslrf.org or in publication (Sixth international symposium on the intraductal approach to breast cancer 2009). The sixth symposium was held in 2009 and was attended by over 120 clinicians, researchers, and advocates who expressed a growing interest and excitement for this field. This basic knowledge of the ductal/lobar systems intraductal approach to breast cancer would appear to be essential if the treatment and prevention of breast cancer is to evolve and to be applied in a more logical and less invasive way.

While the excitement with the new tool of a microcatheter and a novel technique of DL might have led clinicians to jump ahead of the basic knowledge, it does not seem in vain and we have presented the lessons learned in this cautionary tale. It should be apparent that the details of Keynes quote on the degree and constitution of the breast secretions are still elusive and need further exploration.

References

Rochman S, Mills D, Kim J, Kuerer H, Love S State of the Science and the Intraductal Approach for Breast Cancer: Proceedings Summary of the Sixth International Symposium on the Intraductal Approach to Breast Cancer Santa Monica California, 19-21 February 2009 (2009) BMC Proc 3 (Suppl 5):11

Baltzell KA, Moghadassi M, Rice T, Sison JD, Wrensch M (2008) Epithelial cells in nipple aspirate fluid and subsequent breast cancer risk: a historic prospective study. BMC Cancer 19:8–75

Bhandare D, Nayar R, Bryk M, Hou N, Cohn R, Golewale N, Parker NP, Chatterton RT, Rademaker A, Khan SA (2005) Endocrine biomarkers in ductal lavage samples from women at high risk for breast cancer. Cancer Epidemiol Biomarkers Prev 14:2620–2627

Bonser GM, Dossett SA, Jull SW (1961) Human and experimental breast cancer. CC Thomas, Springfield

Brogi E, Robson M, Panageas KS, Casadio C, Ljung BM, Montgomery L (2003) Ductal lavage in patients undergoing mastectomy for mammary carcinoma: a correlative study. Cancer 98:2170–2176

Buehring GC (1979) Screening for breast atypias using exfoliative cytology. Cancer 43:1788–1799

Buehring GC, Letscher A, McGirr KM, Khandhar S, Che LH, Nguyen CT, Hackett AJ (2006) Presence of epithelial cells in nipple aspirate fluid is associated with subsequent breast cancer: a 25-year prospective study. Breast Cancer Res Treat 98:63–70

Cabioglu N, Hunt KK, Singletary SE, Stephens TW, Marcy S, Meric F, Ross MT, Babiera GV, Ames FC, Kuerer HM (2003) Surgical decision making and factors determining a diagnosis of breast carcinoma in women presenting with nipple discharge. J Am Coll Surg 196:354–364

Carruthers CD, Chapleskie LA, Flynn MB, Frazier TG (2007) The use of ductal lavage as a screening tool in women at high risk for developing breast carcinoma. Am J Surg 194:463–466

Chatterton RT Jr (2005) Characteristics of salivary profiles of oestradiol and progesterone in premenopausal women. J Endocrinol 186:77–84

Cooper A (1845) The anatomy and diseases of the breast. Lea and Blanchard, Philadelphia

Danforth DN Jr, Abati A, Filie A, Prindiville SA, Palmieri D, Simon R, Ried T, Steeg PS (2006) Combined breast ductal lavage and ductal endoscopy for the evaluation of the high-risk breast: a feasibility study. J Surg Oncol 94: 555–564

Dooley WC, Ljung BM, Veronesi U, Cazzaniga M, Elledge RM, O'Shaughnessy JA, Kuerer HM, Hung DT, Khan SA, Phillips RF, Granz PA, Euhus DM, Esserman LJ, Haffty BG, King BL, Kelley MC, Anderson MM, Schmit PS, Clark RR, Kass FC, Anderson BO, Troyan SL, Arias RD, Quiring JN, Love SM, Page DL, King EB (2001) Ductal lavage for detection of cellular atypia in women at high risk for breast cancer. J Natl Cancer Inst 93:1624–1632

Dua RS, Isacke CM, Gui GP (2006) The intraductal approach to breast cancer biomarker discovery. J Clin Oncol 24:1209–1216

Dupont WD, Page DL (1985) Risk factors for breast cancer in women with proliferative breast disease. N Engl J Med 312:146–151

Euhus DM, Bu D, Ashfaq R, Xie XJ, Bian A, Leitch AM, Lewis CM (2007) Atypia and DNA methylation in nipple duct lavage in relation to predicted breast cancer risk. Cancer Epidemiol Biomarkers Prev 6:1812–1821

Fabian CJ (2007) Is there a future for ductal lavage? Clin Cancer Res 13:4655–4656

Fackler MJ, Malone K, Zhang Z, Schilling E, Garrett-Mayer E, Swift-Scanlan T, Lange J, Nayar R, Davidson NE, Khan SA, Sukumar S (2006) Quantitative multiplex methylation-specific PCR analysis doubles detection of tumor cells in breast ductal fluid. Clin Cancer Res 12:3306–3310

Going JJ, Moffat DF (2004) Escaping from Flatland: clinical and biological aspects of human mammary duct anatomy in three dimensions. J Pathol 203:538–544

Hartman A, Daniel BL, Kurian AW, Mills MA, Nowels KW, Dirbas FM, Kingham KE, Chun NM, Herfkens RJ, Ford JM, Plevritis SK (2004) Breast magnetic resonance image screening and ductal lavage in women at high genetic risk for breast carcinoma. Cancer 100:479–489

Holland R, Veling SH, Mravunac M, Hendriks JH (1985) Histologic multifocality of Tis, T1-2 breast carcinomas. Implications for clinical trials of breast-conserving surgery. Cancer 56:979–990

Johnson-Maddux A, Ashfaq R, Cler L, Naftalis E, Leitch AM, Hoover S, Euhus DM (2005) Reproducibility of cytologic atypia in repeat nipple duct lavage. Cancer 103:1129–1136

Keynes G (1923) Chronic mastitis. Br J Surg 11:89–121

Khan SA, Wiley EL, Rodriguez N, Baird C, Ramakrishnan R, Nayar R, Bryk M, Bethke KB, Staradub VL, Wolfman J et al (2004) Ductal lavage findings in women with known breast cancer undergoing mastectomy. J Natl Cancer Inst 96:1510–1517

Khan SA, Wolfman JA, Segal L, Benjamin S, Nayar R, Wiley EL, Bryk M, Morrow M (2005) Ductal lavage findings in women with mammographic microcalcifications undergoing biopsy. Ann Surg Oncol 12:689–696

Khan SA, Lankes HA, Patil DB, Bryk M, Hou N, Ivancic D, Nayar R, Masood S, Rademaker A (2009) Ductal lavage is an inefficient method of biomarker measurement in high-risk women. Cancer Prev Res (Phila Pa) 2:265–273

King BL, Love SM (2005) The intraductal approach to the breast: raison d'être. Breast Cancer Res 7:198–204

King EB, Barrett D, King M-C, Petrakis NL (1975) Cellular composition of the nipple aspirate specimen of breast fluid. I. The benign cells. Am J Clin Pathol 64:728–738

King BL, Tsai SC, Gryga ME, D'Aquila TG, Seelig SA, Morrison LE, Jacobson KK, Legator MS, Ward DC, Rimm DL, Phillips RF (2003) Detection of chromosomal instability in paired breast surgery and ductal lavage specimens by interphase fluorescence in situ hybridization. Clin Cancer Res 9:1509–1516

Kurian AW, Mills MA, Jaffee M, Sigal BM, Chun NM, Kingham KE, Collins LC, Nowels KW, Plevritis SK, Garber JE, Ford JM, Hartman AR (2005) Ductal lavage of fluid-yielding and non-fluid-yielding ducts in BRCA1 and BRCA2 mutation carriers and other women at high inherited breast cancer risk. Cancer Epidemiol Biomarkers Prev 14:1082–1089

Leborgne R (1946) Intraductal biopsy of certain pathologic processes of the breast. Surgery 19:47–54

Linder J (2004) Editorial: ductal lavage of the breast. Diagn Cytopathol 30:140–142

Loud JT, Thiébaut AC, Abati AD, Filie AC, Nichols K, Danforth D, Giusti R, Prindiville SA, Greene MH (2009) Ductal lavage in women from BRCA1/2 families: Is there a future for ductal lavage in women at increased genetic risk of breast cancer? Cancer Epidemiol Biomarkers Prev 18:1243–1251

Love SM, Barsky SH (1996) Breast-duct endoscopy to study stages of cancerous breast disease. Lancet 348:997–999

Love SM, Barsky SH (2004) Anatomy of the nipple and breast ducts revisited. Cancer 101:1947–1957

Love SM, Zhang B, Zhang W, Zhang B, Yang H, Rao J (2009) Local drug delivery to the breast: a phase 1 study of breast cytotoxic agent administration prior to mastectomy. BMC Proc 3(Suppl 5):S29

Maddux AJ, Ashfaq R, Naftalis E, Leitch AM, Hoover S, Euhus D (2004) Patient and duct selection for nipple duct lavage. Am J Surg 188:390–394

Mahoney ME (2009) Intraductal therapy of DCIS with liposomal doxorubicin: a preoperative trial in rural California. Sixth international symposium on the intraductal approach to breast cancer. BMC Proc 3((Suppl 5):S26

Mai KT, Yazdi HM, Burns BF, Perkins DG (2000) Pattern of distribution of intraductal and infiltrating ductal carcinoma: a three-dimensional study using serial coronal giant sections of the breast. Hum Pathol 31:464–474

Mendrinos S, Nolen JD, Styblo T, Carlson G, Pohl J, Lewis M, Ritchie J (2005) Cytologic findings and protein expression profiles associated with ductal carcinoma of the breast in ductal lavage specimens using surface-enhanced laser desorption and ionization-time of flight mass spectrometry. Cancer 105:178–183

Mills D, Chia D, Casano A, Tondre J, Nguyen T, Love S (2009) Preliminary exploration into the physiology of the resting breast. BMC Proc 3(Suppl 5):S26

Papanicolaou GN, Holmquist DG, Bader GM, Falk EA (1958) Exfoliative cytology of the human mammary gland and its value in the diagnosis of cancer and other diseases of the breast. Cancer 11:377–409

Patil DB, Lankes HA, Najar R, Masood S, Bryt M, Hou N, Rademaker A, Khan SA (2008) Reproducibility of ductal lavage cytology and cellularity over a six month interval in high risk women. Breast Cancer Res Treat 112:327–333

Petrakis NL (1986) Physiologic, biochemical and cytologic aspects of nipple aspirate fluid. Breast Cancer Res Treat 8:7–19

Petrakis NL, Lowenstein JN, Wiencke JK, Lee MM, Wrensch MR, King EB, Hilton JF, Miike R (1993) Gross cystic disease fluid protein in nipple aspirates of breast fluid of Asian and non-Asian women. Cancer Epidemiol Biomarkers Prev 2:573–579

Ramsay DT, Mitoulas LR, Kent JC, Larsson M, Hartmann PE (2005) The use of ultrasound to characterize milk ejection in women using an electric breast pump. J Hum Lact 21:421–428

Rusby JE, Brachtel EF, Michaelson JS, Koerner FC, Smith BL (2007) Breast duct anatomy in the human nipple: three-dimensional patterns and clinical implications. Breast Cancer Res Treat 106:171–179

Sartorius OW (1973) Breast fluid cells help in early cancer detection. (Medical News). JAMA 224:823, 826–827

Sartorius OW, Smith HS, Morris P, Benedict D, Friesen L (1977) Cytologic evaluation of breast fluid in the detection of breast disease. J Natl Cancer Inst 59:1073–1080

Teboul M, Halliwell M (1995) Atlas of ultrasound and ductal echography of the breast: the introduction of anatomic intelligence into breast imaging. Blackwell Science, Oxford

Tondre J, Nejad M, Brennan M, Rao J, Chatterton R, Pagoda JM, Love SM (2006) Preliminary analysis of hormones and cells in lavage fluid. Distinct ducts in healthy women. In: AACR 2006 international conference on frontiers in cancer prevention research, September 2006

Tondre J, Nejad M, Casano A, Mills D, Love S (2008) Technical enhancements to breast ductal lavage. Ann Surg Oncol 15:2734–2738

Tot T (2005) DCIS, cytokeratins, and the theory of the sick lobe. Virchows Arch 447:1–8

Twelves D, Gui G (2008) The feasibility of nipple aspiration and ductal lavage as a screening tool in healthy women with increased breast cancer risk. Eur J Surg Oncol 34:1156–1157

Visvanathan K, Santor D, Ali SZ, Brewster A, Arnold A, Armstrong DK, Davidson NE, Helzlsouer KJ (2007) The reliability of nipple aspirate and ductal lavage in women at increased risk for breast cancer: a potential tool for breast cancer risk assessment and biomarker evaluation. Cancer Epidemiol Biomarkers Prev 16:950–955

Wrensch MR, Petrakis NL, Miike R, King EB, Chew K, Neuhaus J, Lee MM, Rhys M (2001) Breast cancer risk in women with abnormal cytology in nipple aspirates of breast fluid. J Natl Cancer Inst 93:1791–1798

Yamamoto D, Senzaki H, Nakagawa H, Okugawa H, Gondo H, Tanaka K (2003) Detection of chromosomal aneusomy by fluorescence in situ hybridization for patients with nipple discharge. Cancer 97:690–694

The Distribution of the Earliest Forms of Breast Carcinoma

6

Maria P. Foschini and Vincenzo Eusebi

6.1 Introduction

The pathological workup of breast specimens has dramatically changed in recent years since the increasing use of large (macro) sections (Foschini et al. 2006, 2007; Tot 2003, 2005, 2007a). Large-format histology sections were applied for the first time to human tissue by Cheatle (1921) and by Ingleby and Holly (1939) to visualize the relationship between neoplastic lesions and the surrounding tissue. Subsequently, the method was improved (Wellings and Jensen 1973; Sarnelli and Squartini 1986; Faverly et al. 1992; Foschini et al. 2002) and studies based on large sections have evidenced important correlations between mammography and pathology, first of all regarding tumor extent (Egan and Mosteller 1977; Faverly et al. 1994; Gallager and Martin 1969).

Large sections are also useful in assessing the status of the excision margins and in facilitating the correct measurement of the size of the tumor (Foschini et al. 2002). Accordingly, the issue was addressed by Jackson et al. (1994) who compared two series of operated breast carcinomas, one studied with conventional histology method and the other with large sections. The size of the lesion could be determined in all cases using large sections, while size could be measured in only 63% of the cases studied with conventional small blocks. Further advantages of using large sections are proper assessment of the extent of the tumors, and assessment of the *unifocality* of in situ and invasive lesions and of multiple (multifocal and multicentric) lesions (Foschini et al. 2006, 2007; Tot 2005).

M.P. Foschini
Department of Hematology and Oncology,
Section of Pathology "M. Malpighi"
University of Bologna at Bellaria Hospital, Bologna, Italy
e-mail: mariapia.foschini@ausl.bologna.it

6.2 Mural Spread of Neoplastic Cells

The genesis of ductal carcinoma in situ (DCIS) from terminal ductal lobular unit (TDLU) was proposed by Wellings and Jensen (1973) using large sections. This view has been accepted for decades and only recently challenged by Tot (2005).

Since the seminal papers by Going and Moffat (2004), Mai et al. (2000) and Ohtake et al. (1995), it is well established that the breast is constituted of 11–48 lobes which are independent microanatomic structures. Three dimensionally, breast lobes can be depicted as cones with apex directed toward the nipple and their base, which contain most of the lobules, facing the deep fascia. Some lobes (dominant lobes) can be extremely widespread over more than a quadrant and cannot be individually separated from the other lobes because the branches of the ductal system intermingle with those of adjacent lobes. This is well known to radiologists who frequently observe such spread of injected contrast medium into a collecting duct over more than one quadrant. Ohtake et al. (1995) have suggested the existence of branching anastomoses between different lobes, a view that is not confirmed by radiologists who never see retrograde spreading of the contrast medium into branches of different lobes.

Presence of anastomoses would be relevant as it would imply diffusion of neoplastic cells from one lobe to the next without the necessity of invading the stroma. This is pertinent to the knowledge that neoplastic cells from poorly differentiated carcinomas may climb along the duct walls on their way to the epidermis, which is finally cancerized in the form of Paget's cell carcinoma (Marucci et al. 2002). This phenomenon is mostly evident in cells that express HER-2 and show dendritic features (Fig. 6.1), a morphological hallmark of a cell that is capable of

T. Tot (ed.), *Breast Cancer*, DOI: 10.1007/978-1-84996-314-5_6,
© Springer-Verlag London Limited 2011

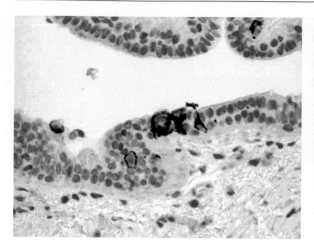

Fig. 6.1 Her-2 positive dendritic cells "climbing" along a galactophore duct. These cells were located between a DCIS/DIN3 present deep in the breast and Paget's cell carcinoma in the nipple

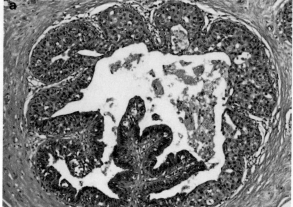

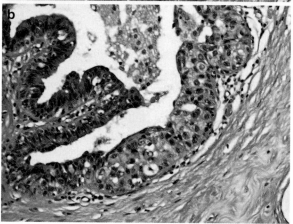

Fig. 6.2 (**a**) Mural spread of neoplastic cells located between the basal lamina and luminal epithelium. (**b**) The neoplastic cells show pleomorphic nuclei (and were Her-2 and e-cadherin positive, which is not illustrated in this figure). A clear-cut DCIS/DIN3 was located nearby

movement (Marucci et al. 2002; Tavassoli and Eusebi 2009). An additional feature of intraductal spread is the so-called pagetoid spread, classically observed in lobular carcinomas in situ (LCIS). This form of "mural" ductal spread was described by Fechner (1973), but is not exclusive to lobular carcinomas being present also in duct carcinomas of poorly differentiated type (Fig. 6.2a and b) as well as in neuroendocrine DCIS (Tsang and Chan 1996). The spread of the cells along duct walls is not unanimously accepted (Tot 2005); nevertheless, it would be difficult to justify the presence of individual neoplastic cells located in the ducts far away from the main DCIS, a phenomenon that would not been explained even by the field effect theory (Slaughter et al. 1953; Braakhuis et al. 2004).

DCIS have been traditionally classified according to their histological architecture and were named clinging, micropapillary, papillary, cribriform and comedo carcinomas (Rosen and Oberman 1993). Such subdivision of DCIS, however, was not practically useful as about 50% of the cases were of mixed type (Patchefsky et al. 1989), and in addition, it did not provide any prognostic or predictive information. After the publication of the seminal paper by Holland et al. (1994), the structural criteria to classify DCIS were abandoned and intraductal neoplasms were mostly classified according to their cytoarchitectural differentiation. This led to establishing the category of well-differentiated DCIS when neoplastic nuclei were monotonous and cells were oriented along

lumina; of poorly differentiated DCIS showing pleomorphic nuclei and no orientation along lumina, and finally, of intermediately differentiated DCIS with irregular pleomorphic nuclei and cells oriented along lumina. Accordingly, well-differentiated DCIS are estrogen receptor (ER) and progesterone receptor (PR) rich, while poorly differentiated DCIS are ER and PR poor with most of the latter showing HER-2 positivity (Bobrow et al. 1994).

After the paper of Holland et al. (1994), as it frequently happens in pathology, classifications of DCIS being mostly variations on the theme of the original proposal flourished, as did the terminological disputes. A classification very similar to the one of Holland et al. (1994) was adopted by WHO (2003) although different terminologies were used, i.e., DCIS/DIN (ductal intraepithelial neoplasia) I, II, and III. This classification was also adopted by the AFIP breast tumor fascicle (2009).

6.3 How to Define In Situ Neoplastic Lesion?

Historically, the first definition of in situ carcinoma was provided by Broders (1932) who illustrated a case of what Foote and Stewart (1941) defined later as in situ lobular carcinoma. The first acceptable description of comedocarcinoma was that of Bloodgood (1934). Cheatle (1921) using large sections in 1921 stated for the first time that carcinomas initially existed within ducts. Dawson (1933) also concluded that the majority of cases arise in the terminal, intralobular ducts, a view further expanded by Wellings and Jensen (1973) who stated that intraductal extension of breast carcinoma is a noninvasive continuous proliferation of neoplastic cells originating in ductal or lobular epithelium of TDLUs preserving the basement membrane (Wellings and Jensen 1973). Nevertheless, in the premammographic era, some cases diagnosed as grade 3 DCIS/DIN3 were accompanied by simultaneous presence of lymph node metastases to such an extent that this led to label the primary breast tumors as "infiltrating comedocarcinoma" (Stewart 1950). Stewart himself stated that "comedocarcinoma is invariably infiltrating when its presence is discovered" (1950) and Sirtori and Talamazzi (1967) that in situ carcinomas of the breast hardly exist.

The current classical view is that in situ lesions are invariably surrounded by a continuous layer of myoepithelial cells and basal lamina whereas invasive lesions show discontinuous or fragmented basal lamina (Azzopardi et al. 1979). To this classical view, exceptions probably exist. It has been shown that myoepithelial elements can be absent in normal breast with apocrine changes (Cserni 2008). If a DCIS originates from such structures, it would be devoid of myoepithelial cells. In a case of DCIS of our own in which the in situ nature was undisputable (both structurally and immunohistochemically, i.e., presence of basal lamina), the myoepithelial differentiation of the basal cells could not be proved (Fig. 6.3a–e). Damiani et al. (1999) in an immunohistochemical study designed to assess whether cases in a series of "comedocarcinoma"

were in situ or invasive, employed at the same time three different markers (actin, laminin ,and collagen IV) as only one was not sufficient to establish the correct diagnosis. The presence of one of these, in conjunction with appropriate structural features, was sufficient to regard the given lesion for being in situ. In spite of that, in two cases it was stated that the authors did not reach any conclusion and considered them as indeterminate for invasion. Intracystic papillary carcinomas of large size frequently do not show any myoepithelial layer. These same lesions are equated to DCIS/DIN as practically never generate nodal metastases. Therefore, it seems that the term "in situ" in the breast is a concept of a nonmetastasizing proliferative intraglandular lesion not strictly related to stringent morphologic features. The same applies to invasion. Nerves and vessels including lymphatics, veins, and arteries are occasionally "invaded" by "benign" glandular structures and no harm to the patient ensues (Davies 1973; Eusebi and Azzopardi 1976; Taylor and Norris 1967).

Neoplastic ductoneogenesis is a proliferative not yet morphologically well-defined process. It is characterized by digitiform newly formed tubules filled by neoplastic cells that sprout from ducts in cases of DCIS, most frequently of poorly differentiated type (Tabár et al. 2004). This is probably the neoplastic counterpart of acinar and tubular proliferation seen physiologically in lobules during pregnancy or in benign lesions such as sclerosing adenosis of acinar and periductal types (Tanaka and Oota 1970). Accordingly, newly formed large tubules clump together; they appear distended and filled by neoplastic cells. Most of "neogenetic" tubules show a myoepithelial cell layer and/or a basal lamina. In some of these, the process is defective and consequently myoepithelial elements and/or basal lamina are lacking, which simulates an "invasive comedocarcinoma." This is so true that in a small series of 11 cases of DIN3 with features suggestive of stromal invasion on hematoxylin–eosin (H&E stain), it was found that immunohistochemistry for smooth muscle actin, collagen IV, and laminin assured the correct diagnosis of DIN3 in four cases, of invasive carcinoma in five cases. In two, it was not possible to establish the diagnosis, in spite of immunohistochemistry. This was due to the fact that the "comedo" nests had very heterogeneous staining being variably positive in adjacent clumps for one or another marker while rare

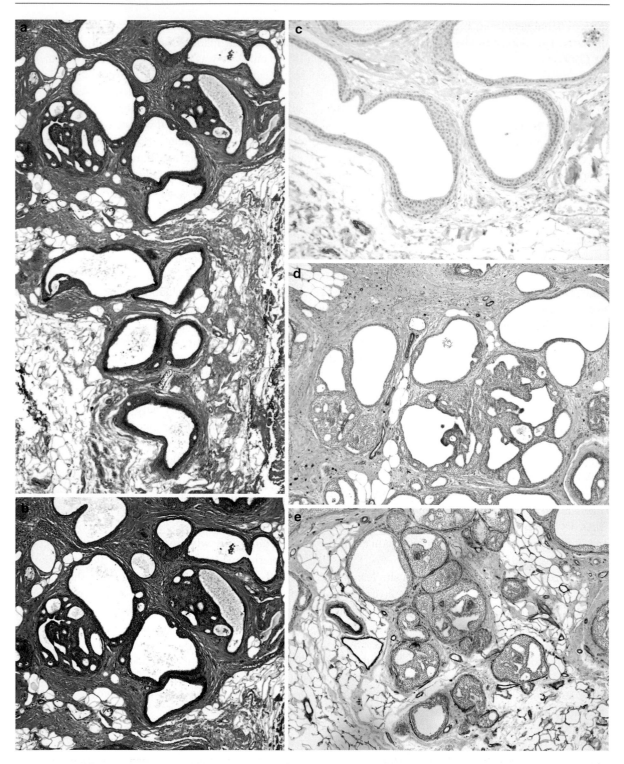

Fig. 6.3 (**a**) Well-differentiated DCIS characterized by flat epithelial atypia and cribriform structures. (**b**) The cells are well oriented; the nuclei are monotonous. A cribriform structure is well evident. (**c**) Keratin 14 immunohistochemistry: The basal cells are present but not expressing keratin 14 (nor p63 or smooth muscle actin, not illustrated in this figure). (**d**) The same case stained on laminin: The glandular neoplastic structures are totally devoid of laminin. (**e**) The same case stained on collagen IV: The neoplastic glandular structures are well outlined by collagen IV

clumps were totally negative for all of them. A final situation is constituted by "blunt invasion" in which carcinoma infiltrates as round or linear nests that simulate ducts distended by carcinoma in situ (Koerner 2009). This type of invasion has probably led Cowen and Bates (1984) to state that the diagnosis of invasion is confounded in some instances as invasive carcinomas can simulate DCIS. Therefore, it is possible to conclude that the diagnosis of in situ lesions, especially in DCIS/DIN3, is occasionally very difficult if not impossible. Immunohistochemistry is often helpful, but the use of large sections is mandatory in order to examine the entire lesion as in these cases the subgross architecture has consistent diagnostic relevance. Ductoneogenesis as described above is a scenario that has not been fully proven; nevertheless, if it is true, it would explain why DCIS forms a lump. One duct only, even if extremely distended by neoplastic cells would hardly be palpable. On the contrary, when several distended neogenetic ducts clump together and are simultaneously distended by neoplastic cells, these would make the lump clinically evident.

6.4 Unifocality, Multifocality, and Multicentricity of DCIS

Faverly et al. (1994) in a seminal paper published in 1994 demonstrated that poorly differentiated DCIS/DIN3 were unifocal proliferations while the opposite was seen in well-differentiated DCIS/DIN1 which were multifocal. Tot (2007a) stratified DCIS in diffuse (24%) (along major ducts), multifocal (40%) (defined as involvement of multiple distant lobules with uninvolved tissue in between), unifocal (32%) (defined as involvement of single or adjacent lobules without uninvolved tissue in between). Tot (2005, 2007b) suggested that the simultaneous and/or asynchronous multiple in situ tumor foci are usually localized in a single lobe of the breast, and he proposed the theory of the sick lobe of one breast stating that the sick lobe itself was genetically malconstructed from birth and that accumulation of genetic changes during the decades following the postnatal period would have led to malignant changes of the epithelial cell in any part of the sick lobe.

Foschini et al. (2006) in a study of 13 cases of lobular intraepithelial neoplasia (LIN) (Tavassoli and

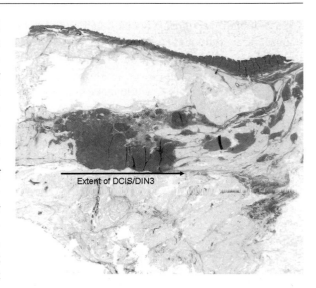

Fig. 6.4 Extent of DCIS/DIN3: This is a nice example of multifocality within the same lobe. Large-format histology slide, H&E stain

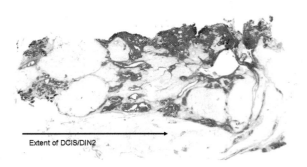

Fig. 6.5 Extent of DCIS/DIN1: The tumor is spread over at least two quadrants. This condition, probably multilobar, might be an example of multicentricity. Large-format histology slide, H&E stain

Eusebi 2009) defined *multifocality* (Fig. 6.4) as multiple foci of LIN present in the same lobe and *multicentricity* (Fig. 6.5) as multiple foci of LIN present in different lobes (Foschini et al. 2006; Tot 2005), a view also shared by Tot (2003). Cases were studied using large sections from mastectomies. The number of neoplastic foci ranged from 2 to 77 (mean 23.92) with 6 cases (46%) showing more than 20 foci. Foschini et al. (2006) also measured the maximum distance among LIN foci which ranged from 5 to 112 mm (mean 35 mm) with 9 cases (69.23%) out of 13 being more than 20 mm. Therefore, it appears that all cases of LIN displayed more than one focus, some foci (30%) clustered within 20 mm, but the majority were scattered through all breast quadrants. A lobe comprises everything between 2% and 23% of the breast volume (Going and Moffat 2004). Some of the cases studied by Foschini et al. (2006) showed foci distant up to 112 mm. This would make highly unlike the fact that more that 60% of LIN arise within a "dominant" large lobe, while it is more plausible that LIN would arise within different lobes being a multifocal and/or multicentric disease.

Foschini et al. (2007) also studied large sections from mastectomies of 45 cases of DCIS/DIN. Thirteen cases were DIN1. The number of DIN1 foci ranged from 1 (one case) to over 100 (mean 35.08). The maximum distance among multiple foci ranged from 12 to 55 mm (mean 35.42 mm). In 10 out of 13 cases (76.9%), the maximum distance was superior to 20 mm. Twelve cases were DCIS/DIN3. The number of foci varied from 1 (one case) to over 100 (one case), mean 24. On the all, DIN3 foci were in lower number than DIN1, being in 4 cases out of 12 (33.3%) the number of foci lower than 20. The range of the maximum distance among foci varied from 2 to 51 mm, the mean distance being 22 mm. Five cases only out of 12 (45.4%) displayed a distance superior to 20 mm. The 20 cases of DCIS/DIN2 were similar to those of DIN3. Therefore, it seems that DIN1 is a widespread condition involving more than a quadrant and hence more than one lobe, whereas DIN2 and DIN3 appear to cluster together, probably confined to one lobe. It also appears that DIN1 and LCIS show more similarities than differences than what has been previously recognized.

The fact that LIN and DIN1 are probably multilobar conditions with very distant neoplastic foci appearing almost simultaneously suggests the existence of a genetic "malconstruction" where the oncogenic factors act. DIN3 seem to be more localized, unilobar conditions (Fig. 6.6). These would be more compatible with an acquired neoplastic transformation where "environmental oncogenic factors" would face the tumor.

6.5 Conclusions

Most of the data obtained indicate that DCIS grade 1 and LIN are very often true multicentric (multilobar) diseases, while DCIS grade 2 and 3 are frequently unifocal or at most multifocal (unilobar) diseases. A more widespread use of large sections in routine pathology will give more accurate knowledge on extent and growth patterns of breast in situ neoplasms.

References

Azzopardi JG, Ahmed A, Millis RR (1979) Problems in breast pathology. W.B. Saunders, London
Bloodgood JC (1934) Comedo carcinoma (comedo-adenoma) of the female breast. Am J Cancer 22:842–853
Bobrow LG, Happerfield LC, Gregory WM, Springall RD, Millis RR (1994) The classification of ductal carcinoma in situ and its association with biological markers. Semin Diagn Pathol 11:199–207
Braakhuis JMB, Leemans RC, Brakenhoff RH (2004) A genetic progression model of oral cancer: current evidence and clinical implications. J Oral Pathol Med 33:317–322
Broders AC (1932) Carcinoma in situ contrasted with benign penetrating epithelium. JAMA 99:1670–1674
Cheatle GL (1921) Benign and malignant changes in duct epithelium of the breast. Br J Cancer 8:306
Cowen PN, Bates C (1984) The significance of intraduct appearances in breast cancer. Clin Oncol 10:67–72
Cserni G (2008) Lack of myoepithelium in apocrine glands of the breast does not necessarily imply malignancy. Histopathology 52:253–254
Damiani S, Ludvikova M, Tomasic G, Bianchi S, Gown AM, Eusebi V (1999) Myoepithelial cells and basal lamina in poorly differentiated in situ duct carcinoma of the breast. An immunocytochemical study. Virchows Arch 434:227–234
Davies JD (1973) Neural invasion in benign mammary dysplasia. J Pathol 109:225–231
Dawson EK (1933) Carcinoma of the mammary lobule and its origin. Edinb Med J 40:57–82
Egan RL, Mosteller RC (1977) Breast cancer mammography patterns. Cancer 40:2087–2090
Eusebi V, Azzopardi JG (1976) Vascular infiltration in benign breast disease. J Pathol 118:9–16

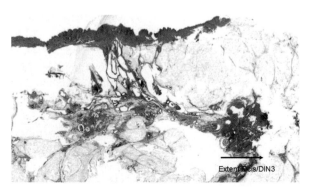

Fig. 6.6 Unilobar, unifocal DCIS/DIN3. Large-format histology slide, H&E stain

Faverly DRG, Holland R, Burgers L (1992) An original stereo-microscopic analysis of the mammary glandular tree. Virchows Arch A Pathol Anat Histopathol 421:115

Faverly DRG, Burgers L, Bult P, Holland R (1994) Three dimensional imaging of mammary ductal carcinoma in situ: clinical implications. Semin Diagn Pathol 11:193–198

Fechner RE (1973) Epithelial alterations in the extralobular ducts of breast with lobular carcinoma. Arch Pathol 93: 164–171

Foote FW, Stewart FW (1941) Lobular carcinoma in situ. Am J Pathol 17:491–500

Foschini MP, Tot T, Eusebi V (2002) Large-section (macrosection) histologic slides. In: Silverstein MJ (ed) Ductal carcinoma in situ of the breast. Lippincott, Philadelphia, pp 249–254

Foschini MP, Righi A, Cucchi MC, Ragazzini T, Merelli S, Santeramo B, Eusebi V (2006) The impact of large sections and 3D technique on the study of lobular in situ and invasive carcinoma of the breast. Virchows Arch 448:256–261

Foschini MP, Flamminio F, Miglio R, Calò DG, Cucchi MC, Masetti R, Eusebi V (2007) The impact of large sections on the study of in situ and invasive duct carcinoma of the breast. Hum Pathol 38:1736–1743

Gallager HS, Martin JE (1969) Early phases in the development of breast cancer. Cancer 24:1170–1178

Going JJ, Moffat DF (2004) Escaping from Flatland: clinical and biological aspects of human mammary duct anatomy in three dimensions. J Pathol 203:538–544

Holland R, Peterse JL, Millis RR, Eusebi V, Faverly D, van de Vijver M, Zafrani B (1994) Ductal carcinoma in situ: a proposal for a new classification. Semin Diagn Pathol 11:167–180

Ingleby H, Holly C (1939) A method for the preparation of serial slices of the breast. Bull Int Assoc Med Museums 19:93–96

Jackson PA, Merchant W, McCormick CJ, Cook MG (1994) A comparison of large block macrosectioning and conventional techniques in breast pathology. Virchows Arch 425: 243–248

Koerner FC (2009) Diagnostic problems in breast pathology. Saunders, Philadelphia

Mai KT, Yazdi HM, Burns BF, Perkins DG (2000) Pattern of distribution of intraductal and infiltrating ductal carcinoma: a three-dimensional study using serial coronal giant sections of the breast. Hum Pathol 31:464–474

Marucci G, Betts CM, Golouh R, Peterse JL, Foschini MP, Eusebi V (2002) Toker cells are probably precursors of Paget cell carcinoma: a morphological and ultrastructural description. Virchows Arch 441:117–123

Ohtake T, Abe R, Kimijima I, Fukushima T, Nomizo T, Kimijma I (1995) Intraductal extension of primary invasive breast carcinoma treated by breast conservative surgery. Cancer 76:32–45

Patchefsky AS, Shwartz GF, Finkelstein SD, Prestipino A, Sohn SE, Singer SS, Feig SA (1989) Heterogeneity of intraductal carcinoma of the breast. Cancer 63:731–741

Rosen PP, Oberman HA (1993) Tumors of the mammary gland. Armed Forces Institute of Pathology, Washington

Sarnelli R, Squartini F (1986) Multicentricity in breast cancer: a submacroscopic study. Pathol Annu 21:143–158

Sirtori C, Talamazzi F (1967) Il carcinoma intraduttale della mammella non è mai un carcinoma in situ. Tumori 53: 641–644

Slaughter DP, Southwick HW, Smeejkal W (1953) Field cancerization in oral stratified squamous epithelium; clinical implications of multicentric origin. Cancer 6;963–968

Stewart FW (1950) Tumors of the breast. Armed Forces Institute of Pathology, Washington

Tabár L, Chen HH, Yen MF, Tot T, Tong TN, Chen LS, Chiu YH, Duffy SW, Smith RA (2004) Mammographic tumor features can predict long-term outcomes reliably in women with 1–14-mm invasive breast carcinoma. Cancer 101: 1745–1759

Tanaka Y, Oota K (1970) A stereomicroscopic study of the mastopathic human breast. II. Peripheral type of duct evolution and its relation to cystic disease. Virchows Arch A Pathol Anat Histopathol 349:215–228

Tavassoli FA, Devili P (eds) (2003) World Health Organization classification of tumors. Pathology & genetics. Tumours of the breast and female genital organs. IARC, Lyon

Tavassoli FA, Eusebi V (2009) Tumors of the breast. American Registry of Pathology/Armed Forces Institute of Pathology, Washington

Taylor HB, Norris HJ (1967) Epithelial invasion of nerves in benign disease of the breast. Cancer 20:2245–2249

Tot T (2003) The diffuse type of invasive lobular carcinoma of the breast: morphology and prognosis. Virchows Arch 443:718–724

Tot T (2005) DCIS, cytokeratins, and the theory of the sick lobe. Virchows Arch 447:1–8

Tot T (2007a) Clinical relevance of the distribution of the lesions in 500 consecutive breast cancer cases documented in large format histologic sections. Cancer 110:2551–2560

Tot T (2007b) The theory of the sick breast lobe and the possible consequences. Int J Surg Pathol 15:369–375

Tsang WYW, Chan JKC. (1996) Endocrine ductal carcinoma in situ (E-DCIS) of the breast. Am J Surg Pathol 20(8): 921–943

Wellings SR, Jensen HM (1973) On the origin and progression of ductal carcinoma in the human breast. J Natl Cancer Inst 50:1111–1118

The Implications of the Imaging Manifestations of Multifocal and Diffuse Breast Cancers

7

László K. Tabár, Peter B. Dean, Tibor Tot, Nadja Lindhe, Mats Ingvarsson, and Amy Ming-Fang Yen

7.1 Introduction

Mammographic screening of asymptomatic women leads to the detection of an unprecedented number of in situ and nonpalpable 1–9 mm and 10–14 mm invasive breast cancers. Detecting breast cancer at an earlier phase in its development and at a smaller tumor size is, however, no guarantee that the disease will be localized to a small, confined volume in every case. In fact, multifocal and/or diffuse breast cancers comprise the majority of breast cancers in every size range (Holland et al. 1985; Tot 2007). These studies have also shown that the frequency of unifocal and multifocal breast cancers is unaffected by tumor size at detection (Table 7.1).

The unfortunately frequent multifocal/diffuse nature of breast cancer defines the roles of the interdisciplinary breast team members:

1. The *radiologist* needs to assess the volume of breast tissue that has been affected by the disease, after having detected the lesion at screening and reached a diagnosis using a multimodality imaging workup.
2. Since breast cancer is not a systemic disease in its earliest detectable phase, it is primarily a *surgical* disease when nonpalpable and detected at screening. The benefit of early detection depends upon complete surgical removal of the disease. The full extent of each breast cancer, as outlined by imaging, should guide the surgical approach.
3. The all-too-frequent multifocality and lobar distribution of breast cancer require the routine use of modern large-section *pathology* technique, which provides the most comprehensive correlation with the imaging findings. The high-resolution, three-dimensional imaging techniques (MRI and ultrasound examination of the breast) expose the limitations inherent to the currently used small histologic glass slides. Failure to confirm the nature of lesions detected by imaging leads to underestimation of true disease extent and unjustified claims of overdiagnosis by imaging.
4. The risk-benefit and cost-benefit ratios for the use of *adjuvant therapeutic regimens* on women with screen-detected, 1–14 mm breast cancer are highly unfavorable, as demonstrated in Diagrams 7.1–7.6. The 26-year survival of 576 women with 1–14 mm invasive breast cancer, who were subjected to breast-conserving surgery and postoperative irradiation, was 88% (Diagram 7.1), while the corresponding figure for 384 women who received breast-conserving surgery without postoperative irradiation, Tamoxifen, or chemotherapy was 89% (Diagram 7.2). These survival curves are, however, a summation of several, diverse survival curves, a reflection of the heterogeneous nature of breast cancer within the same tumor size range. Separation of cases having casting type calcifications on the mammogram from the remainder identifies cases having a poor versus a very good long-term outcome. Diagrams 7.3 and 7.4 show the outcome of these two groups with

L.K. Tabár (✉)
Department of Mammography, Central Hospital Falun, Falun, Sweden
e-mail: laszlo@mammographyed.com

T. Tot (ed.), *Breast Cancer*, DOI: 10.1007/978-1-84996-314-5_7,
© Springer-Verlag London Limited 2011

and without postoperative irradiation (Diagrams 7.3 and 7.4). The use of all five mammographic tumor features enables a more precise discrimination between subgroups with good and poor outcome, again with and without postoperative adjuvant therapy (Diagrams 7.5 and 7.6). We can conclude that adjuvant therapeutic regimens offer little or no demonstrable benefit to the 1–14 mm nonpalpable screen-detected breast cancers. A similar conclusion was reached by Cady and Chung: "The reduction in need for radiation and systemic adjuvant chemotherapy, which are both expensive and toxic, is made possible by detecting highly curable T1a and T1b breast cancers" (Cady and Chung 2005).

Table 7.1 The frequency of unifocal versus combined multifocal breast cancers by tumor size in 565 cases diagnosed in Falun 2005–2007

	Unifocal	Nonunifocal	All
In situ	29% (23/79)	71% (56/79)	79
1–9 mm	37% (33/90)	63% (57/90)	90
10–19 mm	46% (103/225)	54% (122/225)	225
20–29 mm	36% (36/100)	64% (64/100)	100
30+ mm	18% (13/71)	82% (58/71)	71
All	37% (208/565)	63% (357/565)	565

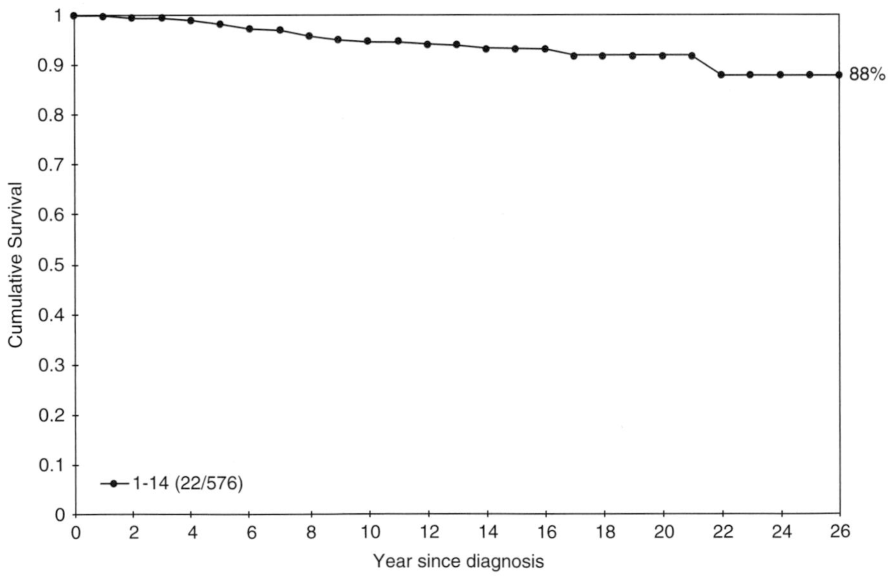

Diagram 7.1 Twenty-six-year cumulative survival of 576 consecutive women with 1–14 mm invasive breast cancer. Women aged 40–69 at diagnosis, who received breast-conserving surgery and postoperative irradiation. Dalarna County, Sweden

Diagram 7.2 Twenty-six-year cumulative survival of 384 consecutive women aged 40–69 at diagnosis with 1–14 mm invasive breast cancer who received breast-conserving surgery but no chemotherapy, Tamoxifen or postoperative irradiation. Dalarna County, Sweden

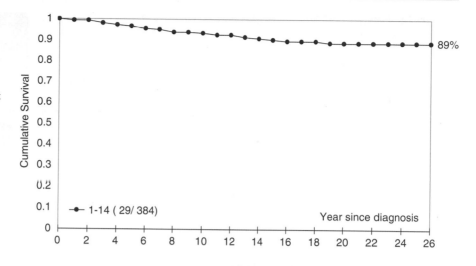

Diagram 7.3 Twenty-six-year cumulative survival of 576 consecutive women with 1–14 mm invasive breast cancer according to the presence or absence of casting type calcifications on the mammogram. Women aged 40–69 at diagnosis, who received breast-conserving surgery and postoperative irradiation. Dalarna County, Sweden

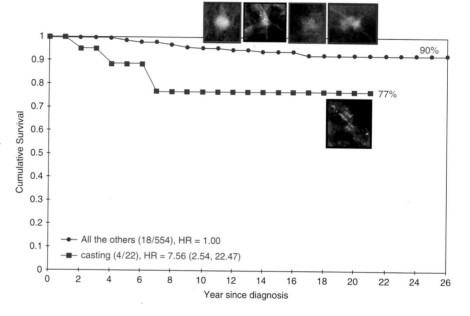

Diagram 7.4 Twenty-six-year cumulative survival of 384 consecutive women aged 40–69 at diagnosis with 1–14 mm invasive breast cancer according to the presence or absence of casting type calcifications on the mammogram. These women received breast-conserving surgery but no chemotherapy, Tamoxifen or postoperative irradiation. Dalarna County, Sweden

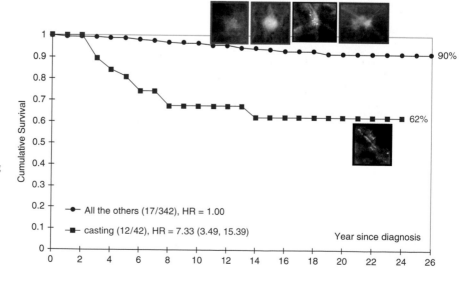

100%
100%
1
0.9
0.8
0.7
0.6
0.5
0.4
0.3
0.2
0.1
0
92%
93%
77%
Cumulative Survival
Stellate without calcifications (11/350), HR = 1.00
Circular/oval without calcifications (6/134), HR = 1.41 (0.52, 3.82)
Powdery calcifications +- tumor mass (0/30), HR = 0.00 (.,.)
Crushed stone-like calcifications +- tumor mass (0/39), HR = 0.00 (.,.)
Casting type calcifications +- tumor mass (4/22), HR = 8.04 (2.54, 25.45)
0 2 4 6 8 10 12 14 16 18 20 22 24 26
Year since diagnosis

Diagram 7.5 Twenty-six-year cumulative survival of 567 consecutive women with 1–14 mm invasive breast cancer according to the five mammographic tumor features. Women aged 40–69 at diagnosis, who received breast-conserving surgery and postoperative irradiation. Dalarna County, Sweden

100%
1
0.9
0.8
0.7
0.6
0.5
0.4
0.3
0.2
0.1
0
92%
86%
62%
Cumulative Survival
Powdery calcifications +- tumor mass (0/18), HR = 0.00 (.,.)
Stellate without calcifications (8/204), HR = 1.00
Crushed stone-like calcifications +- tumor mass (2/37), HR = 1.34 (0.28, 6.30)
Circular/oval without calcifications (6/79), HR = 1.79 (0.62, 5.15)
Casting type calcifications +- tumor mass (12/42), HR = 9.26 (3.78, 22.70)
0 2 4 6 8 10 12 14 16 18 20 22 24 26
Year since diagnosis

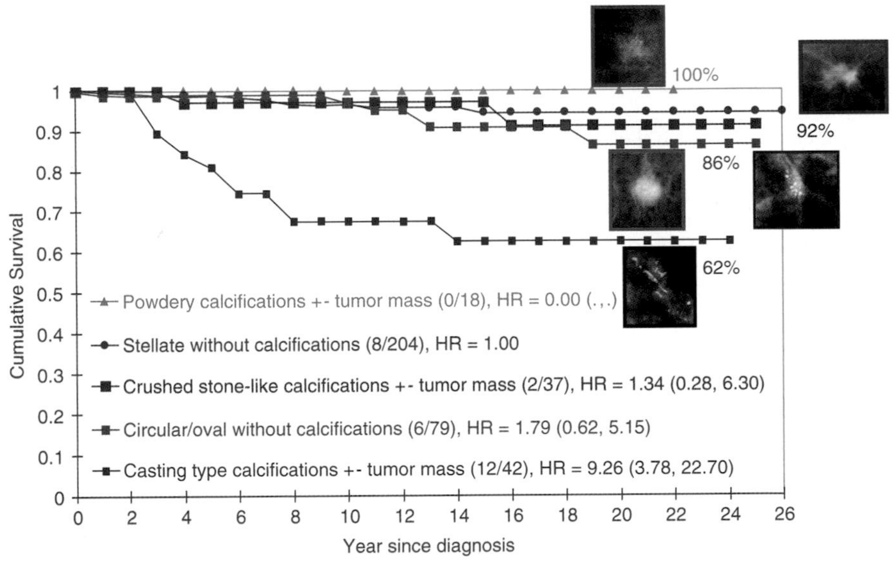

Diagram 7.6 Twenty-six-year cumulative survival of 384 consecutive women aged 40–69 at diagnosis with 1–14 mm invasive breast cancer according to the five mammographic tumor features on the mammogram. These women received breast-conserving surgery but no chemotherapy, Tamoxifen or postoperative irradiation. Dalarna County, Sweden

1
0.9
0.8
.7
.6
.5
.4
0.3
0.2
0.1
0
90%
74%
Cumulative survival
p<0.0001
Unifocal (30/311)
MF+D (36/148)
Time since diagnosis (year)
0 1 2 3 4 5 6 7 8 9 10

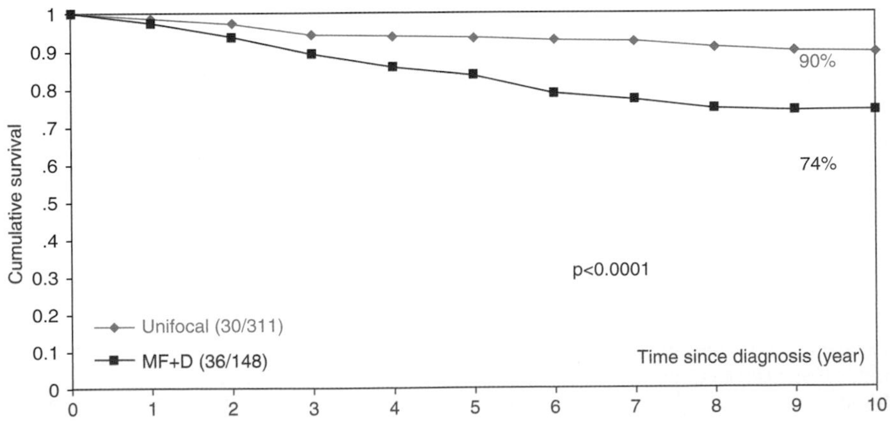

Diagram 7.7 Ten year cumulative survival of 311 women with unifocal invasive breast cancer (with or without associated in situ) versus 148 women with multifocal and diffuse invasive breast cancer, diagnosed in Dalarna county, Sweden during the years 1996–1998

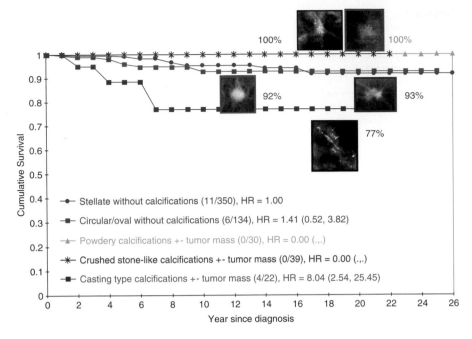

Diagram 7.8 Ten-year
cumulative survival of women
with 1–9 mm unifocal
invasive breast cancer (with
or without associated in situ)
versus women with multifocal and diffuse invasive breast
cancer, diagnosed in Dalarna
county, Sweden during the
years 1996–1998

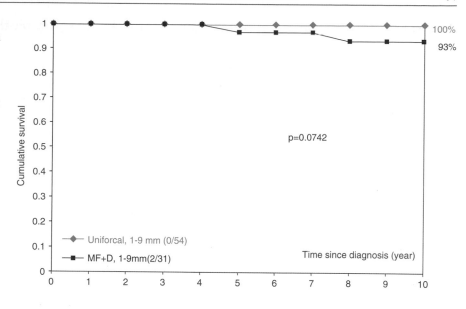

Diagram 7.9 Ten-year
cumulative survival of women
with 10–14 mm unifocal
invasive breast cancer (with or
without associated in situ)
versus women with
10–14 mm multifocal and
diffuse invasive breast cancer,
diagnosed in Dalarna county,
Sweden during the years
1996–1998

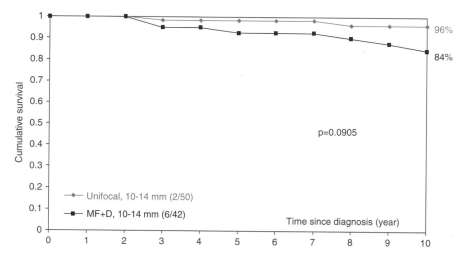

Diagram 7.10 Ten-year
cumulative survival of
women with >15 mm
unifocal invasive breast
cancer (with or without
associated in situ) versus
women with >15 mm
multifocal and diffuse
invasive breast cancer,
diagnosed in Dalarna county,
Sweden during the years
1996–1998

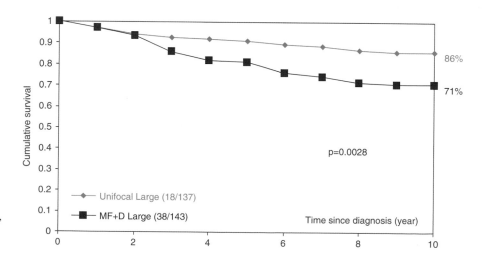

7.2 The Multifocal Nature of Breast Cancer and the Imaging Methods of Choice

The two comprehensive histopathologic analyses of the extent and distribution of breast cancer published from two separate institutions 2 decades apart (Holland et al. 1985. Tot 2007) arrived at the same conclusion that multifocal and diffuse breast cancers account for approximately 60% of the cases. According to the recent study of Tot, based on large-section histology, approximately 40% of breast cancers are unifocal, irrespective of tumor size; 20% are multifocal, but limited to a region measuring less than 40 mm; 40% of breast cancers are either multifocal or diffuse, when the invasive and/or in situ foci occupy a region larger or equal to 40 mm. The arbitrary cutoff point of 40 mm has been adopted to guide the choice between breast-conserving surgery and mastectomy.

Multimodality breast imaging has been developed over the past 2 decades for the following reasons:

- The heterogeneous and often multifocal nature of breast cancer
- The difficulty of detecting small breast cancers in dense breasts
- The need to describe the true extent of the disease for appropriate surgical management

Each imaging method reflects the underlying normal anatomy and pathology, but with its own capabilities and limitations. The method or combination of methods chosen for imaging benign and malignant breast diseases will depend upon which method or combination of methods will be able to visualize:

- The nature of the underlying disease
- The extent of the pathologic tissue
- The lesion in question against the background of breast parenchyma

Mammography is at its best in demonstrating all forms of pathology in the fatty replaced breast as well as demonstrating microcalcifications, irrespective of the mammographic parenchymal pattern (Tabar et al. 2005). However, the majority of breast cancers do not present with calcifications on the mammogram, and there is a high priority for detecting invasive, noncalcified breast cancers, when smaller than 15 mm, also in dense breasts (Yen et al. 2003). *Breast ultrasound*, while inferior in revealing calcifications, excels in demonstrating invasive tumors regardless of the nature of the surrounding tissue, and has thus become an invaluable complementary imaging tool. Ultrasound is also the most convenient method for image-guided percutaneous biopsy. *Galactography* retains its unique ability to image the underlying cause of spontaneous bloody or serous breast discharge, especially in the absence of mammographic or palpatory findings. *Magnetic resonance imaging* adds the new aspect of functional imaging, which is particularly useful for describing the full extent of the disease. MRI can also detect additional ipsi/contralateral tumor foci not detected by mammography. Other functional imaging methods using *radioactive isotopes* are under evaluation.

7.3 The Diverse Imaging Appearances and Long-Term Outcome of Unifocal, Multifocal, and Diffuse Breast Cancers

The histologic diversity of breast cancer is reflected in the diversity of its imaging appearance at mammography, ultrasound, and MRI. The individual and/or combined imaging findings are illustrated with representative examples (Examples 7.1–7.15).

Unifocal breast cancers, accounting for approximately 40% of all breast cancer cases, are invasive in most cases and may appear as a solitary stellate (spiculated) or circular/oval density (Examples 7.1 and 7.2). In our material, in situ carcinoma was unifocal in 29% of all in situ cases. In some of these cases, a single TDLU is distended by the accumulating cancer cells, central necrosis, and associated amorphous calcifications (Example 7.3). In the absence of calcifications, unifocal in situ breast cancer may present as a tumor mass (Examples 7.4 and 7.5). *Multifocal/diffuse breast cancers* are categorized as either *limited* (approx. 20%) (Examples 7.6–7.9) or *extensive* (approx. 40%) (Examples 7.10–7.15). Their imaging appearance is similar in nature but differs in extent, the cutoff point being arbitrarily set at 40 mm.

Four of our survival curves demonstrate the *survival advantage* inherent to tumor unifocality regardless of tumor size range (Diagrams 7.7–7.10). These data quantify the *deleterious effect of multifocality* and emphasize the importance of detecting this entity. The thorough preoperative multimodality imaging approach, including mammography, breast ultrasound and especially breast MRI, offers the best opportunity for detecting the unifocal/multifocal/diffuse nature and describing the true extent of breast cancer. Multifocality is a negative prognostic factor, independent of tumor size, although its effect becomes more significant with increasing tumor size.

Example 7.1 A 69-year-old asymptomatic woman, screening examination

Figs. 7.1.1 and 7.1.2 Right and left breasts, details of the MLO projections. The mammograms show adipose breasts. There is a tiny asymmetric density in the axillary tail of the right breast (within the rectangle)

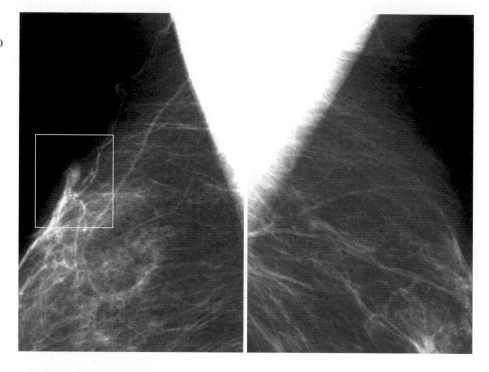

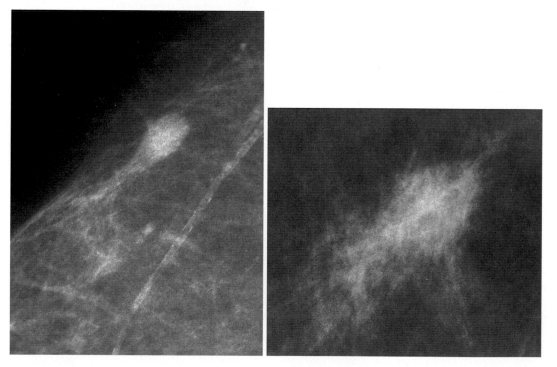

Figs. 7.1.3 and 7.1.4 Photographic magnification of the region in the right MLO projection containing the tiny ill-defined lesion (1.3). Microfocus magnification: the mammographic finding consists of a <10 mm solitary, ill-defined, mammographically malignant tumor with no associated calcifications (1.4)

Figs. 7.1.5–7.1.7 Breast ultrasound: The lesion measures about 6 mm (1.5). Image taken during ultrasound-guided 14-g core biopsy (1.6)

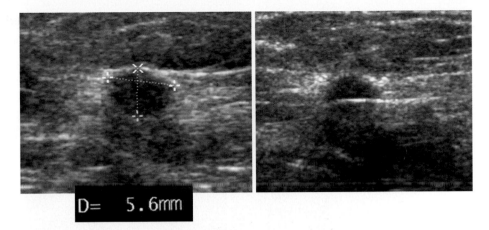

Figs. 7.1.8–7.1.13 Series of breast MRI images confirm the solitary nature of the lesion

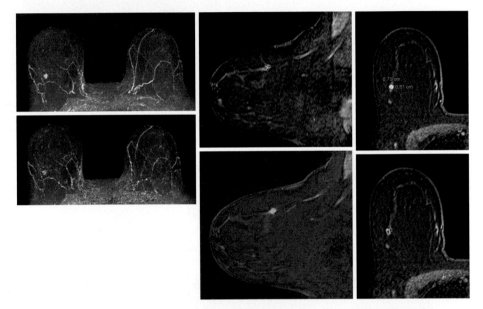

Figs. 7.1.14 and 7.1.15 Operative specimen radiograph (7.1.14). The lesion is centrally located in the specimen. Low-power histologic image (7.1.15) of the solitary 6 × 7 mm well-differentiated invasive ductal carcinoma

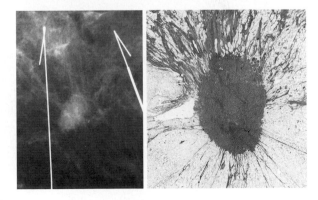

Comment: This case is representative of unifocal invasive breast cancers, which account for approximately 40% of all breast cancer cases.

Example 7.2 A 64-year-old asymptomatic woman, called back from screening for further assessment of the mammographically detected tiny, solitary, ill-defined lesion in the upper inner quadrant of her left breast

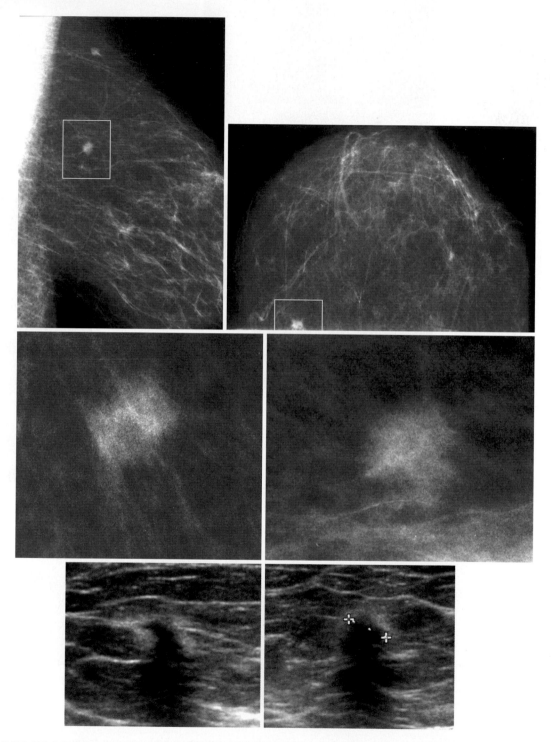

Figs. 7.2.1–7.2.6 Left breast, mediolateral (7.2.1) and craniocaudal (7.2.2) projections. There is a <10 mm lesion in the upper inner quadrant. Microfocus magnification images (7.2.3, 7.2.4) show a solitary, spiculated, mammographically malignant tumor. Breast ultrasound examination (7.2.5, 7.2.6) confirms the mammographic diagnosis

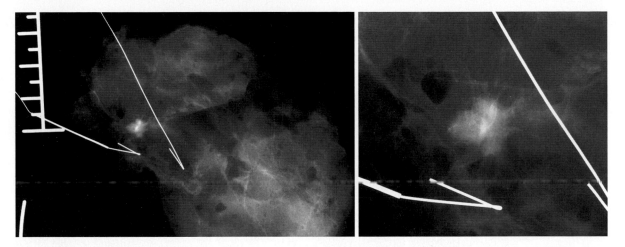

Figs. 7.2.7 and 7.2.8 Radiograph of the surgical specimen following preoperative localization using the bracketing technique

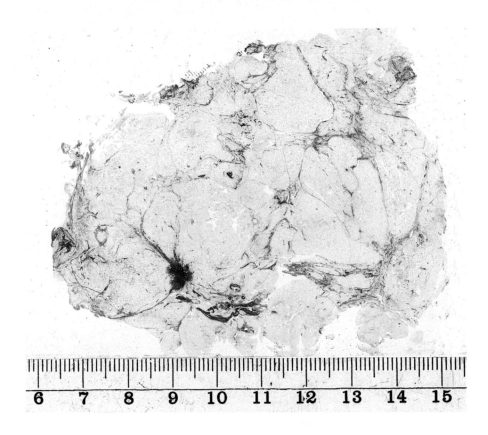

Fig. 7.2.9 Large-section histology. The solitary stellate invasive tumor measures 9 mm

Comment: This case is representative of unifocal stellate invasive breast cancers. Stellate/spiculated tumor shape is the most frequent mammographic appearance of invasive breast cancers in the tumor size category 1–14 mm.

Example 7.3 A 54-year-old asymptomatic woman, screening examination. She was called back to the assessment center for further workup of the cluster of microcalcifications detected on the screening mammograms of the left breast

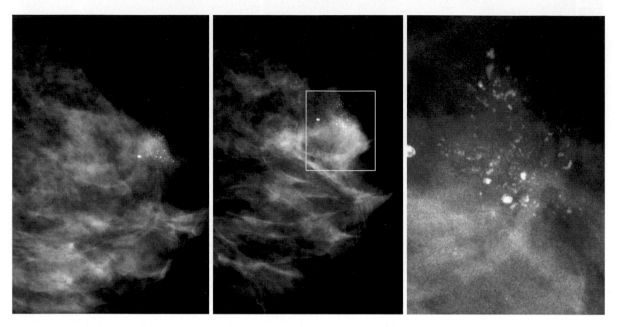

Figs. 7.3.1–7.3.3 Left breast MLO projection (3.1), lateromedial horizontal projection (3.2), and microfocus magnification (3.3): The 15X10 mm solitary cluster of malignant-type microcalcifications vary in shape, density, and size. No associated tumor mass is demonstrable

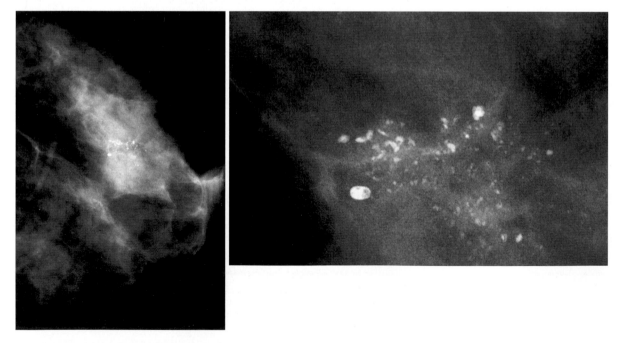

Figs. 7.3.4 and 7.3.5 Left breast craniocaudal projection (3.4) and microfocus magnification (3.5): There is a mixture of crushed stone-like and short casting-type, mammographically malignant-type microcalcifications in a large cluster

Figs. 7.3.6 and 7.3.7 Breast MRI: There is a 15x10 mm focal area with contrast enhancement in the lateral portion of the left breast, suggesting malignancy

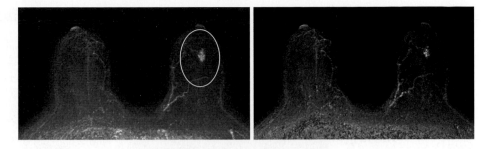

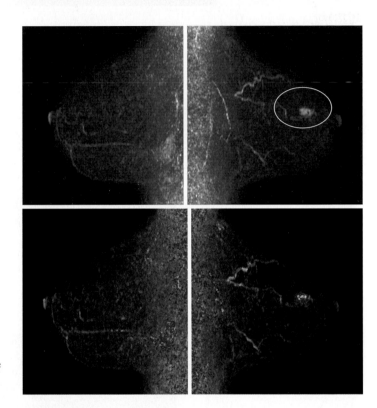

Figs. 7.3.8–7.3.11 Breast MRI, sagittal views: The contrast enhancement is localized in the upper outer quadrant and measures 13x10x7 mm

Figs. 7.3.12 and 7.3.13 Breast ultrasound: Corresponding to the mammographically detected region with the malignant-type calcifications, ultrasound examination shows a hypoechoic, ill-defined lesion measuring 15 mm. The lesion also contains tiny calcifications. A tiny simple cyst is seen adjacent to the tumor

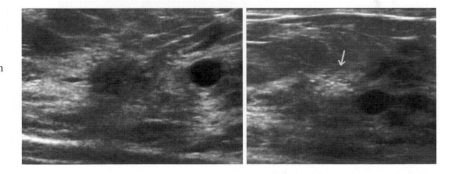

Figs. 7.3.14–7.3.17 Image
taken during ultrasound-
guided 14-g biopsy (7.3.14)
and radiographs of the
percutaneous biopsy
specimen (7.3.15, 7.3.16).
Histology of the core
specimen, immunohis-
tochemistry, smooth muscle
actin: In situ carcinoma
(7.3.17)

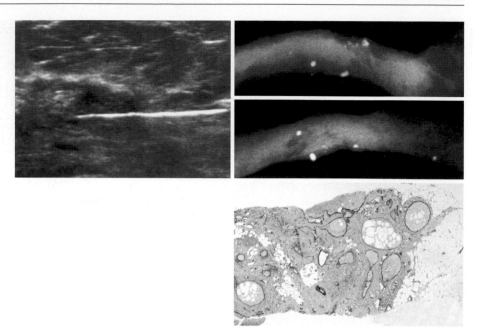

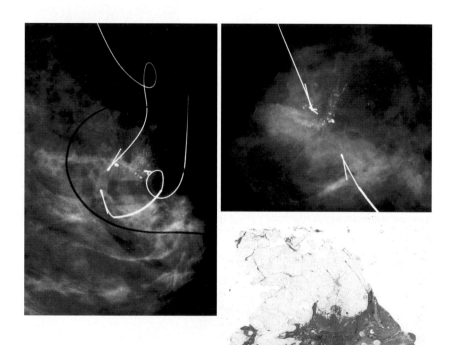

Figs. 7.3.18–7.3.20 Preoperative
localization using the bracketing
technique (7.3.18). Specimen
radiograph containing the microcalcifications (7.3.19) and large-section
histology (7.3.20). The pathologic
area measures 15 x 10 mm at
histology

Figs. 7.3.21 and 7.3.22 Microfocus magnification of one of the specimen slices. Both casting-type and crushed stone-like calcifications are seen within the cluster (7.3.21). The histologic image demonstrates the cancer-filled, extremely distended acini with central necrosis and amorphous calcifications (7.3.22)

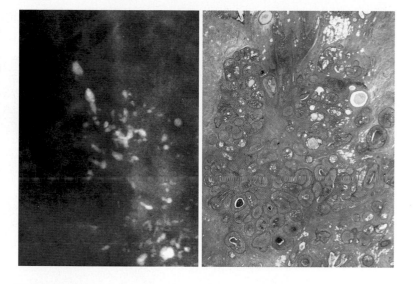

Figs. 7.3.23–7.3.26 Specimen radiographs show a large cluster of malignant-type calcifications (7.3.23, 7.3.24). Low- and high-power histology images of the solitary, 15 x 10 mm TDLU distended and deformed by Grade 2 in situ carcinoma (7.3.25, 7.3.26)

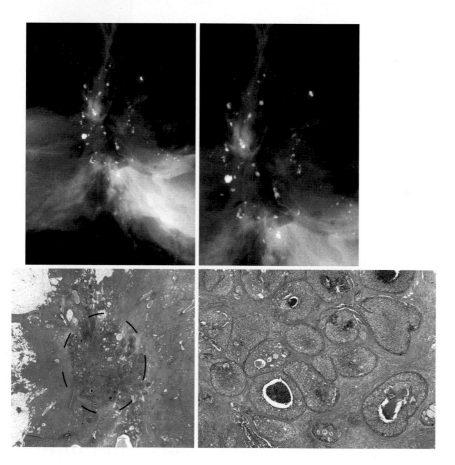

Comment: This case is typical of unifocal in situ carcinoma, where the TDLU is dilated by the accumulating cancer cells, central necrosis, and amorphous calcifications.

Example 7.4 A 47-year-old asymptomatic woman, screening case. She was called back for further assessment of the right retroareolar lesion

Fig. 7.4.1 Right breast, details of the CC projection. There is a low density, circular lesion with no associated calcifications in the retroareolar region

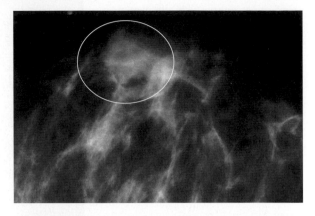

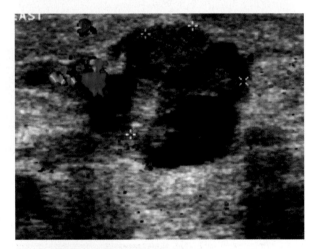

Figs. 7.4.2 and 7.4.3 Breast ultrasound (7.4.2) shows an intracystic papillary growth. Low-power large-section histology image (7.4.3): The intracystic papillary carcinoma in situ is surrounded by a thick fibrous capsule

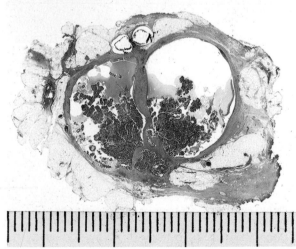

Comment: This case is typical of unifocal in situ carcinoma, where the mammographic finding is a dominant mass; however, ultrasound examination reveals an intracystic papillary growth which proves to be an intracystic in situ carcinoma at histologic examination.

Example 7.5 A 64-year-old woman, called back from screening for evaluation of the tiny asymmetric density in the lower portion of the left breast

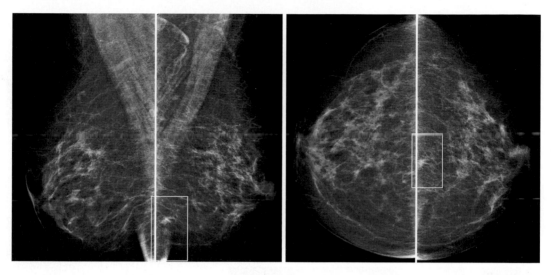

Figs. 7.5.1–7.5.4 Right and left breasts, MLO (7.5.1, 7.5.2) and CC (7.5.3, 7.5.4) projections. There is a tiny, low density, nonspecific asymmetric lesion in the lower portion of the left breast at the 6 o'clock position. No calcifications are associated with the asymmetric density

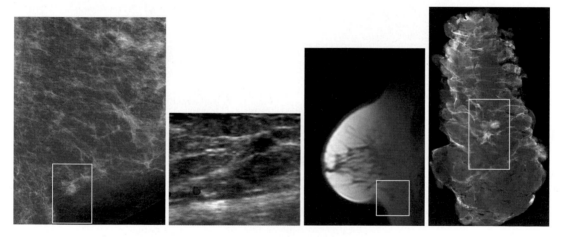

Figs. 7.5.5–7.5.8 Microfocus magnification, MLO projection (7.5.5) of the ill-defined, mammographically malignant density. Ultrasound (7.5.6) and MRI (7.5.7) images and specimen radiograph (7.5.8)

Figs. 7.5.9 and 7.5.10 Microfocus magnification of the specimen slice containing the tiny ill-defined tumor (7.5.7). Histology (immunostaining on estrogen receptors) of the TDLU distended by the 12-mm Grade 2 in situ carcinoma (7.5.8) Histology examination courtesy: Pia Boström, M.D., Department of Pathology, Turku University Hospital, Turku, Finland

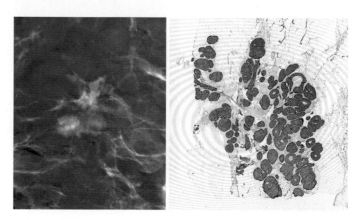

Example 7.6 A 71-year-old asymptomatic woman, screening examination. Called back for assessment of the microcalcifications found on the mammograms of her right breast

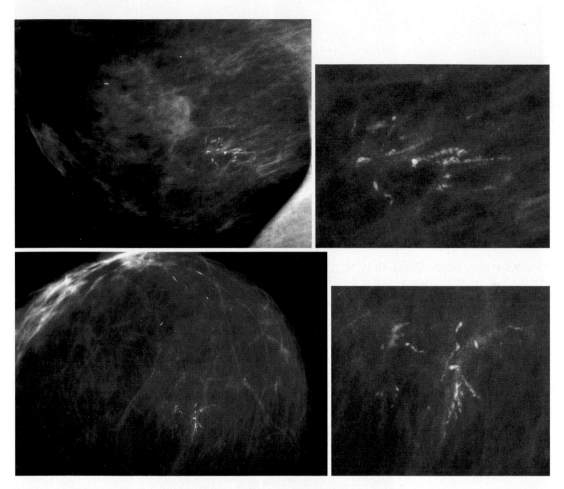

Figs. 7.6.1–7.6.4 Detail of the right MLO (7.6.1) and craniocaudal projections (7.6.3). There is a cluster of calcifications with no associated tumor mass in the lower inner quadrant. Microfocus magnification images (7.6.2, 7.6.4) show a mixture of fragmented and dotted casting-type, mammographically malignant-type calcifications

Figs. 7.6.5 and 7.6.6 Microfocus magnification of one of the surgical specimen slices demonstrating the fragmented and dotted casting-type calcifications (7.6.5). Large-section histology (7.6.6) image of the surgically removed tissue

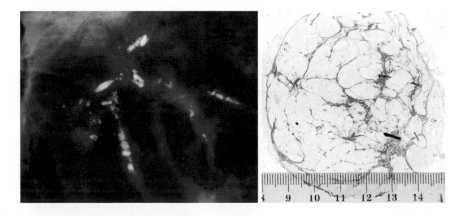

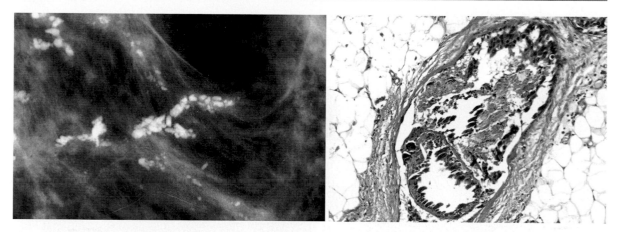

Figs. 7.6.7 and 7.6.8 Mammographic–histologic correlation: The amorphous calcifications, corresponding to the dotted casting-type calcifications on the mammogram are localized within a duct distended by cancer cells and necrosis

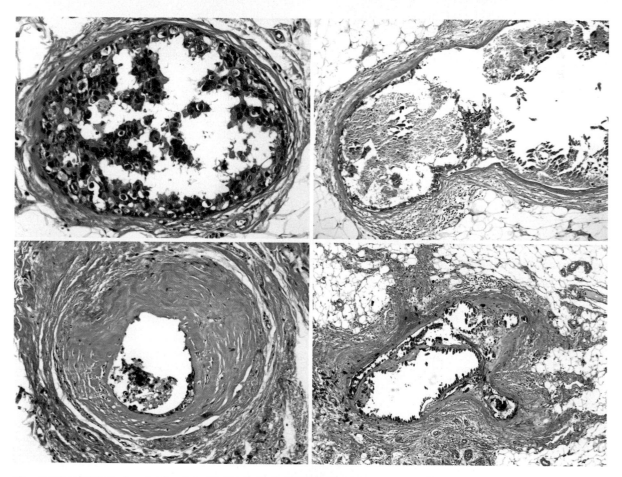

Figs. 7.6.9–7.6.12 Further details of the histologic findings: Grade 3 micropapillary cancer in situ (7.6.9), a duct-like structure distended by necrosis and amorphous calcifications (7.6.10), cross section of a duct with an incomplete layer of malignant cells and with periductal fibrosis (7.6.11) and extensive desmoplastic reaction surrounding a duct (7.6.12) containing a few cancer cells and a large, fragmented amorphous calcification

Final histology: 15 x 10 mm Grade 3 in situ carcinoma with no signs of invasion.

Comment: This case represents a <40 mm high-grade in situ carcinoma. The corresponding mammographic image shows casting-type calcifications.

Example 7.7 A 54-year-old asymptomatic woman, called back from screening for assessment of the multiple cluster crushed stone-like calcifications in the lower portion of the right breast

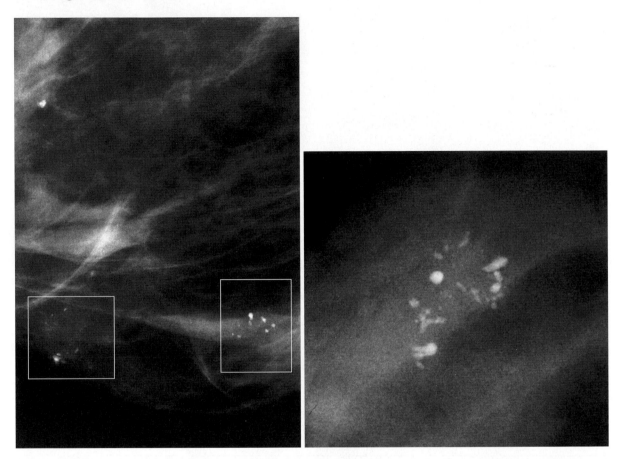

Figs. 7.7.1and 7.7.2 Detail of the right MLO projection (7.7.1) shows multiple cluster crushed stone-like calcifications (in rectangles). No associated tumor mass is demonstrable. Microfocus magnification image of one of the clusters (7.7.2). The calcifications are of the mammographically malignant type

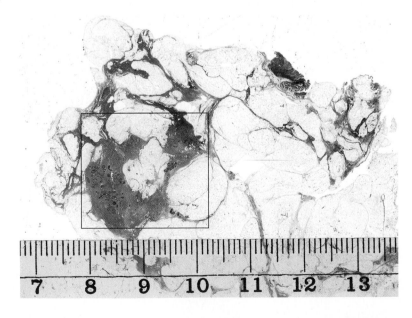

Fig. 7.7.3 Large-section histology. The multiple foci of in situ carcinoma are localized within the rectangle

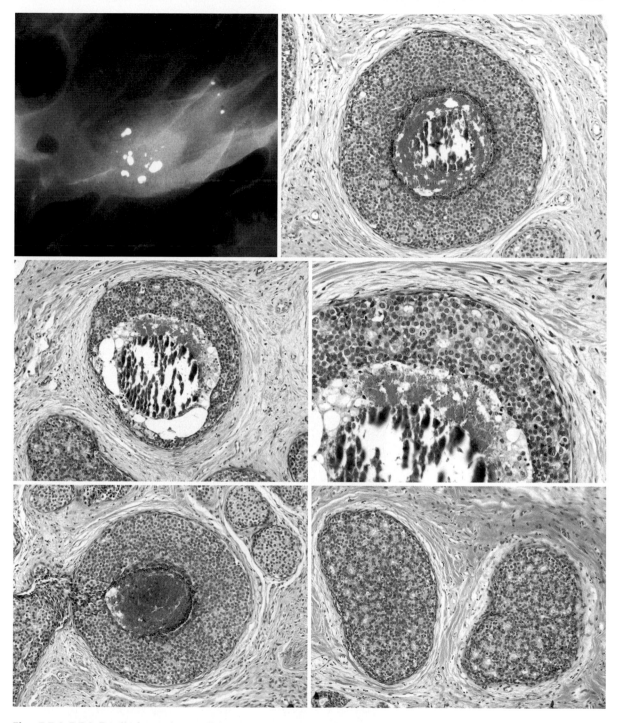

Figs. 7.7.4–7.7.9 Detail of a specimen radiograph with two clusters of crushed stone-like calcifications (7.7.4). Details of the histologic examination (H&E) (7.7.5–7.7.9): Grade 2 in situ carcinoma distends the acini. Central necrosis and amorphous calcification are seen in some of the acini

Comment: In this case the multiple cluster, crushed stone-like calcifications represent a multifocal but limited-extent (<40 mm) intermediate grade in situ carcinoma.

Example 7.8 A 66-year-old asymptomatic woman who attended mammography screening. She was called back for further assessment of the microcalcifications detected on the mammograms of her left breast

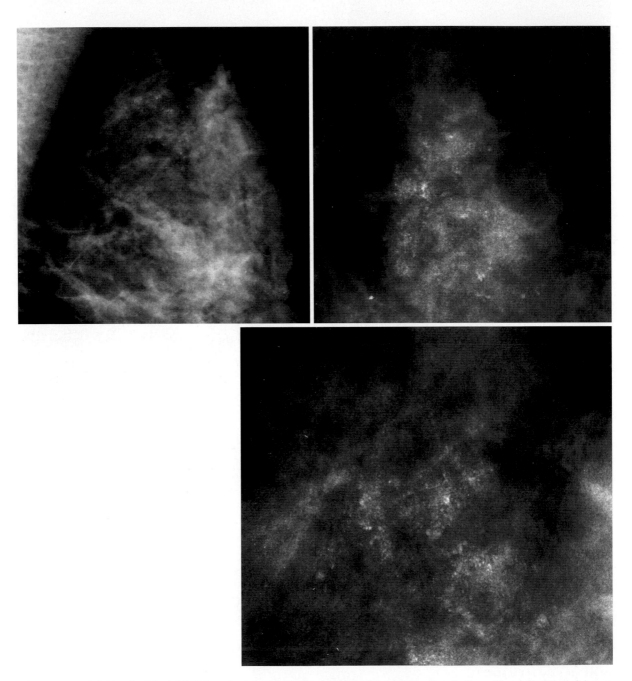

Figs. 7.8.1–7.8.3 Detail of the left MLO projection (7.8.1). There are very faint calcifications in the axillary tail of the left breast. Microfocus magnification images (7.8.2, 7.8.3) reveal multiple clusters of powdery/cotton ball-like calcifications without an associated tumor mass

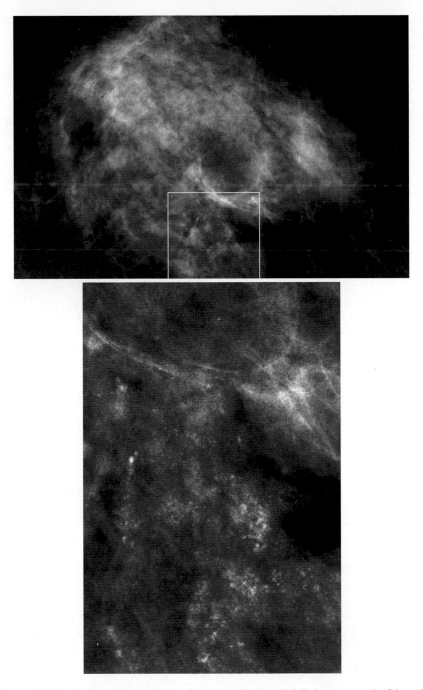

Figs. 7.8.4 and 7.8.5 Left CC projection (7.8.4) and microfocus magnification (7.8.5) demonstrate the faint calcifications near the chest wall

Fig.7.8.6 Breast ultrasound examination does not show an invasive tumor, only a simple cyst hidden in the dense fibrous tissue

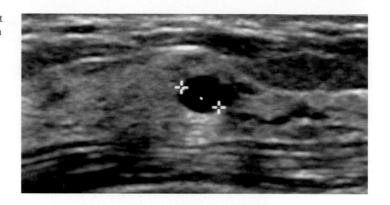

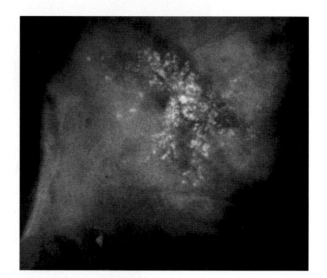

Fig. 7.8.7 Specimen radiograph following large-bore percutaneous needle biopsy using radio frequency. The specimen contains tissue including some of the calcifications

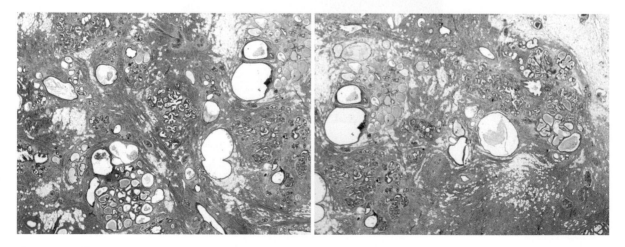

Figs. 7.8.8 and 7.8.9 Low-power histology images of the percutaneous biopsy: Several terminal ductal-lobular units (TDLUs) are involved by a Grade 1 in situ carcinoma of clinging and micropapillary type

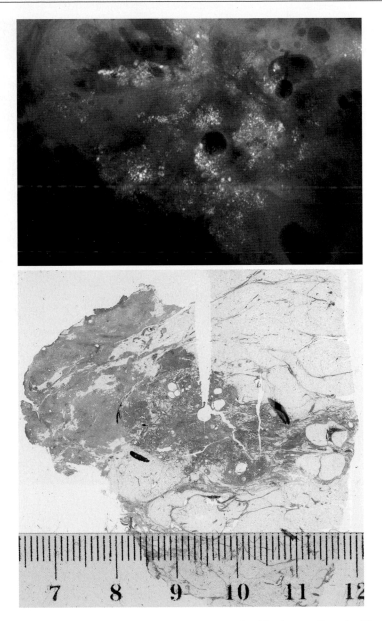

Figs. 7.8.10 and 7.8.11 Surgical specimen radiograph (7.8.10). Large-section histology outlines the 30 x 20 mm region with the mammographically detected calcifications (7.8.11)

Figs. 7.8.12 and 7.8.13 Microfocus magnification images of the surgical specimen showing the cotton ball-like calcifications

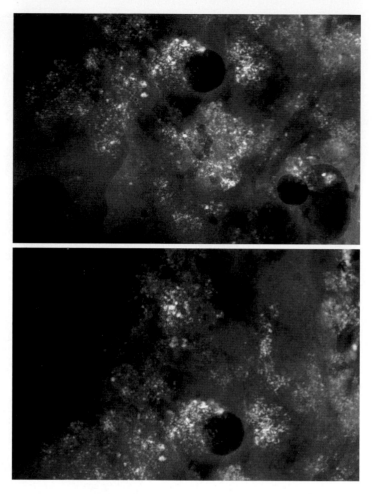

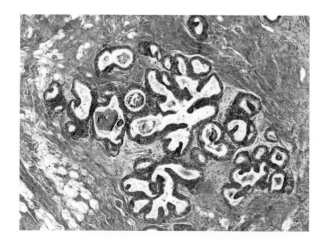

Fig. 7.8.14 Histology image with a single TDLU with clinging and micropapillary Grade 1 in situ carcinoma

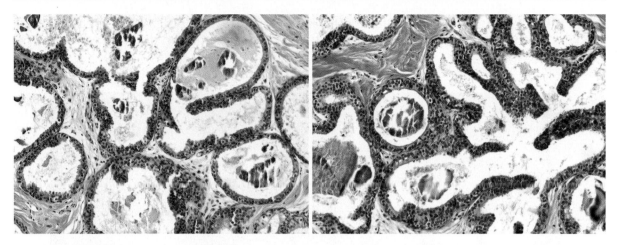

Fig. 7.8.15 and 7.8.16 Higher power histology images demonstrating dilated acini with clinging in situ carcinoma and intraluminal microcalcifications

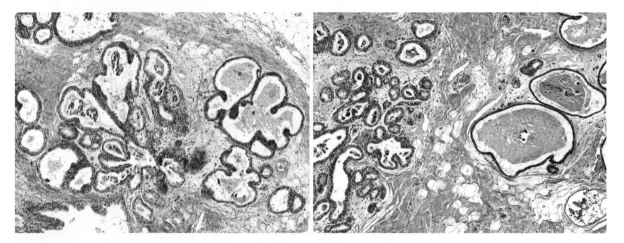

Figs. 7.8.17 and 7.8.18 Histology images of cystically dilated TDLUs containing secretion and microcalcifications

Final histology: 30 X 20 mm area with Grade 1 micropapillary/cribriform/clinging carcinoma in situ. No invasive focus was found.

Comment: This case represents a <40 mm low grade in situ carcinoma. The corresponding mammographic image shows powdery, cotton ball-like calcifications.

Example 7.9 A 68-year-old asymptomatic woman, screening examination. She was called back for further assessment of the asymmetric density detected on the mammograms of her left breast

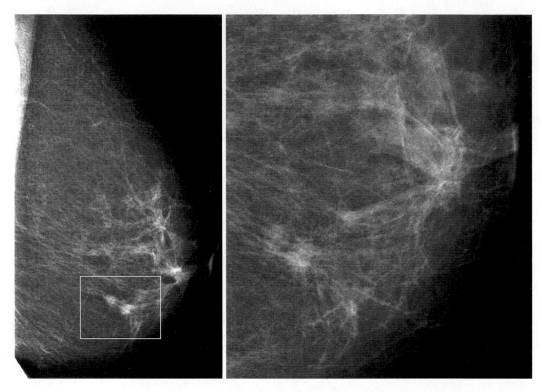

Figs. 7.9.1 and 7.9.2 Lateromedial horizontal projection (7.9.1) and microfocus magnification (7.9.2). There are two mammographically malignant spiculated tumors adjacent to each other in the lower portion of the left breast. No associated calcifications are seen

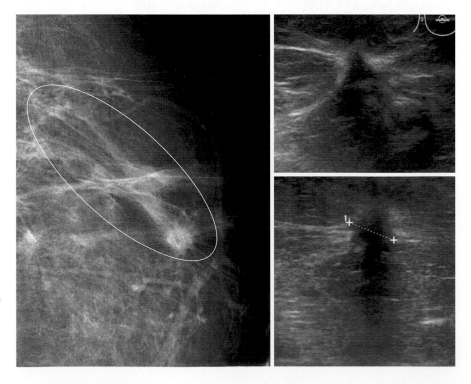

Figs. 7.9.3–7.9.5 Microfocus magnification image (7.9.3) on the CC projection. A bridge connects the two stellate lesions. Ultrasound examination (7.9.4, 7.9.5) confirms the mammographic diagnosis

Fig. 7.9.6 Radiograph of the surgical specimen slice demonstrates the two small tumors and the interconnecting bridge

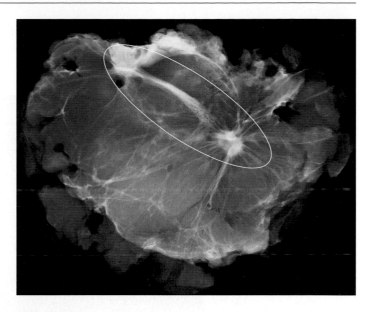

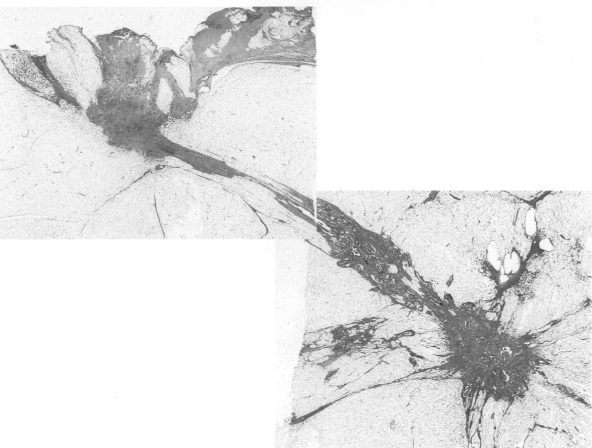

Figs. 7.9.7 and 7.9.8 Histology: Two invasive ductal carcinoma foci (10 and 8 mm) are connected with a fibrous tissue containing Grade 2 in situ carcinoma. Histology examination courtesy: Associate Professor Pauliina Kronqvist, M.D., Department of Pathology, Turku University Hospital, Turku, Finland

Comment: This case represents multifocal invasive cancers limited to a <40 mm region in the breast.

Example 7.10 An 86-year-old woman referred to mammography for a palpable thickening in her left breast

Fig. 7.10.1 Left breast, detail of the craniocaudal projection. Against a fibrous background a large number of clusters of crushed stone-like and casting-type calcifications are seen with no associated tumor mass

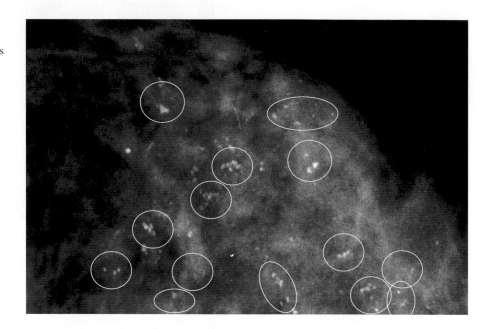

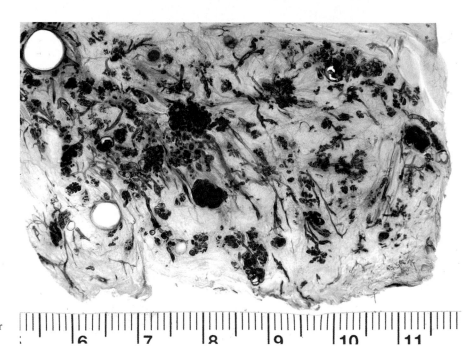

Fig. 7.10.2 The crushed stone-like calcifications are localized in cancer-filled terminal ductal lobular units (TDLUs), demonstrated on this subgross (3D) histology image. Also, some of the ducts are distended by cancer cells

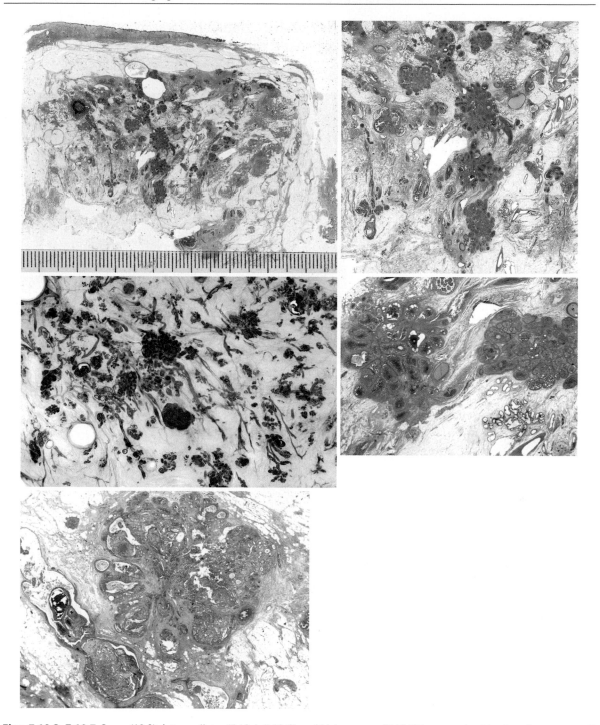

Figs. 7.10.3–7.10.7 Low- (10.3), intermediate- (7.10.4–7.10.6), and higher power (7.10.7) large-section histology images as well as the detail of a subgross (3D) histology slide (7.7.5) demonstrate multiple cancerous TDLUs and ducts occupying an entire lobe

Histologic diagnosis: 6 x 5 cm area with multiple foci of in situ carcinoma having solid/cribriform and micro-papillary architecture.

Comment: This case is an example of extensive (>40 mm) in situ breast cancer with a large number of cancer-filled TDLUs spread throughout a large lobe. Interconnecting ducts are also filled with cancer cells, necrotic debris, and amorphous calcifications, corresponding to the mammographically detected crushed stone-like and casting-type calcifications.

Example 7.11 A 58-year-old woman, called back from mammography screening for assessment of the asymmetric density associated with microcalcifications in the upper outer quadrant of the right breast

Figs. 7.11.1 and 7.11.2 Right breast, MLO (7.11.1) and lateromedial horizontal (7.11.2) projections. The two small ill-defined, mammographically malignant tumors (7.11.1, 7.11.2) are associated with malignant-type calcifications

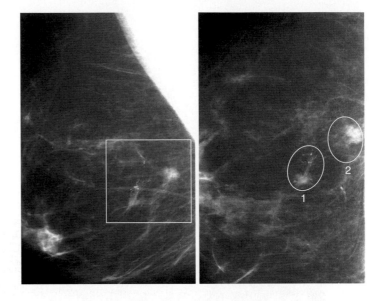

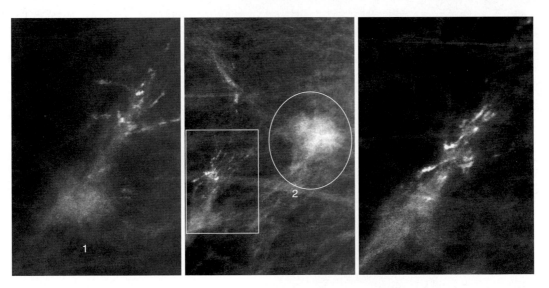

Figs. 7.11.3–7.11.5 Microfocus magnification of invasive tumor # 1 and the associated casting-type calcifications (7.11.3), invasive tumor # 2 (7.11.4) and the associated casting-type calcifications (7.11.5)

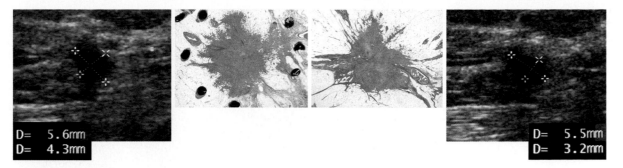

Figs. 7.11.6–7.11.11 Ultrasound images (7.11.6, 7.11.10) and low power histology images of the tiny invasive tumors (7.11.8, 7.11.9)

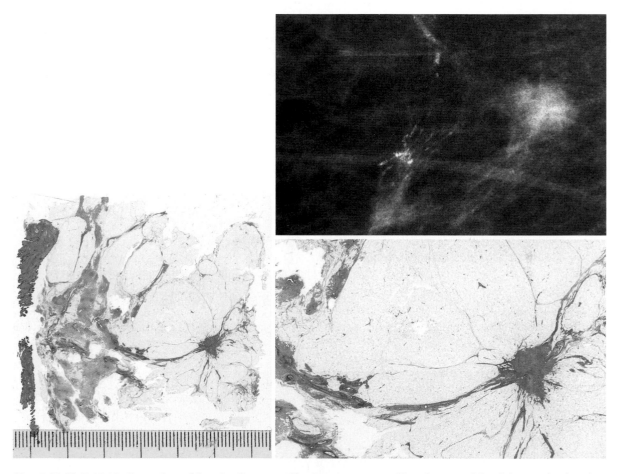

Figs. 7.11.12–7.11.14 Comparison of the microfocus magnification mammogram of invasive tumor # 2 and the associated casting-type calcifications (7.11.12) with low-power large-section histology images (7.11.13, 7.11.14)

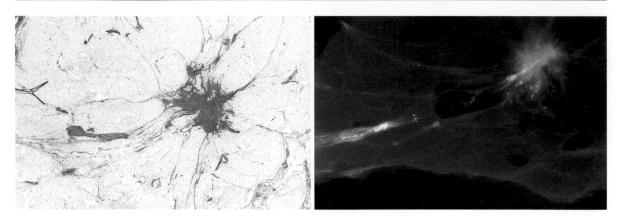

Figs. 7.11.15 and 7.11.16 Comparison of the large-section histology image of invasive tumor # 2 and the associated Grade 3 in situ carcinoma (7.11.15) with the specimen slice radiograph (7.11.16)

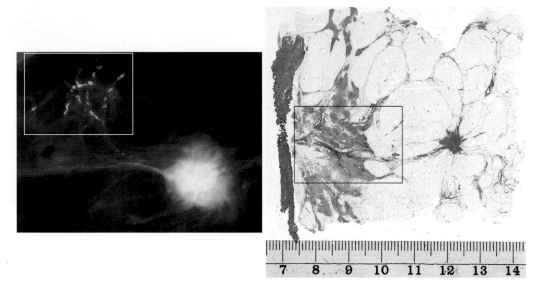

Figs. 7.11.17 and 7.11.18 Comparison between an additional specimen slice radiograph (7.11.17) and a low-power large-section histology image (7.11.18)

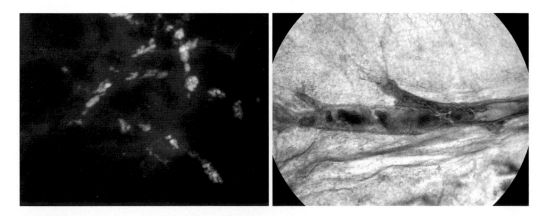

Figs. 7.11.19 and 7.11.20 Comparison between dotted casting-type calcifications on the mammogram (7.11.19) and subgross, 3D histology (7.11.20)

Figs. 7.11.21–7.11.23 3D histology images of additional cancer-filled ducts with solid and cribriform cell architecture

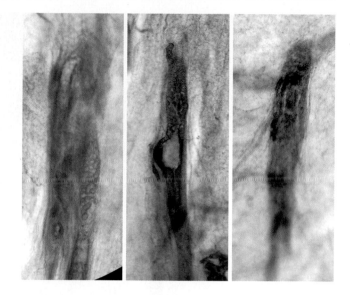

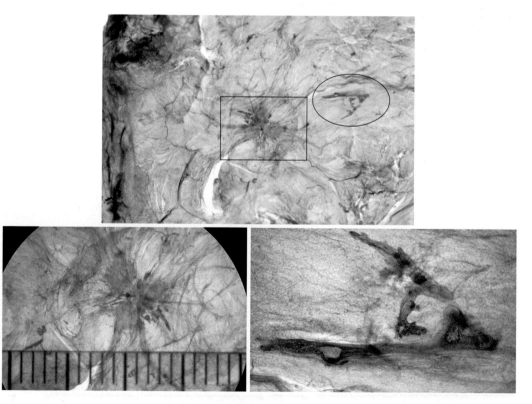

Figs. 7.11.24–7.11.26 Large thick-section (3D) histology showing both the tiny invasive cancer (rectangle) and the in situ component (ellipse) (7.11.24). Photographic magnification of the invasive (7.11.25) and the in situ components (7.11.26)

Figs. 7.11.27–7.11.30 Detail of
the surgical specimen slice
radiograph (7.11.27), low-power
histology of the associated Grade
3 in situ carcinoma (7.11.28) and
the moderately differentiated
invasive ductal carcinoma
(7.11.29, 7.11.30)

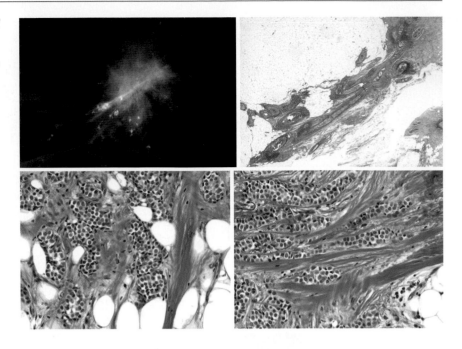

Final histology: Two moderately differentiated invasive ductal carcinomas measuring 9 x 8 mm and 8 x 8 mm. Grade 3 invasive carcinoma coexists with Grade 3 in situ carcinoma, which is seen both within the invasive tumors and also surrounding them. The total extent of the malignant tumors is 60 x 50 mm. There were 5/13 affected axillary lymph nodes, as well as lymph vessel invasion (LVI).

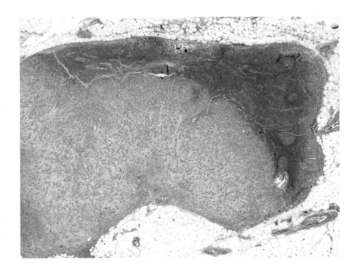

Fig. 7.11.31 Lymph node metastases

Fig. 7.11.32 Lymph vessel invasion (H&E staining)

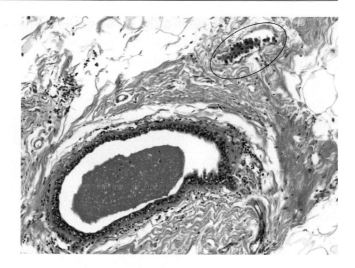

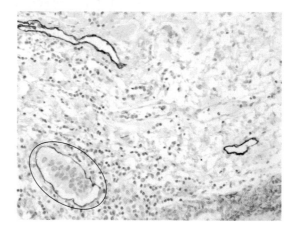

Fig. 7.11.33 Lymph vessel invasion (D2-40 immunostaining)

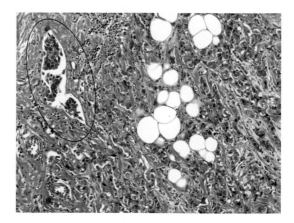

Fig. 7.11.34 Lymph vessel invasion (H&E staining)

Comment: This extensive, metastatic malignant process spread over most of a lobe is nevertheless given a TNM classification of T1b, as if it were a single focus measuring from 6 to 10 mm. A full evaluation of the true extent of the disease is necessary to guide appropriate therapy.

Example 7.12 A 66-year-old woman who had her last mammogram 20 years ago. At that time, she was examined for extremely large, bilateral cysts that have been emptied on several occasions

Figs. 7.12.1 and 7.12.2 Left breast MLO (7.12.1) and CC (7.12.22) projections. These mammograms were taken 20 years before the current examination and show large cysts that were drained several times

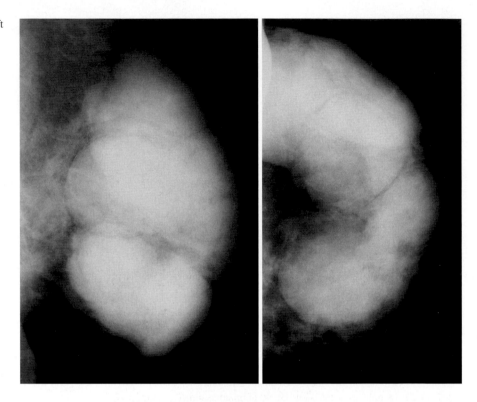

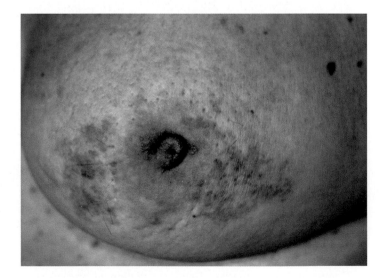

Fig. 7.12.3 A few weeks before the current examination, 20 years after her previous mammogram, she noticed a considerable change in the appearance of her left areola and periareolar region. She also felt a thickening in the upper outer quadrant of her left breast

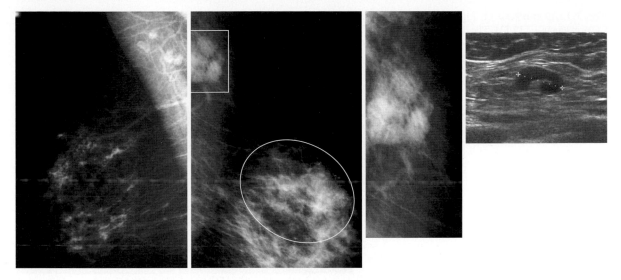

Figs. 7.12.4–7.12.7 Right (4) and left MLO projections (7.12.5), microfocus magnification of the left axillary lymph nodes (7.12.6) and ultrasound examination of one of the pathologic axillary lymph nodes (7.12.7)

Figs. 7.12.8 and 7.12.9 Microfocus magnification images show extensive casting-type, mammographically malignant-type calcifications occupying most of the upper outer quadrant

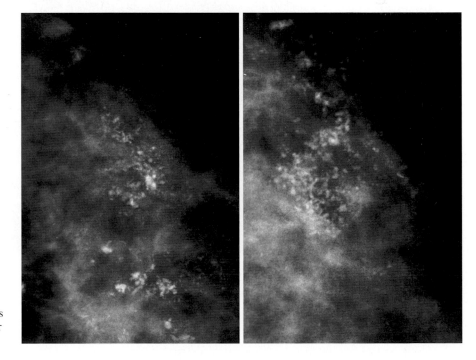

Figs. 7.12.10 and 7.12.11 Right (7.12.10) and left CC projections (7.12.11). The malignant-type calcifications are seen in the lateral portion of the left breast (*rectangle*). There is also a focus of architectural distortion in the medial portion of the right breast (*circle*)

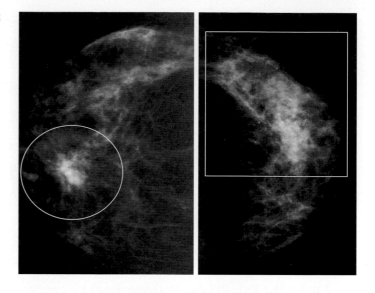

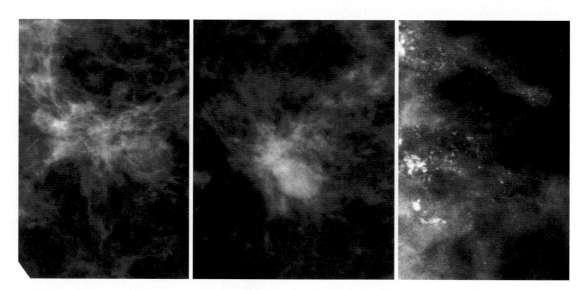

Figs. 7.12.12–7.12.14 Right CC (7.12.12) and MLO (7.12.13) microfocus magnification images of the architectural distortion. Microfocus magnification image in the left CC projection (7.12.14)

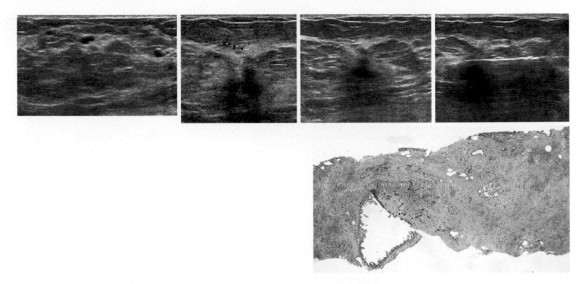

Figs. 7.12.15 The ultrasound image (7.12.15) of the right breast lesion combined with the microfocus magnification images (7.12.12, 7.12.13) suggest hyperplastic breast changes rather than malignancy. Figs. 7.12.16 and 7.12.17. Ultrasound examination of the left upper outer quadrant reveals several invasive cancer foci. Figs. 7.12.18 and 7.12.19. Ultrasound-guided core needle biopsy confirms the diagnosis of invasive ductal carcinoma associated with the in situ component

Figs. 7.12.20–7.12.22 This series of 2-mm thick, reconstructed coronal 3D ultrasound sections through the left breast demonstrate multiple irregular, hypoechoic foci corresponding to individual invasive tumors

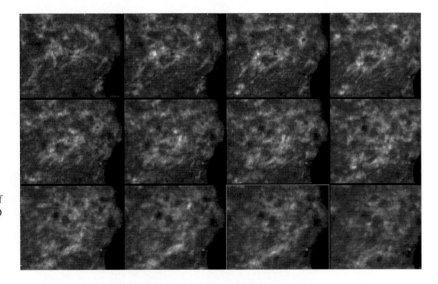

Figs. 7.12.20–7.12.22 (continued)

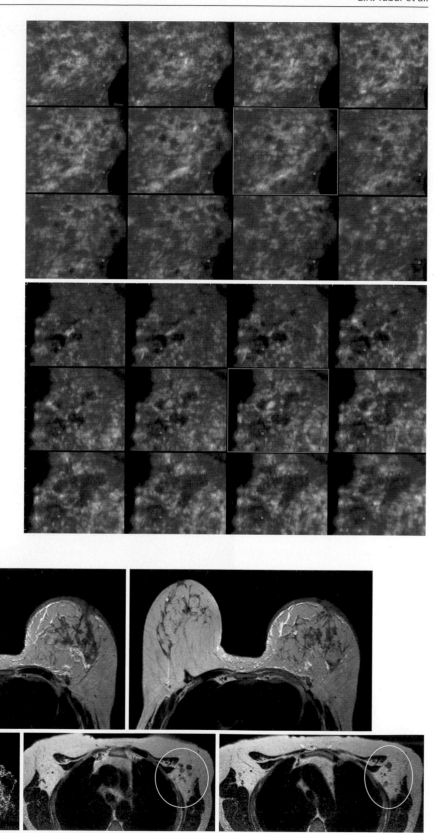

Figs. 7.12.23–7.12.27 Breast MRI demonstrates alteration of the breast shape. The extensive malignant process occupies much of the breast. The thickened skin is due to lymphatic obstruction in the axilla

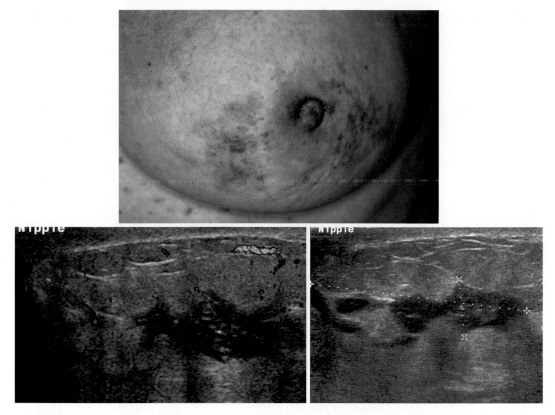

Figs. 7.12.28–7.12.30 The clinical and ultrasound manifestation of the lymph stasis in the peri- and subareolar region

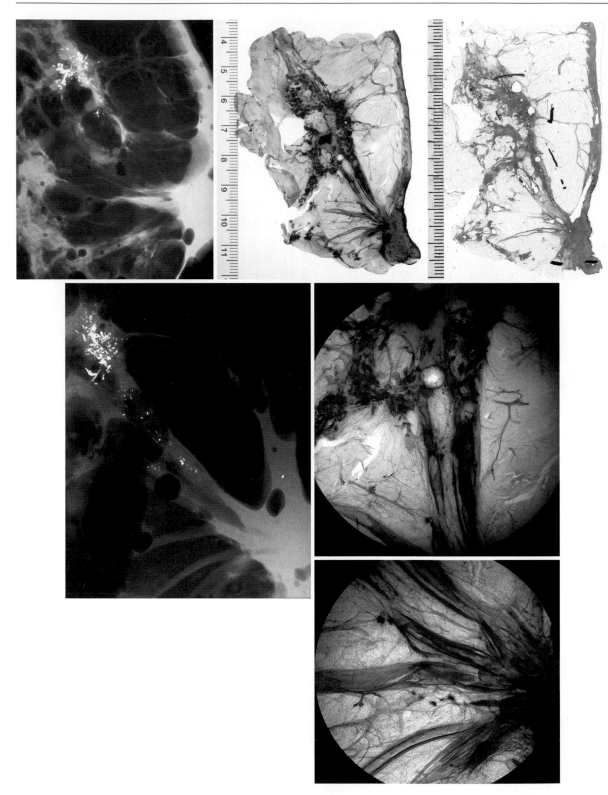

Figs. 7.12.31–7.12.36 Correlative mastectomy specimen radiograph, large-section subgross (3D), and conventional histologic images

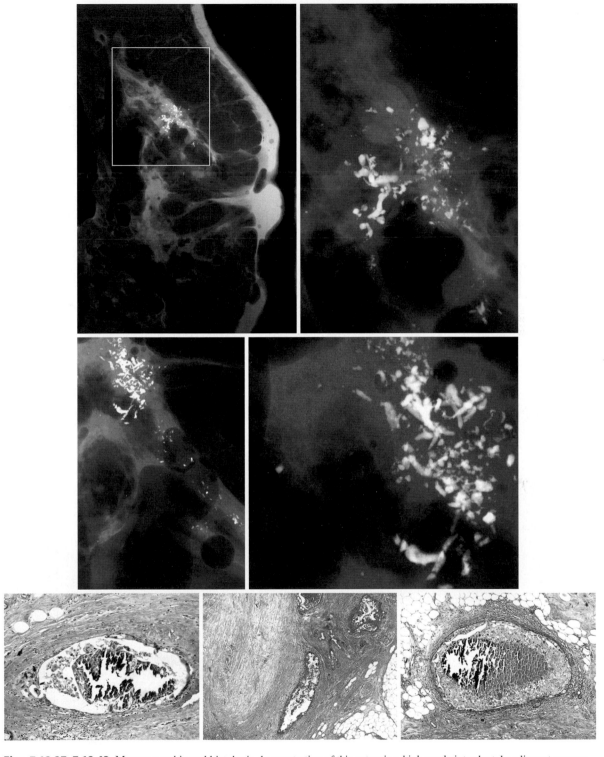

Figs. 7.12.37–7.12.43 Mammographic and histologic demonstration of this extensive, high-grade intraductal malignant process

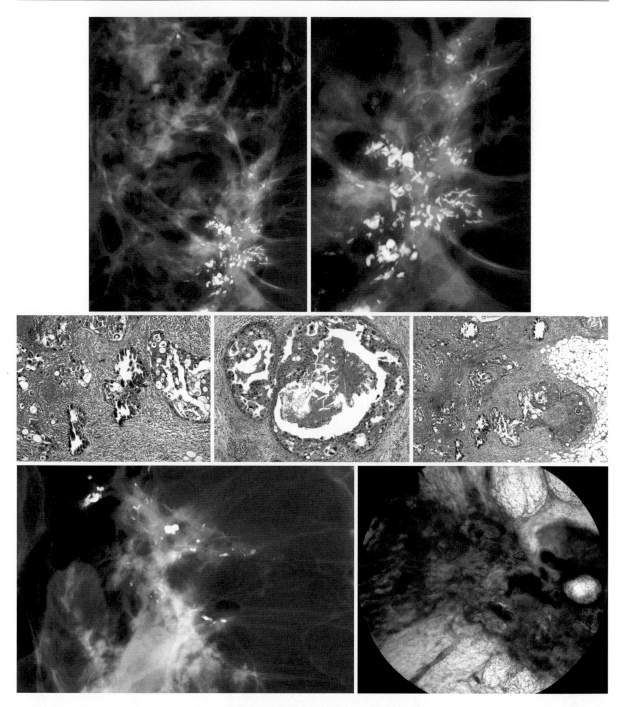

Figs. 7.12.44–7.12.50 Radiographs of additional slices from the mastectomy specimen (7.12.44, 7.12.45, 7.12.49) demonstrate architectural distortion, corresponding to invasive foci. Histology (7.12.46–7.12.48, 7.12.50) shows the combination of in situ and invasive foci

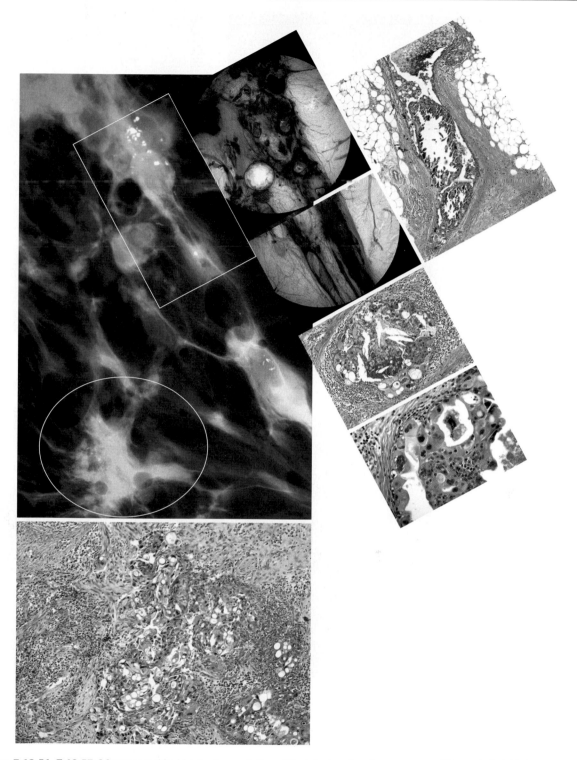

Figs. 7.12.51–7.12.57 Mammographic–histologic correlation of the intraductal malignant process. The encircled, ill-defined density with a radiating structure corresponds to a poorly differentiated invasive ductal carcinoma on histology (7.12.57)

Figs. 7.12.58–7.12.62 The extensive malignancy also infiltrates the skin and subareolar tissue

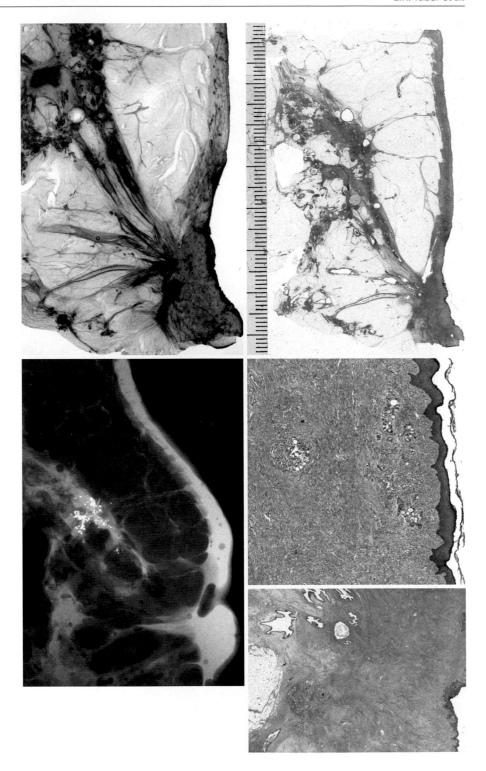

Histology of the left breast: Multifocal poorly differentiated breast cancer (5 x 5, 3 x 3, 1 x 1 mm) associated with Grade 3 in situ carcinoma on an area measuring 70x60 mm. Total disease extent: 70 x 60 mm pN 6/7. LVI

Figs. 7.12.63–
7.12.67 Mammographic, ultrasound, breast MRI, fine needle aspiration cytology, and low-power histologic demonstration of the axillary node metastases

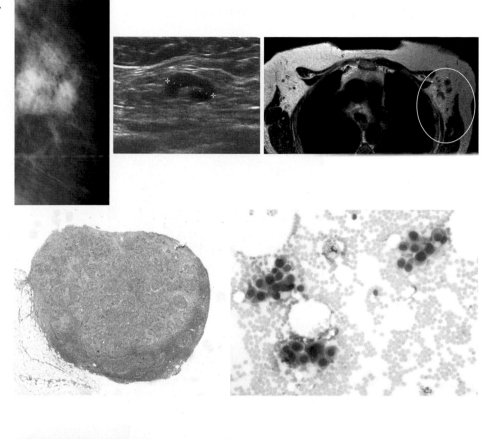

Figs. 7.12.68–
7.12.70 Right breast, CC projection (7.12.68), and microfocus magnification (7.12.69) of the focus of architectural distortion. Histology (7.12.70): Radial scar and fibrocystic change

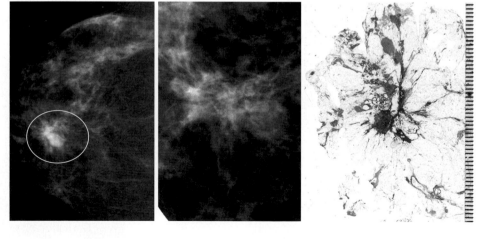

Comment: Extensively multifocal and diffuse breast cancers currently provide the greatest challenge for both diagnosis and therapy. Despite all our efforts, these cancers account for most breast cancer deaths.

Unfortunately, the tumor burden in these cases is systematically underestimated by the current classification system. Multimodality imaging can accurately map the true disease extent.

Example 7.13 A 61-year-old woman with bloody nipple discharge from the right breast. No tumor mass was palpable at physical examination

Figs. 7.13.1 and 7.13.2 Right and left MLO projections: There is an asymmetric density with no associated microcalcifications, occupying the upper portion of the right breast

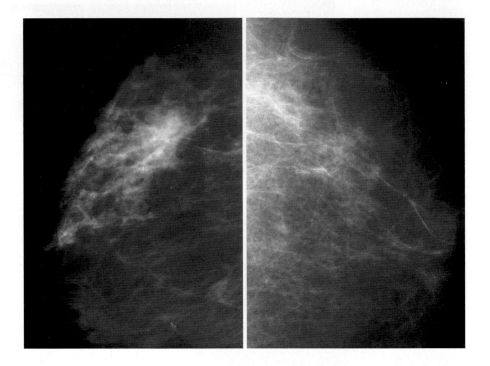

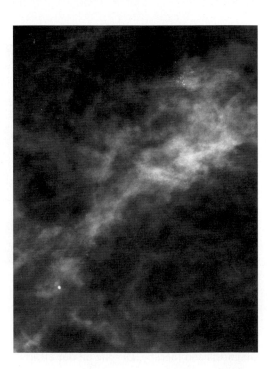

Fig. 7.13.3 Right breast, MLO projection, microfocus magnification: The asymmetric density has some architectural distortion

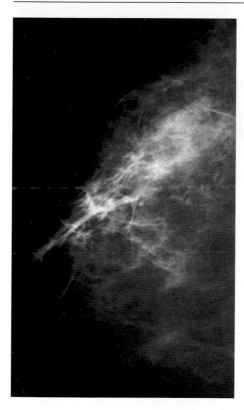

Fig. 7.13.4 Right breast, galactography: The main duct and its branches are filled with contrast media. There is an abnormally large number of duct branches close to the chest wall

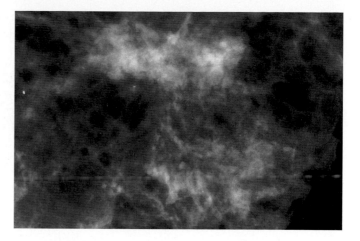

Fig. 7.13.5 Specimen slice radiograph demonstrating the tortuous, distended ducts

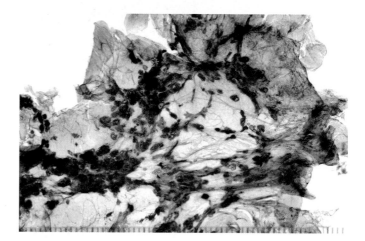

Fig. 7.13.6 Subgross (3D) histology. The unexpectedly large number of ducts are distended and crowded together

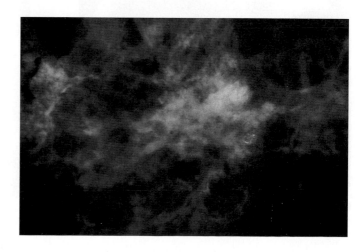

Fig. 7.13.7 Specimen radiograph. The mammographic image is a good reflection of the tightly packed, cancer-filled, distended ducts shown on the subgross (3D) histology image

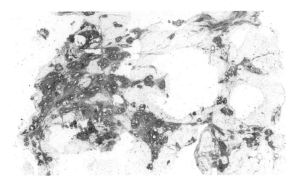

Fig. 7.13.8 Large thin-section histology, low power. The cancerous ducts are packed closely together as in neoduct-genesis cases

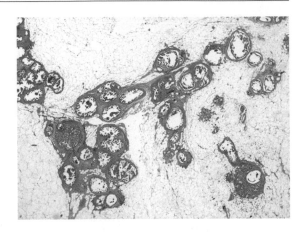

Fig. 7.13.10 Higher power magnification histology image: micropapillary cancer in situ with a thick periductal desmoplastic reaction

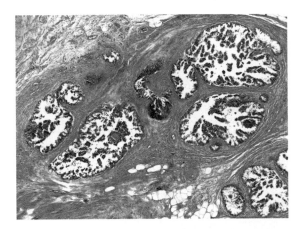

Fig. 7.13.9 Intermediate magnification of the cancerous ducts

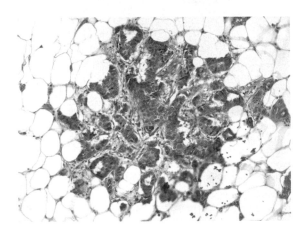

Fig. 7.13.11 Tiny invasive ductal carcinoma focus associated with the extensive micropapillary in situ process

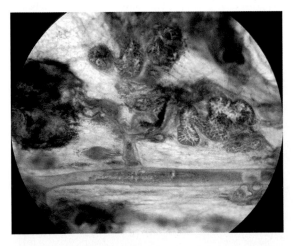

Fig. 7.13.12 Subgross (3D) histology image. The ducts are filled with micropapillary cancer in situ and with fluid produced by the cancer cells

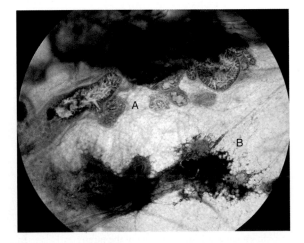

Fig. 7.13.13 The in situ component is marked (A) and the small invasive focus is marked (B)

Final histology: Many microinvasive cancer foci, the largest focus measuring 5 mm (moderately differentiated invasive ductal carcinoma). In addition, micropapillary cancer in situ over a large area (>70 mm). pN 0/2

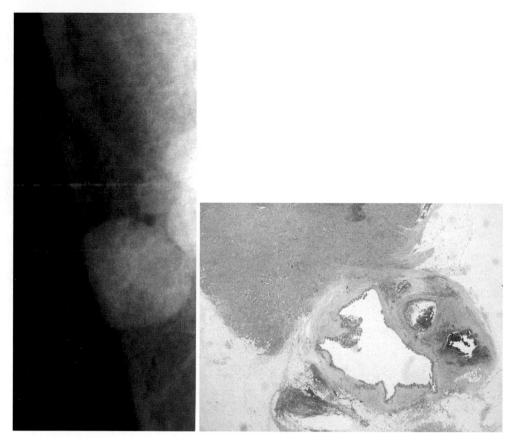

Fig. 7.13.14 Three years following mastectomy multiple foci of recurrent tumor are demonstrated on the MLO projection from the site of the mastectomy. Fig. 7.13.15. Histology image of the invasive and in situ components of the recurrent carcinoma

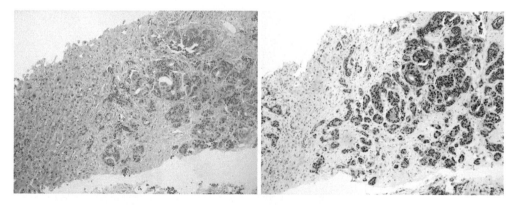

Fig. 7.13.16 and 7.13.17 Core needle biopsy showed liver metastases 10 years following treatment. The patient died of breast cancer 11 years after treatment

Comment: Although the primary tumor was classified as a T1a carcinoma, in reality the tumor burden was enormous, as it involved the entire lobe. In addition to the multiple invasive foci, each <5 mm, the entire lobe was filled with a malignant, micropapillary process, which can be considered to be neoductgenesis.

Example 7.14 A 67-year-old woman, called back from mammography screening for an assessment of the asymmetric density in the upper outer quadrant of her left breast. The patient noticed slight skin retraction over the left upper outer quadrant, and intended to seek care for it, but an invitation to screening arrived at about the same time

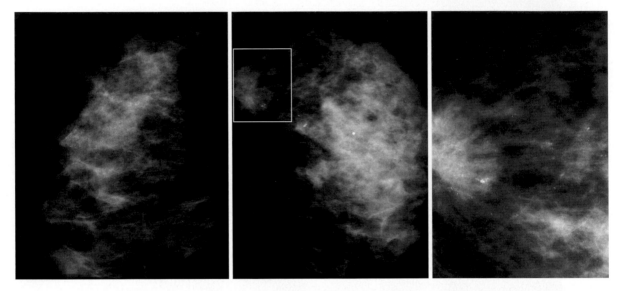

Figs. 7.14.1–7.14.3. Detail of the right and left MLO projections (7.14.1, 7.14.2) and microfocus magnification of the area marked with the rectangle (7.14.3). The spiculated tumor is mammographically malignant. It also contains malignant-type calcifications

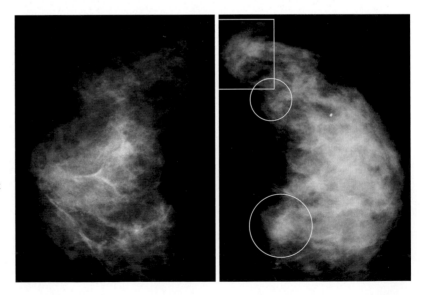

Figs. 7.14.4 and 7.14.5. Right and left craniocaudal projections. The spiculated tumor demonstrated on images 2 & 3 is localized in the upper outer quadrant (rectangle). There are two additional lesions with convex, ill-defined contours, suspicious for malignancy (marked with circles)

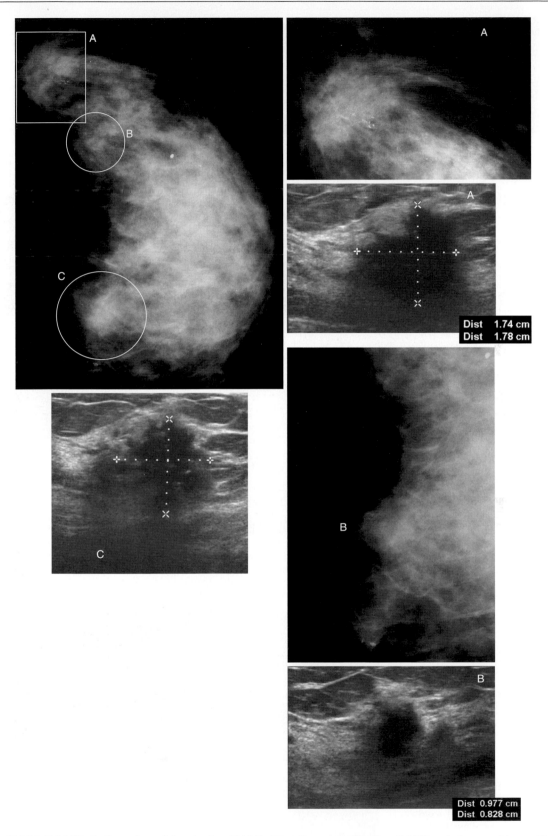

Figs. 7.14.6–7.14.13. Left craniocaudal projection (7.14.6). Microfocus magnification (7.14.7) and ultrasound image (7.14.8) of the spiculated tumor (A) marked with the rectangle. Microfocus magnification (7.14.10) of the region containing the second tumor focus (B). Ultrasound images (7.14.11, 7.14.13) of the second (B) and third tumor foci (C)

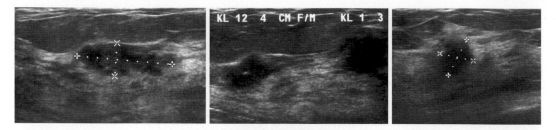

Figs. 7.14.14–7.14.16. Additional cancer foci detected in the left breast with hand-held ultrasound

Figs. 7.14.17–7.14.18 14-g core biopsy of two separate tumor foci

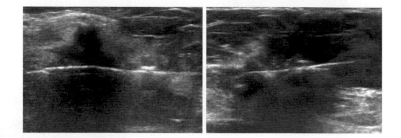

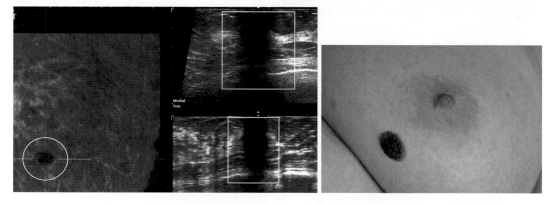

Figs. 7.14.19 and 7.14.20 3D automated coronal ultrasound image, skin level (7.14.19). The encircled, hypoechoic finding is seen as shadowing at the skin level in the conventional ultrasound images (rectangles). The large wart (7.14.20) causes the shadowing

Fig. 7.14.21 This series of 2-mm thick, 3D automated coronal ultrasound slices in multiview format demonstrate the presence of a large number of hypoechoic cancer foci, some of which are encircled

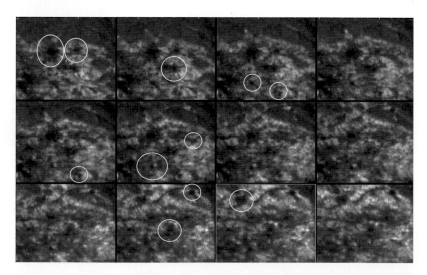

Figs. 7.14.22–7.14.25 The crosshairs indicate the selected hypoechoic lesion on the 3D coronal ultrasound image. The orthogonal conventional ultrasound images in the axial and sagittal planes correspond to the position of the crosshairs and provide the ultrasound diagnosis

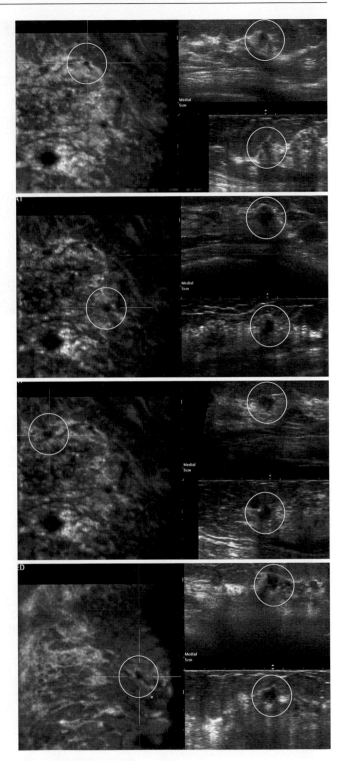

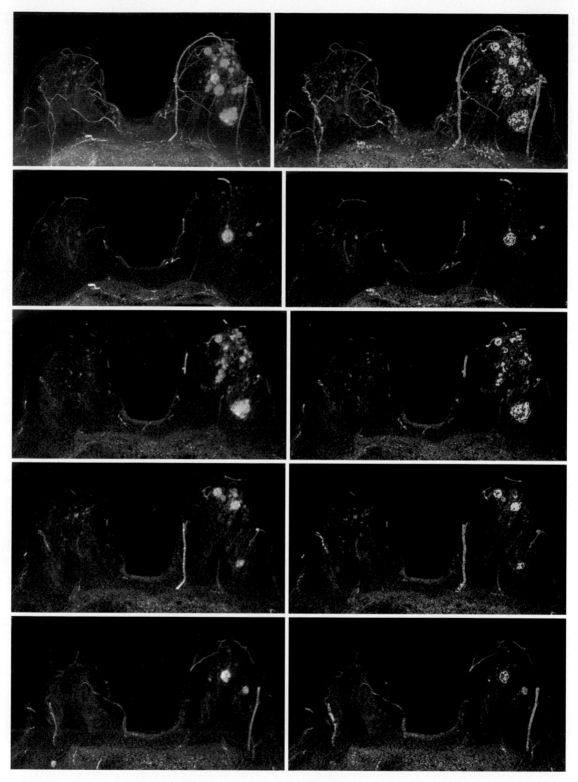

Figs. 7.14.26–7.14.35 Breast MRI image series demonstrate the large number of breast cancer foci spread over a region measuring 100 x 75 x 45 mm. (7.14.26, 7.14.27): Maximal intensity projections (MIP) without (left image) and with (right image) angiomap. (7.14.28–7.14.35): Thin MIP images without (*left image*) and with (*right image*) angiomap

Figs. 7.14.36–7.14.39 Breast MRI images, sagittal views. The large number of breast cancer foci spread over a region measuring 100 x 75 x 45 mm

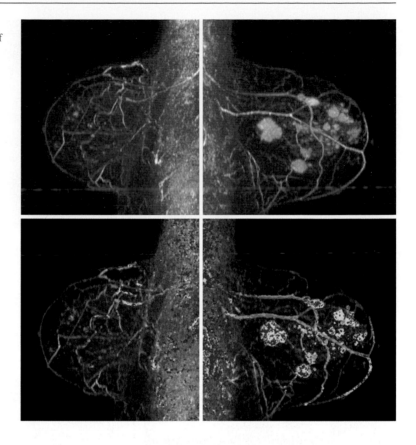

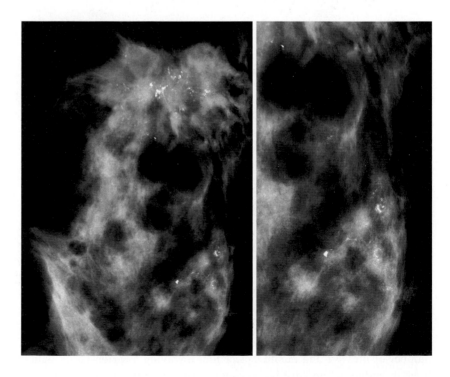

Figs. 7.14.40 and 7.14.41 Specimen radiographs of two mastectomy specimen slices. Casting-type calcifications can be seen both within the large stellate tumor (7.14.40) and in the slice without an associated tumor mass (7.14.41)

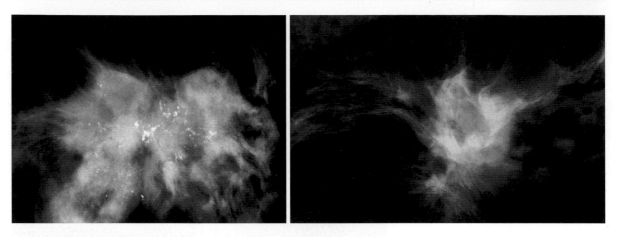

Figs. 7.14.42 and 7.14.43 Specimen radiographs, detailed view of two of the many cancer foci

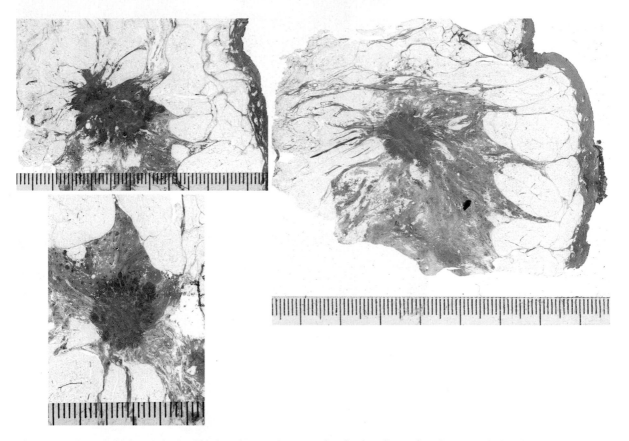

Figs. 7.14.44–7.14.46 Large-section histology images demonstrating the three largest invasive tumor foci

Final histology: Multiple poorly differentiated invasive and Grade 3 in situ ductal carcinoma foci were found over a region measuring 180 X 60 mm. The largest invasive foci measured 24 X 15, 15 X 12, 14 X 11 mm. Four of the nine surgically removed axillary lymph nodes had metastases at histologic examination.

Comment: This case is an example of breast cancers with significant multifocal invasive tumors where the multimodality imaging technique and the subsequent large-section histologic examination demonstrate a large number of invasive and in situ cancer foci involving a region larger than 40 mm. The tumor burden will be large in multifocal invasive breast cancer cases, despite the small size of the individual tumors.

Example 7.15 A 73-year-old woman who felt a hard tumor in her left breast and was referred to mammography

Figs. 7.15.1–7.15.4 Right and left MLO (7.15.1, 7.15.2) and CC (7.15.3, 7.15.4) projections. One cannot distinguish a tumor mass corresponding to the palpatory finding, due to the extensive homogenous fibrosis

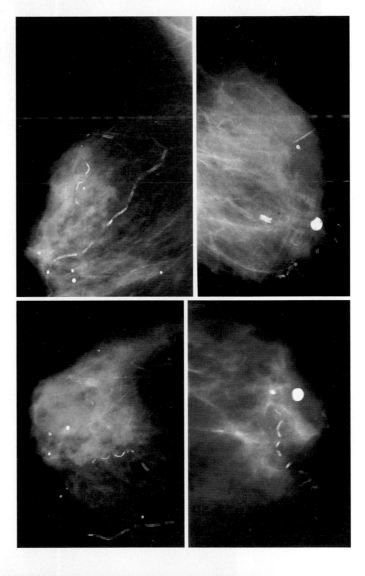

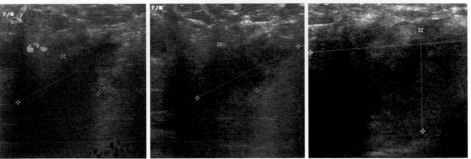

Figs. 7.15.5–7.15.7 Breast ultrasound demonstrates a large, irregular, hypoechoic lesion, suggesting malignancy

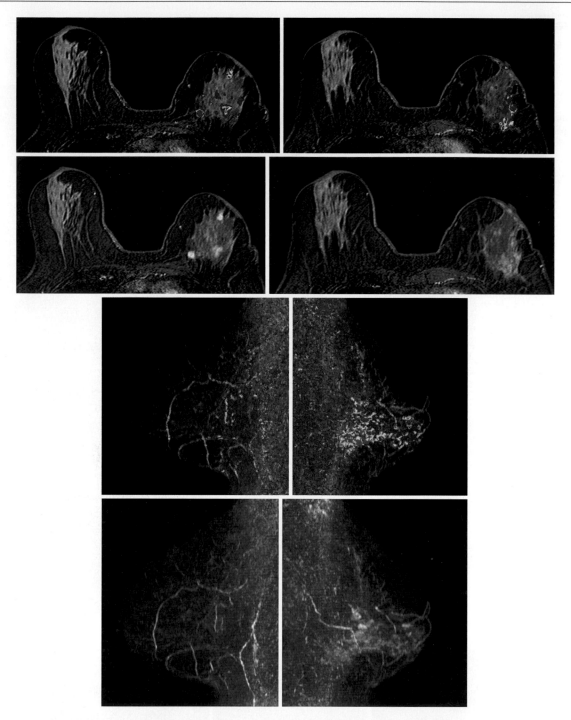

Figs. 7.15.8–7.15.15 A series of axial and sagittal breast MRI images. The left breast is grossly deformed by the extensive, diffuse malignant process

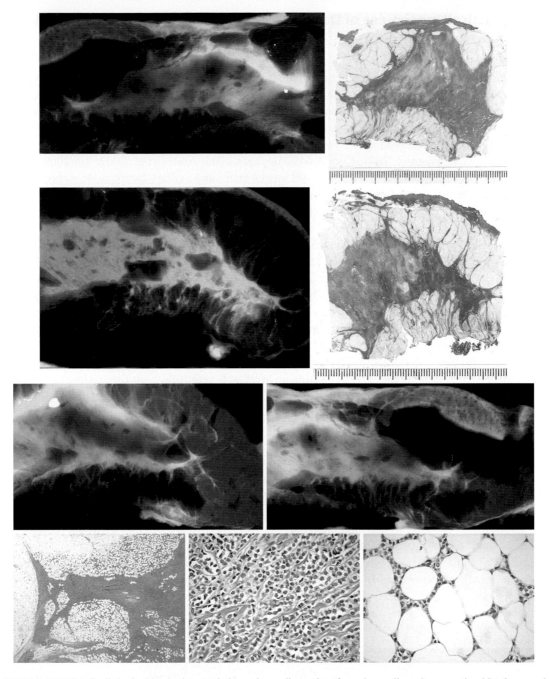

Figs. 7.15.16–7.15.24 Radiologic–histologic correlation using radiographs of specimen slices, large-section histology, and low-power histologic images

Comment: The most common and challenging example of diffusely infiltrating breast cancer is the classic form of invasive lobular carcinoma. Mammography consistently underestimates or even misses this subtype of breast cancer, even when palpable. However, breast ultrasound and MRI provide excellent visualization of this deceptive breast cancer subtype.

7.4 The Practical Importance of Determining the Unifocal Versus Multifocal/Diffuse Nature of Breast Cancer

The TNM classification system relies upon the diameter of the largest tumor focus when describing multifocal breast cancer cases. Thus, a solitary, 10×10 mm invasive carcinoma will belong to the same size category as a case with multiple tumor foci, provided that the largest focus measures no more than 10×10 mm. But, the tumor burden of the multifocal case may be many times greater, contributing to a significantly higher frequency of lymph node and lymph vessel involvement than observed with unifocal tumors within the same tumor size category (Chua et al. 2001; Coombs and Boyages 2005; Andea et al. 2002; Tot 2009). The study by Tot described the presence of LVI (lymph vessel involvement) and axillary lymph node metastases according to tumor size categories and found a linear relationship in both multifocal and unifocal tumors, but the risk of LVI and lymph node metastases was approximately double for the multifocal tumors in each tumor size category (Table 7.2).

In addition, the local recurrence rate was only 3% in unifocal in situ carcinoma cases, whereas multifocal and diffuse in situ carcinomas had local recurrence rates of 13% and 12%, respectively (17% in those showing signs of neoductgenesis and 8% in cases without the histologic signs of neoductgenesis) (Tot and Tabar 2005). In clinical practice, these histologic tumor characteristics have an important prognostic role and influence patient management (Woo et al. 2002). Indeed, a higher rate of LVI and axillary lymph node positivity is associated with poor long-term patient outcome; Egan observed 15% annual fatality rate in multifocal cases compared with a 2.5% annual fatality rate in unifocal cancers (Egan 1982). These observations have been recently confirmed by Tot, who found a 1% fatality rate among the unifocal in situ and 1–14 mm invasive carcinoma cases (2/134) during an average 5-year follow-up time, while the corresponding figure was 5% in the multifocal carcinoma group of the same size category (6/108). These data (Table 7.3) emphasize the importance of diagnosing the multifocal nature of breast cancer using the multimodality approach, with particular emphasis on breast MRI.

In diffuse invasive breast cancer cases, such as large invasive lobular carcinomas, there is an even higher frequency of lymph node metastases and poorer long-term outcome than in extensive multifocal invasive breast cancers. Another subset of diffuse breast cancer with a surprisingly poor prognosis is characterized by casting type calcifications of the mammogram. In these tumors, there is a striking discrepancy between the TNM classification (1–9 mm, 10–14 mm tumor size) and the poor long-term outcome. This discrepancy is best explained by the presence of neoductgenesis or duct-forming invasive carcinoma, which produces a large tumor burden and frequent vascular invasion (Tabar et al. 2007). Although this diffuse breast cancer mimics the characteristics of an in situ process at histology, it often behaves like an advanced invasive breast cancer with difficult local control and highly unpredictable long-term prognosis.

Table 7.2 The frequency of lymph vessel involvement and lymph node invasion in 704 breast cancer cases diagnosed at Falun Central Hospital, Sweden

	Vascular Invasion			Lymph Node Macrometastasis		
	Unifocal	Multifocal or Diffuse	Sum	Unifocal	Multifocal or Diffuse	Sum
1–9 mm	13% (8/61)	17% (16/93)	16% (24/154)	3% (2/61)	14% (13/93)	10% (15/154)
10–14 mm	15% (11/71)	27% (26/95)	22% (37/166)	11% (8/71)	29% (28/95)	22% (37/166)
15–19 mm	33% (20/61)	43% (35/82)	38% (55/143)	26% (16/61)	37% (30/82)	32% (46/143)
20–29 mm	26% (14/53)	51% (47/92)	42% (61/145)	23% (12/53)	53% (49/92)	42% (61/145)
30+ mm	40% (8/20)	53% (40/76)	50% (48/96)	45% (9/20)	64% (49/76)	60% (58/96)
Sum	23% (61/266)	37% (164/438)	32% (225/704)	18% (47/266)	39% (169/438)	31% (217/704)

Table 7.3 Proportional breast cancer death in unifocal, limited, and extensive multifocal as well as in diffuse breast cancers according to tumor size. Breast cancer cases diagnosed at Falun Central Hospital, Sweden in 1996–1998. 43 cases had unknown tumor size 26/82 cases had unknown tumor size because either the patients were not operated or they had preoperative adjuvant chemotherapy

Invasive In situ	Unifocal Unifocal	Unifocal Nonunifocal	MF Inv Any In situ	Diffuse Inv Any In situ	All
In situ	0%(0/35)	5%(2/43)	n.a.	n.a.	3%(2/78)
1–9 mm	0%(0/52)	0%(0/14)	8%(1/13)	0/0	1%(1/79)
10–14 mm	4%(2/47)	11%(2/19)	5%(1/19)	0/0	6%(5/85)
15–19 mm	2%(1/55)	20%(2/10)	15%(4/27)	0/0	8%(7/92)
20–29 mm	16%(9/57)	25%(5/20)	33%(11/33)	0/0	23%(25/110)
30+ mm	24%(5/19)	20% (1/5)	25%(6/24)	26%(6/23)	25%(18/71)
Unknown	n.a.	n.a.	n.a.	n.a.	60%(26/43)
All	6%(17/265)	11%(12/111)	20%(23/116)	26%(6/23)	15%(82/558)

7.5 Conclusions: A Flaw Inherent to the Current TNM Classification of Malignant Tumors

The current TNM classification system, which predates the screening era, uses the size of the largest invasive focus as a major descriptive factor, and fails to take multifocality into account. However, treatment planning, including the surgical approach, should be determined by the extent of the tumor, but this essential information is not included in the TNM classification. The preoperative imaging workup using the multimodality approach has the capability of describing the full extent of the disease. The best way of assessing tumor burden is to describe the overall tumor volume and also estimate the tumor surface area (Andea et al. 2004). Application of this information during the treatment planning process of each individual case will help to ensure complete removal of the malignant tissue. The use of dogmatic treatment guidelines, such as "lumpectomy and postoperative irradiation" for most breast cancer cases, has led to overtreatment of unifocal cases and undertreatment of multifocal cancers. Also, the failure of taking multifocality into account places the unifocal tumor with excellent long-term prognosis and the multifocal tumors with the same maximum individual tumor size, but with poor prognosis, into the same TNM category. To offset this deficiency, we propose that a quantitative evaluation of the tumor burden, in terms of total tumor volume and tumor surface area, be integrated into Cancer Registry databases. The resulting information will provide a more reliable outcome measure and will also serve as a solid database for therapeutic guidelines.

References

Andea AA, Wallis T, Newman LA, Bouwman D, Dey J, Wisscher DW (2002) Pathologic analysis of tumor size and lymph node status in multifocal/multicentric breast carcinoma. Cancer 94:1383–1390

Andea AA, Bouwman D, Wallis T, Wissher DW (2004) Correlation of tumor volume and surface area with lymph node status in patients with multifocal/multicentric breast carcinoma. Cancer 100:20–27

Cady B, Chung M (2005) Mammographic screening: no longer controversial. Editorial. Am J Clin Oncol 28:1–4

Chua B, Ung O, Taylor R, Boyages J (2001) Frequency and predictors of axillary lymph node metastases in invasive breast cancer. ANZ J Surg 71:723–728

Coombs NJ, Boyages J (2005) Multifocal and multicentric breast cancer: does each focus matter? J Clin Oncol 23:7497–7502

Egan RI (1982) Multicentric breast carcinomas: clinical-radiographic-pathologic whole organ studies and 10-year survival. Cancer 49:1123–1130

Holland R, Veling SHJ, Mravunac M, Hendriks JHCL (1985) Histologic multifocality of Tis, T1-2 breast carcinomas. Implications for clinical trials of breast conserving surgery. Cancer 56:979–990

Tabar L, Tot T, Dean PB (2005) Breast cancer: the art and science of early detection with mammography. Thieme, Stuttgart/New York

Tabar L, Tot T, Dean PB (2007) Breast cancer. Early detection with mammography. Carting type calcifications: sign of a subtype with deceptive features. Thieme, Stuttgart/New York

Tot T (2007) Clinical relevance of the distribution of the lesions in 500 consecutive breast cancer cases documented in large-format histologic sections. Cancer 110:2551–2560

Tot T, Tabar L (2005) Mammographic-pathologic correlation of ductal carcinoma in situ of the breast using two- and three-dimensional large histologic sections. Semin Breast Dis 8:144–151

Tot T (2009) The metastatic capacity of multifocal breast carcinomas: extensive tumors versus tumors of limited extent. Hum Pathol 40:199–205

Woo CS, Silberman H, Nakamura SK, Ye W, Sposto R, Colburn W, Waisman JR, Silverstein MJ (2002) Lymph node status combined with lymphovascular invasion creates a more powerful tool for predicting outcome in patients with invasive breast cancer. Am J Surg 184:337–340

Yen MF, Tabar L, Vitak B, Smith RA, Chen HH, Duffy SW (2003) Quantifying the potential problem of overdiagnosis of ductal carcinoma in situ in breast cancer screening. Eur J Cancer 39:1746–1754

Lobar Ultrasound of the Breast

8

Dominique Amy

8.1 Introduction

The radiological diagnosis of breast carcinoma is based on three different techniques today: mammography, magnetic resonance imaging (MRI), and breast ultrasound (echography). A major disadvantage of mammography is the lack of precise anatomical references. In fact, the radiologist using this technique makes a global analysis of the connective and fatty tissues containing the fibro-glandular block but the lobes of the breast are not outlined on the normal mammogram. MR mammography is based on contrast enhancement dependent on angiogenesis and as such gives no opportunity to relate the lesions to lobar anatomy of the breast. Conventional breast echography with orthogonal vertical and horizontal scanning is only a transcript of the mammographic findings from the radiologist's point of view. It does not allow viewing anatomical structures, and only a limited part of the breast volume can be studied. Description of lobes, lobules, and ducts, or the localization of specific terminal ductal-lobular unit (TDLUs) groups never appears in an echography report.

As the first consequence of these observations, one could ask whether the mammary gland is the only organ of the human body which radiological images should not be interpreted relying on the knowledge of its normal anatomy. The second question is how to detect a "millimetric" (a few millimeters in size) lesion if one does not know how to search for it and where and how it develops. For these purposes, we aimed to introduce a new concept taking large-format histology sections of the breast as a model (Fig. 8.1). This concept was termed ductal echography. The accuracy and the reproducibility of the results using this approach give us a new alternative for breast imaging, improve our diagnostic skills, and allow better understanding of the lobar breast morphology and its physiologic variations.

First of all, we will underline the complexity and variability of the lobes regarding their origin, their size, and shape, raised and discussed previously in this book. The possibility of detecting "millimetric" lesions increases parallel to improved understanding of the modifications of lobar morphology at the earliest phases of breast cancer natural history. It all becomes simple if we understand where exactly the cancer could appear, how it would evolve, and which method should be used for detecting it.

After many years of utilizing ductal echography in diagnostic routine and thousands of analyzed cases,

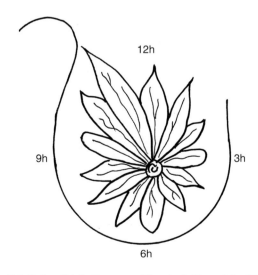

Fig. 8.1 Lobar distribution around the nipple like petals of daisy with horary (clockwise) location

D. Amy
Centre de Radiologie,
Aix-En-Provence, France
e-mail: domamy@wanadoo.fr

T. Tot (ed.), *Breast Cancer*, DOI: 10.1007/978-1-84996-314-5_8,
© Springer-Verlag London Limited 2011

153

we can postulate that we have been able to enhance our diagnostic accuracy, particularly in detecting multifocal, multicentric, and diffusely growing cancers. The detection rates for these tumors are superior to those of mammography itself or mammography combined with conventional echography. Tumors can also be detected earlier this way as the stromal reaction, which facilitates the detection with mammography, is initially absent. In the meantime, it is important to recall that ductal echography is not an anatomo-pathology technique and that it does not allow detecting all the "millimetric" lesions, a few of them will still be missed.

The multimodality radiological approach combining mammography with ductal echography (and doppler sonography, elastography, 3D ultrasound images) is the best possible approach today in routine diagnosis of early breast carcinomas. MR mammography is a valuable complement to these techniques in some precisely defined indications.

8.2 Anatomical Background

Detailed analysis of the large-format histology image in Fig. 8.2a–c gives us the basis for comparing anatomical structures with findings on ductal echography. Beginning from the surface of the skin and proceeding toward the chest wall, we will find the nipple, the areola, and the other structures of the skin (from left to right side of the image) with a thin layer of subcutaneous fatty tissue below. Next, we can see the linear connective structure of the superficial layer of the subcutaneous fascia (fascia superficialis). The typical fatty lobes are interrupted by the Cooper's ligaments, which connect the fascia and the upper surface of the breast lobe. The lobe itself is a very well-defined structure being in connection with the nipple in the upper left part of the section, and ending up at the right margin of the image (partially represented in the image). The ductal axis and lobular groups are also visible within the lobe. The inferior surface of the lobe is bristled up by the inferior Cooper's ligaments (giving a mirror pattern of the front lobe surface), which cross the fatty tissue on their way to the deep layer of the fascia (fascia inferior).

Our aim was to image breast anatomy in details as perfectly as this exceptional histology section. We asked whether it is possible to completely or at least partially reproduce this model with echography. Breast

is an external organ particularly well suitable for ultrasound examination. However, the choice of the ultrasound technique proved to be crucial. Should we use orthogonal scanning of all the breast quadrants from the top to the bottom, from internal to external zones, or, alternatively, radial scanning around the areola with the objective of rediscovering the lobar and ductal architecture? Which ultrasound probe is best adapted to the analysis of the different lobes and to exploration of the axillary tissue?

8.3 Ductal Echography

As described for a long time ago, the breast has 15 to 20 lobes organized all around the nipple just like the daisy petals. The importance of this description remained for a long time purely theoretical as none of the imaging techniques could reveal such a disposition. The anatomical variations that the length of some of the lobes can be 14–16 cm indicated that only the use of the longest possible echography probe could image all the lobes. Since a dedicated probe of 9.5 cm has been designed, using 10 MHz frequency and an adapted water-bag, imaging of all the breast lobes has become a reality. Concentric scanning and/or a translation probe movements along the ductal axis and the axillary areas are required to image the largest lobes.

Using this approach, we can present all the lobes in equal echography projections on the same way, irrespective to the variations in their size and shape and to their localization within the breast. Indicating their position clockwise allows us to localize them very precisely (for example R.10 corresponds to the lobe at 10 o'clock in the right breast, L.6 indicates its position in the left breast at 6 o'clock).

This echographic presentation gives the opportunity to analyze breast tissue on the same way as using the large-format histology image in Fig. 8.2. Viewing from the skin toward the chest wall and from the left hand side to the right, the nipple (with some ducts within it) is seen at the upper left part of the images in Fig. 8.2b and c, the areola, and the skin right to it. The hyperechogenic fibrous tissue of the superior Cooper's ligaments connects fascia superior and the front of the lobar surface, with a hyperechogenic small cone implantation. Likewise, the inferior Cooper's ligaments connect the lower lobe surface, through the fatty lamina, to the inferior fascia, which itself parallels the

Fig. 8.2 (**a–c**) Large-format histology section (**a**) showing a cross section of an entire breast lobe (Courtesy of Dr. Tibor Tot, Falun Sweden). Inverted (**b**) and original (**c**) ductal echography images produced with radial lobar scanning; note the perfect correlation of the echographic image and the histology image in Fig.8.2a

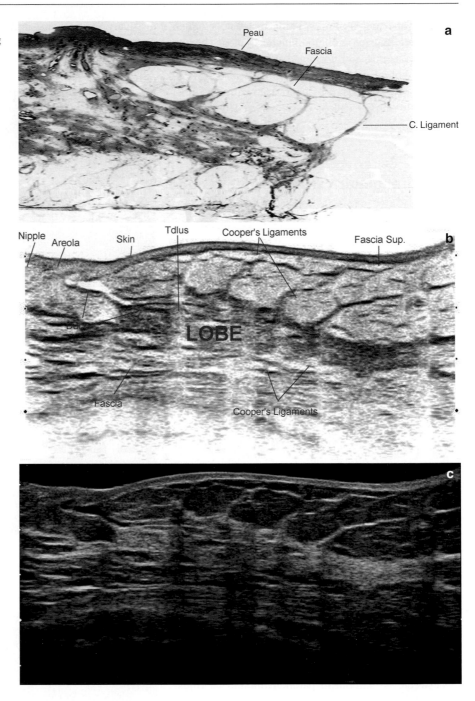

surface of the pectoralis muscle. The lobe corresponds to a hyperechogenic area with different ductal axis visible within it, the largest one at the top of the lobe, the smallest in its depth. The lobules correspond to small hypoechogenic structures located along and mainly at the front part of the ducts.

The comparison of the histology and echography images resulted obviously in perfect matching proving that ductal echography is the method of choice among the noninvasive approaches for studying breast anatomy. No other imaging modality can generate comparable information. Getting more experienced, exploring the advantages of using appropriate equipment, and following Dr. Teboul's teaching (Teboul 2004; Teboul and Halliwell 1995), we have become able to better understand the variations of the lobar breast morphology regarding the topographic position of the lobes, their age-related physiologic modifications, their changes under therapeutic and hormonal influences as well as under pathological conditions. We have also realized that our observations are concordant with the lobar character of breast cancer conceptualized by Dr. Tot (2007b).

8.4 Morphologic Variations of the Lobes

The sonographic variations of lobar breast anatomy are numerous, and some of them may be difficult to analyze. Using a strict and reproducible protocol allows us to visualize all the lobes with the same accuracy irrespective to their dimensions or localization, to minimize the technical difficulties, and also to slightly reduce the examination time. The protocol makes the method less dependent of the skills of the examiner; larger number of cases can be analyzed this way but the results are dependent on thorough knowledge of the anatomic variations.

There are three main echographic types of the breast lobes:

- The mainly fibrous lobe, which is hyperechogenic and contains only very few detectable epithelial structures
- The mainly epithelial lobe, which is hypoechogenic, with much less connective tissue
- The intermediate lobe with approximately equal amount of epithelial and fibrous tissue

The age-related variations of the lobar morphology are also numerous with two basic extremes:

- The young women's breast lobes rich in glandular tissue, with minimal amount of fatty tissue (illustrated in Fig. 8.3), and
- The adult type breast lobe of women with a balance between the amount of parenchyma and fat (illustrated in Fig. 8.4)

Most of the lobes undergo involution, which is only partial in premenopausal women (Fig. 8.5) and more advanced in postmenopausal women. With progression of the involution, structures of the lobe may disappear leaving behind delicate residual connective structures, the lobar "skeleton" (illustrated in Fig. 8.6) or may be totally lost. As underlined above, the lobes

also vary in their size and topographic localizations. The lobes in the medial quadrants of the breast and in the lower quadrants are smaller, the largest are the

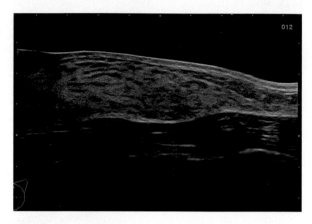

Fig. 8.3 Ductal echography image of a large breast lobe in a young woman showing signs of physiological epithelial proliferation within the lobules and in ductal axis

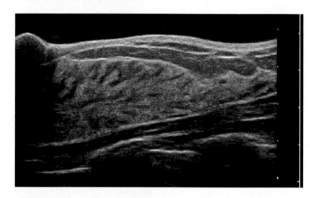

Fig. 8.4 Echographic section of an adult woman's lobe with some hypoechogenic lobules and ducts in the hyperechogenic background of the lobe

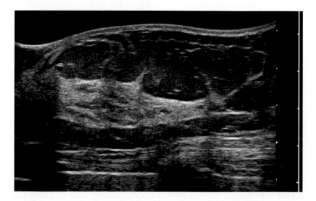

Fig. 8.5 Premenopausal echographic pattern of the breast with reduced lobar size and increased amount of fatty tissue

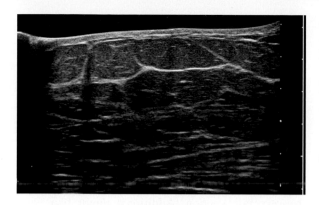

Fig. 8.6 Echographic image showing global lobar involution with small duct axis in a residual hyperechogenic lobe and some Cooper's ligaments

lobes in the upper outer quadrants; some of them may reach the axilla.

Variations also occur regarding the origin of the lobes. The largest lobes are first to develop during the adolescence in the upper outer quadrants, while the smaller ones in the medial inner quadrants appear later during the young women's life. On the opposite, the smaller lobes are the first to disappear during and after the menopause, while those developing earlier located in the upper outer quadrants remain active for a longer time.

Additional variations can be observed regarding the orientation and the distribution of the periareolar lobes. Most of them are well orientated all around the nipple in radial fashion, but some of them have a circuitous way of approaching the nipple and they may overlap each other. This partial superposition of some of the lobes may give the false impression of existence of interlobar connections (anastomoses), and may lead to over- or underestimation of the real dimensions of the observed lobe. It is also difficult to separate the lobes within the retro-areolar area because of their short connection to the nipple. However, studying the mammary gland in adolescents, the partially involuted lobes in postmenopausal women, or in male gynecomastia, demonstrates that the lobes are totally independent of and well separated from each other and represent individual units.

Ductal echography represents an ideal tool of visualizing lobar breast anatomy; however, the normal ducts and lobules are hardly visible because of their small size. Proliferation of the epithelium inside the ducts and lobules causes local or diffuse distension as well as distortion of these structures, and modifies their

acoustic impedance. Then they become "echo-detectable": The hypoechogenic structures correspond to the luminal content of ducts and lobules; the walls of these structures remain invisible. Pathological processes lead to echographic changes that replace the echographic signs of the epithelial proliferation.

8.5 Lobar Implications in Mammary Pathology

The major target in ducto-radial echography is the modification of the normal patterns inside the ductal and lobular structures as well as in the surrounding connective tissue elements of the lobe. Nakama (1991) described the migration of the malignant cells accompanied by lymphocytes, histiocytes, and fibroblasts toward the skin inside the Cooper's ligaments and fascia superficialis. These connective structures are then involved in cancer development at an early stage. (We illustrated the concept with a drawing in Fig. 8.7) This publication confirms Dr. Gallager's conclusions in his article published in December 1969, particularly his conclusion number 2 that "the supportive connective tissue of the breast is also affected by carcinogenic agent" (Gallager and Martin 1969). Teboul (2004); Teboul and Halliwell (1995), as well as Stavros (2006) have also described involvement of the connective tissue and ligaments in cancer development at early stages. They have also underlined the multifocal nature of breast cancer in certain cases. Thanks to the precise echographic anatomy background, Teboul (2004) identified the specific ducto-lobular terminal unit groups, their localization as well as their involvement in the initial steps of the pathological alterations. As he stressed out,

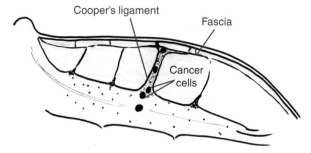

Fig. 8.7 Our drawing illustrating the migration of the cancer cells from the TDLUs into the Cooper's ligament, to the fascia superficialis, and to the skin

the cross section of the ductal axis and the axis of the ligament is the key zone where these groups are located and where our attention should be focused if aiming to study the early pathological modifications of the epithelial structures and of the connective tissue.

These observations are essential in the history of breast echography: radial echographic sections, lobar analysis, search for ductal axis, identification of ligamental ways, and analysis of fascia and skin element alterations. Understanding the origin of the lesion and their development is essential for this analysis. The concept of ductal echography has radically changed the way of examination of the breast. One should not focus on to discover the lesion(s) itself using systematic orthogonal echographic projections in different breast quadrants. Instead, the observer should carry out a lobar analysis (according to the well-established protocol above). The lesions are then usually detectable within the expected structures, within the expected areas, and their development will follow the expected pattern.

The abnormalities should be studied in comparison to the normal lobar anatomy. All the epithelial lesions (both anechogenic/liquid and hypoechogenic/solid) are linked either to a duct, or to a lobule: for example, to a duct in case of ductal ectasia/dilatation and papillomas and to lobules in supraductal alterations. Differentiation between ductal and lobular microcysts will become possible this way. Intralobular localization of fibroadenomas will also become evident. Overlapping of many small fibroadenomas developed in lobules close to each other explains the lobulated silhouette of larger fibroadenomas. Similarly, detection of ductal dilatation due to epithelial proliferation will be possible routinely as well as discovering multifocal lesions near the specific TDLUs. It is crucial to underline that the indirect ligamental signs, often associated with cancer, are absent in benign lesions. These delicate early echographic signs precede the radiological signs related to stromal reaction and, of course, they also precede the clinical signs.

A typical case is demonstrated in Figs. 8.8a–d. The initial diagnosis of breast cancer has been made with mammography regarding a palpable nodule. Echographic examination and MR mammography detected five additional foci of invasive carcinoma. The multifocal and multicentric character of the tumor indicated mastectomy, which was analyzed by Professor Di Marino (Anatomic Laboratory, Marseille Medical University). The specimen was also documented using a large-format histological section by Dr. Rojat-Habib on the Pathology Department of the same University. The pathohistological section corresponded to a 10 cm long radial echography sections. The comparison of the histology section and the echography sections reveals a perfect correlation between these two techniques. Analysis of the different ductal axis shows the signs of duct ectasia. At the distal part of the lobe, two cancer foci are seen (one centimetric and the other millimetric), localized in connection to the Cooper's ligaments. Some ligaments are difficult to study at histology because they are partially represented in the very thin section. Additional tumor foci were detected in other cutting levels, not shown in Fig. 8.8. Like mammography, ductal echography allows a quick, precise, and cheap analysis of multifocal and multicentric lesions. The method allowed a real progress in diagnosing early breast cancer.

8.6 Multifocality, Multicentricity, and Diffuse Lesions

Breast radiology has imaged breast carcinoma for decades like a lesion being most often unifocal and sometimes multifocal. Multifocal and multicentric lesions were distinguished on the basis of the distance between two foci (4 cm). With introduction of ductal echography, a new definition of multiple lesions has become possible: Multifocal cancers should now be defined as those developing within the same lobe along the ductal axis, while multicentric cancers develop in different lobes (they can also be solitary or multifocal). This definition is in agreement with histologic studies.

Figures 8.9a and b illustrate a unifocal breast cancer. Multifocal cancer correspond to hypoechogenic foci, taking place along the ductal axis (picture of a string of pearls), located in the specific TDLUs (Figs. 8.10 and 8.11). Their size depends on their age, and they are more or less associated with indirect anatomic (ligamentary) or echographic (posterior absorption shadow) signs. Although identifying many foci, ductal echography may still underestimate their real number because the smallest ones (most recently appeared) could possibly not be seen. Discovering multiple cancers has become possible through technology progress and practicing using fully digital machines with dedicated probes and through improvement in our way of examination followed by increase of our knowledge.

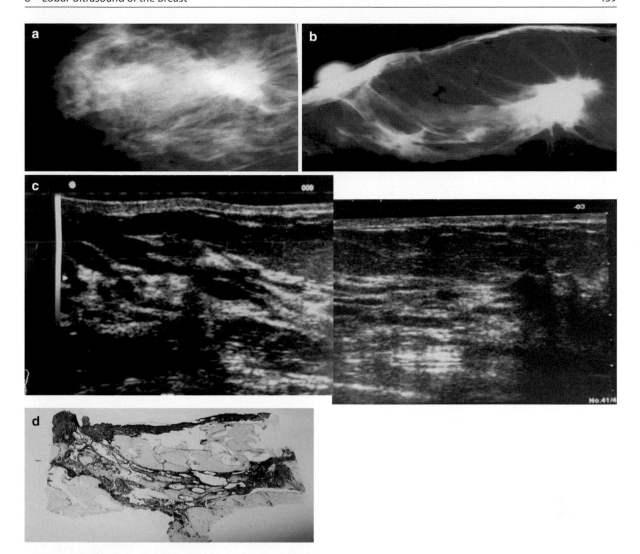

Fig. 8.8 (**a–d**) Mammography (**a** and **b**) and ultrasound (**c**) images of a multifocal breast carcinoma. Note the perfect correlation with the large-format histology section (**d**) (Courtesy of Professor Di Marino and Dr. Rojat Habib, Marseille, France)

The rate of detecting multifocal and multicentric breast cancer cases started with very low values to reach 10–20% a few years ago and to get up to as impressive numbers as 45% nowadays (Tot 2007a). These numbers were surprising, as we were so far away from them in our classical views regarding breast carcinoma. However, the numbers are real as they have been confirmed by other ductal echography specialists and, most of all, by breast pathologists. It seems to us that the "sick lobe theory" (Tot 2007b) reflects the reality we daily observe "in vivo."

Diffuse cancers represent a separate and special group of lesions (Tot 2003). They are difficult to detect and very difficult if not impossible to be differentiated from epithelial proliferation zones. Their characterization often represents the limits of this method and may result in failure of diagnosing (Fig. 8.12).

8.7 Surgical Aspects

The end-result of breast mammographic-echographic examination should be a report giving the maximum of information considering the presence of abnormalities, the biological nature of the abnormalities, their number, and their exact location. A precise mapping of the lesions (with an exact clockwise localization)

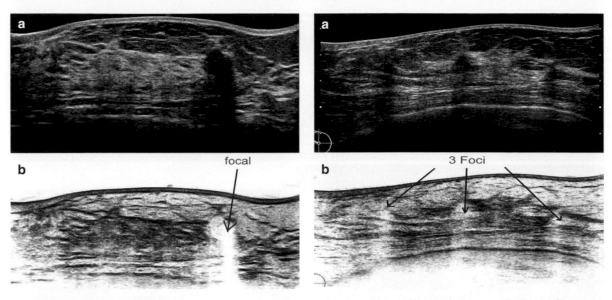

Fig. 8.9 (**a** and **b**) Echography image (**a**) and inverted echography image (**b**) of a few mm large unifocal carcinoma located at the interface of the Cooper's ligament and the rest of the lobe

Fig. 8.11 (**a** and **b**) Echography image (**a**) and inverted echography image (**b**) of a multifocal carcinoma with foci located in different TDLUs along the duct axis (like a string of pearls)

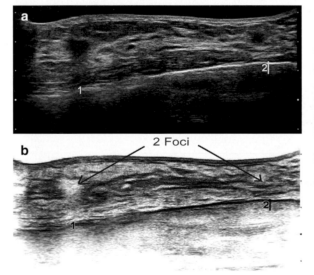

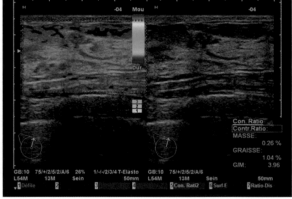

Fig. 8.12 Diffuse invasive lobular carcinoma, hardly detectable in the Cooper's ligament cone with the corresponding elastography, score 2

Fig. 8.10 (**a** and **b**) Echography image (**a**) and inverted echography image (**b**) of a bifocal carcinoma with a proximal and a distal focus at 5 cm distance from each other located within the same lobe

will allow the therapists to choose the best treatment. Notably, eventual recurrences are not the surgeons' responsibility if the preoperative diagnostic information was suboptimal. The role of the diagnostician is crucial and the information he or she generates may have serious consequences. Surgeons such as Professor

Dolfin (Dolfin et al. 2008) or Professor Durante (2006) have been able to develop a specific surgical procedure of lobectomy technique thanks to this background of ducto-radial echography (with pre- and postoperative but also, if necessary, peroperative control examinations). This is an absolutely innovating way of breast surgery. Close collaboration of radiologists, surgeons, oncologists, therapeutics, and the other members of the breast team is mandatory to achieve the best results.

8.8 Conclusion

Ductal echography represents in our opinion an irreplaceable innovation and a major progress in breast carcinoma diagnosis. The concept is based on analyzing lobar anatomy, understanding the morphologic and physiologic variations of the lobes and understanding the appearance and natural history of benign and malignant pathological lesions within the breast structures. The perfect correlation between the echographic and histologic observations is the best proof of the many advantages of ductal echography. Highlighting each lobe individually allows appropriate analysis (in contrast to the conventional echography looking at single lesion inside a quadrant). In our experience, the number of the lobes in most of the breasts is 12 to 15 (less than the 15 to 20 originally described by Going and Mohun 2006). Particular attention should be paid to specific TDLUs and the zones of their localization as this is a very important phase of examination. Subtle alterations in connective tissue structures (seemingly accessories, like the Cooper's ligament, the fascias, and the subcutaneous elements) allow early detection of breast carcinoma hardly ever seen with conventional methods (Amy 2005; Amoros et al. 2009).

The modern echographic approach still remains limited because of the limited probe resolution as well as the availability of special echographic machines. Nevertheless, all the thousands of the lobules within the breast can never ever be properly examined. But the fact that those of them showing the signs of epithelial proliferation or pathological alterations are currently detectable seems to us to be satisfactory. Histological confirmation we had in more or less half of the examined cancer cases, also multifocal or multicentric, is fundamental. Further development is needed for accurate differentiation of breast cancer subtypes, like ductal, lobular, and mixed ducto-lobular.

It is debatable whether we will ever be able to detect the earliest changes in cancer development using echography, but we are already able to observe alterations of the normal morphological constituents of the breast during the disease. Multifocality/multicentricity is often explained by migration of the malignant cells, a phenomenon that cannot be echographically followed; however, observing lesions of different size and age within the same lobe may be a consequence of local cell migration (Fig. 8.13). Finding early bifocal or multifocal cancer foci separated by a distance of

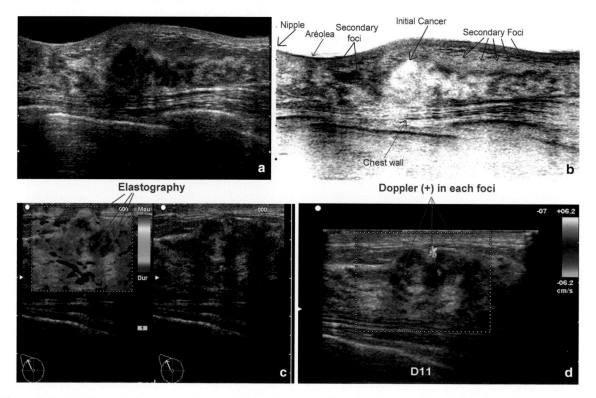

Fig. 8.13 (**a–d**) Echography image (**a**) and inverted echography image (**b**) illustrating a sick breast lobe with a large initial cancer and several additional new foci on both sides of the ductal axis. Elastography score 4 (**c**) and Doppler positivity (**d**) in each of the new multiple millimetric foci within the distal part of the same lobe

several centimeter within a single lobe (Figs. 8.10 and 8.11.) as well as the presence of lesions of the same size within the same and/or in different lobes leads us to the conclusion that multiple malignant foci may develop independently from each other as a result of simultaneous and/or asynchronous malignant process.

The entire new concept presented in this chapter and in this book opens interesting perspectives of surgical and therapeutic character: multifocal, progressive, and extensive lobar involvement should not be treated the same way as a unifocal cancer. The therapeutic strategy should be different at the very early stage of breast cancer development and in the advanced stage, as well.

The diagnostic improvements achieved with introduction of ductal echography, with using large-format histology section, performing controlled breast lobectomy in surgery, introducing new molecular targets in oncology, or peroperative contact radiotherapy and cryotherapy will only be successful if the synergic effects between all these modalities continue. This interdisciplinary approach is more important than ever before. The progress of all this disciplines depends on improvements of the others.

Regarding echography, new equipment (digital machines, new generation of dedicated probes Doppler echography, elastography, three-dimensional reconstruction) have allowed the best of diagnostic performances. But it is also crucial to have dedicated and competent personnel continuously. Ductal echography has become a necessity in specialized breast centers. This is the way and the price of being able to give our patients the best chances for their recovery.

References

Amoros J, Dolfin G, Teboul M (2009) Atlas de Ecografia de la Mama. Ananke, Torino

Amy D (2005) Millimetric breast carcinoma ultrasonic detection. In: Leading Edge conference Pr. Goldberg B. USA

Dolfin G, Chebib A, Amy D, and Tagliabue P (2008) Carcinome mammaire et chirurgie conservatrice. 30e Seminaire Franco-Syrien d'Imagerie Médicale. Tartous, Syrie

Durante E (2006) Multimodality imaging and interventional techniques. IBUS Course Abstracts, Ferrara, Italy

Gallager HS, Martin JE (1969) Early phases in the development of breast cancer. Cancer 24:1170–1178

Going JJ, Mohun TJ (2006) Human breast duct anatomy, the 'sick lobe' hypothesis and intraductal approaches to breast cancer. Breast Cancer Res Treat 97:285–291

Nakama S (1991) Comparative studies on ultrasonogram with histological structure of breast cancer: an examination in the invasive process of breast cancer and the fixation to the skin. In: Kasumi F, Ueno E (eds) Topic in breast ultrasound. Shinohara, Tokyo

Stavros T (2006) Breast ultrasound. Lippincott, Philadelphia

Teboul M, Halliwell M (1995) Atlas of ultrasound and ductal echography of the breast. Blackwell Science, Oxford

Teboul M (2004) Practical ductal echography. Medgen, S.A. Madrid, Spain

Tot T (2003) The diffuse type of invasive lobular carcinoma of the breast: morphology and prognosis. Virchows Arch 443:718–724

Tot T (2007a) Clinical relevance of the distribution of the lesions in 500 consecutive breast cancer cases documented in large–format histologic sections. Cancer 110:2551–2560

Tot T (2007b) The theory of the sick breast lobe and the possible consequences. Int J Surg Pathol 1:68–71

The Lobar Distribution of the Lesions in Breast Carcinoma: Ductoscopy and Surgery

9

William C. Dooley

9.1 Introduction

Breast ductoscopy is an evolving field of surgical technical expertise and a new method of access to the earliest premalignant and malignant lesions for breast cancer researchers. Clinical endoscopy has rapidly improved over the last 40 years and offered researchers and clinicians access to many epithelial surfaces at risk for cancer. In the early 1990s, with the advent of submillimeter endoscopes, this approach could finally be used to examine the breast ductal epithelium. In a period of less than 2 decades, we have through clinical use been able to make direct observations of anatomy and the relationship of anatomy to the processes of breast cancer carcinogenesis. Whether unifocal or multifocal, breast cancers seem to arise within only a single ductal tree. The grade and presence or absence of angiogenesis seem to be associated with lesions in radically different regions of the ducto-lobular tree. Currently, our biopsy tools are rudimentary, but as these improve, the ability to genetically map the sequence of events during carcinogenesis up and down the ductal tree offers perhaps one of the most exciting avenues for increasing understanding or breast cancer carcinogenesis.

9.2 History of Early Ductoscopy

Early in the 1990s, Okazaki and others began to attempt breast ductoscopy for symptomatic pathologic nipple discharge using the first endoscopes less than 2 mm in diameter (Okazaki et al. 1991; Okazaki et al. 2007). As the technology improved and scopes about 1 mm in diameter could be fashioned, they met with greater success at actually canulating the offending orifice and successfully navigating to the lesion of interest present as a polyp or change in the intraluminal surface of the breast duct (Shen et al. 2000; Shao and Nguyen 2001; Matsunaga et al. 2001; Yamamoto et al. 2001a; Yamamoto et al. 2001b). In the Oriental population, nipple fluid abnormalities were a more common presenting symptom of breast cancer and these new scopes offered a way to superficially localize a lesion for diagnostic biopsy. Problems relating to poor image quality and glare/refraction related to air insufflation of the duct limited this new technology's use. Further, since most identified lesions could only be removed via open surgical biopsy, the ductoscopy was only serving as the equivalent of needle localization for a mammographic abnormality.

Important understandings of ductal involvement by cancer and the anatomy of these changes were however being revealed. Dr. Love and her colleagues went on to attempt ductoscopy using the Japanese scopes in the first US trial (Love and Barsky 1996; Love and Barsky 2004). This directly led to recognition of the ability to wash cells from intraductal proliferative lesions and the beginnings of modern attempts of ductal lavage. It was out of the evaluation trial of a ductal lavage system where I got involved. Quickly in the ductal lavage trial participants at my institution, we accumulated several with frankly malignant or suspicious cells reproducibly being lavaged from a single duct orifice. In spite of our best available imaging modalities, we were unable to identify the source of the cells more precisely. I searched for available submillimeter scopes and found one made by an American manufacturer. Using this scope and the principles of

W.C. Dooley
Division of Surgical Oncology, Department of Surgery,
The University of Oklahoma Health Sciences Center,
Oklahoma City, OK, USA
e-mail: william-dooley@ouhsc.edu

T. Tot (ed.), *Breast Cancer*, DOI: 10.1007/978-1-84996-314-5_9,
© Springer-Verlag London Limited 2011

saline ductal distension developed during the ductal lavage trial, I was able to identify the lesion of interest in each of these cases (Dooley 2000). A short series of scope use in patients having surgery with pathologic nipple discharge abnormalities quickly demonstrated ductoscopy's potential value to a breast surgeon in diagnostic and therapeutic planning (Yamamoto et al. 2001a).

9.3 Ductoscopy in Breast Cancer Cases – Lessons Learned

When I first began ductoscopy in the routine management of early-stage breast cancer where a fluid-producing duct could be identified, I quickly learned some important anatomy of the breast and how to identify ducts and positions within the ductal tree containing cancer (Dooley 2002; Dooley 2003). First was the ductal anatomy and duct distribution, as has been described in Dr. Love's chapter. Most upper outer quadrant lesions would be associated with a large branching lobar-ductal complex with a single orifice on the periphery of the nipple papilla plateau from 8:00 to 2:00 o'clock positions. Lesions greater than 2 cm in size clinically or radiographically rarely had ducts that could be identified by breast massage and compression to contain fluid unless they were associated with extensive intraductal component. In general, these lesions with a large halo of peripheral proliferative changes were the easiest ducts to identify as fluid producing. Core biopsy or open biopsy could lead to difficulty in identifying the correct orifice of the lobar-ductal unit by fluid production on the nipple surface.

Once the target duct had been chosen for endoscopy, I used intraductal distension with local anesthetic. The ductal branches of the lobar unit, which dilated the most under this topical anesthetic use were almost always associated with the most proliferative subsegments of ductal breast tissue. Scoping the largest branches would take you to the cancer and precancerous changes quickly. Small side branches rarely if ever were found to have significant proliferative changes. Often invasive cancers would seemingly purse-string the duct shut but tapping the obstruction with the scope – the palpable or ultrasound visible tumor could be seen to move. Some invasive tumors would have grossly ulcerated lesions visible but this was rarer.

Over 40% of early-stage breast cancers had significant intraluminal growths arising in the region of the known tumor and extending well beyond 1 cm beyond the known radiographic and or clinical target cancer (Dooley 2002). Most of these cases had frank extensive intraductal component (EIC) but some would have only multiple foci of atypical ductal hyperplasia (ADH) or of florid usual ductal hyperplasia. Unfortunately, the visual appearance of the intraductal growths on endoscopy did not perfectly correlate to the eventual histologic findings if that region was entirely removed.

In general, intraluminal growths fell into several categories, large spongiform lesions with a distinct stalk were usually solitary papillomas (Shen et al. 2000; Khan et al. 2002; Dooley 2005; Moncrief et al. 2005; Sauter 2005; Sauter et al. 2005; Valdes et al. 2005). Ridging and furrowing of the ductal wall usually occurred only in the larger and more central ducts. These abnormalities usually were either low-grade ductal carcinoma in situ (DCIS) or columnar or florid ductal hyperplasia. Intraductal growths that were peripheral and had evidence of angiogenesis by localized hyperemia were likely to be ADH or DCIS (solid or with comedonecrosis). Exophytic growths fitting these categories only occurred very distally in the ductal tree. Occasionally, sessile hyperemic patches were visible in larger ducts – where few and widely scattered ones were associated with ADH. In general, if lesions were numerous in a region, there was a high chance of diagnosis of DCIS when the entire region was excised. Rare patients had small frond like growths – usually white – resembling sea anemones. These could be either micropapillomas, micropapillary hyperplasia, or micropapillary DCIS. When present again, the multiplicity of lesions greatly increased the chances of DCIS diagnosis. Invasive ductal grade 3 cancers seemed always isolated to a small distal ductal branch. In contrast, grade 1 ductal, tubular, colloid, etc. seemed much more likely to be associated with a large central main ductal trunk.

For the purposes of lumpectomy, I mapped the proliferative activity and resected the known cancer and all intraluminal growths associated with it under ductoscopic guidance (Dooley et al. 2004). Most cancers were peripheral, and all visible proliferative activity was limited to a ductal subbranch, which could be easily resected to the periphery of the breast tissue. Some cancers had associated proliferative changes in several ductal subunits of the same lobar system. Usually, the extent and type of proliferative change was quite different in each subunit. I theorized from this that there were stem cells scattered throughout the lobular unit having the same initiation events but responding locally differently to progression events. I saw a number of patients described radiographically as either multifocal or multicentric on mammography and MRI imaging. In over 1,500 cases, I have never found a single early-stage breast cancer where additional non-contiguous cancers were not endoscopically shown to be connected to the same lobar-ductal tree. This may be an important observation (Okazaki et al. 1991; Dooley 2002; Kapenhas-Valdes et al. 2008) supporting an alternative breast carcinogenesis model such as the lobar theory.

In follow-up of patients managed by endoscopically directed segmental lumpectomy removing all diseased branches of the same lobar-ductal tree as the primary cancer, I have been able to drop local recurrence to less than 1/10 that of traditional breast conservation in those patients without lympho-vascular invasion (LVI). This now actually leaves me with this subcategory of breast conservation patients approximating the local failure rates of mastectomy patients who also lack LVI.

German ductoscopists have been able to reproduce findings similar to mine in breast cancer lumpectomies (Hünerbein et al. 2006a; Hünerbein et al. 2006b; Hünerbein et al. 2007; Grunwald et al. 2007; Jacobs et al. 2007a; Jacobs et al. 2007b). Some American groups have not but each made I believe a classic assumption error (Louie et al. 2006; Kim et al. 2004). These groups believed that if routine pathology did not find either DCIS or invasive cancer – the other proliferative activity was unimportant. Their basis seemed reasonable in that older pathology series suggest that positive margins for ADH or usual ductal hyperplasia are unimportant to local recurrence. Unfortunately, pathologists are not examining but minute fractions of the epithelial surfaces of the ductal tree. Routine pathology then greatly underestimates coexistent proliferative disease so as to confuse these other series conclusions. Many times I find and photograph intraductal lesions and have to send my pathologist back several times for recuts before the visual findings I make can be histologically explained adequately. More recent studies suggesting the sinister nature of widespread noncontiguous ADH for future ipsilateral breast cancer events suggest that my endoscopically driven assumptions may be closer to reality.

9.4 Conclusions

Using the lobar hypothesis, data are now being generated, which would substantially change our approach to breast lumpectomy. When there is a field defect, there may be value in resection of the entire lobar unit or subunit involved. This cannot be defined well using mere pathologic distance measurements to prove adequacy of lumpectomy. We may need to genetically map the extent of carcinogenic changes within the lobe to develop the most rational approach to anatomic correct lumpectomy.

References

Dooley WC (2000) Endoscopic visualization of breast tumors. JAMA 284:1518

Dooley WC (2002) Routine operative breast endoscopy for bloody nipple discharge. Ann Surg Oncol 9:920–923

Dooley WC (2003) Routine operative breast endoscopy during lumpectomy. Ann Surg Oncol 10:38–42

Dooley WC (2005) The future prospect: ductoscopy-directed brushing and biopsy. Clin Lab Med 25:845–850

Dooley WC, Spiegel A, Cox C, Henderson R, Richardson L, Zabora J (2004) Ductoscopy: defining its role in the management of breast cancer. Breast J 10:271–272

Grunwald S, Heyer H, Paepke S, Schwesinger G, Schimming A, Hahn M, Thomas A, Jacobs VR, Ohlinger R (2007) Diagnostic value of ductoscopy in the diagnosis of nipple discharge and intraductal proliferations in comparison to standard methods. Onkologie 30:243–248

Hünerbein M, Raubach M, Gebauer B, Schneider W, Schlag PM (2006a) Intraoperative ductoscopy in women undergoing surgery for breast cancer. Surgery 139:833–838

Hünerbein M, Raubach M, Gebauer B, Schneider W, Schlag PM (2006b) Ductoscopy and intraductal vacuum assisted biopsy in women with pathologic nipple discharge. Breast Cancer Res Treat 99:301–307

Hünerbein M, Dubowy A, Raubach M, Gebauer B, Topalidis T, Schlag P (2007) Gradient index ductoscopy and intraductal biopsy of intraductal breast lesions. Am J Surg 194:511–514

Jacobs VR, Paepke S, Ohlinger R, Grunwald S, Kiechle-Bahat M (2007a) Breast ductoscopy: technical development from a diagnostic to an interventional procedure and its future perspective. Onkologie 30:545–549

Jacobs VR, Paepke S, Schaaf H, Weber BC, Kiechle-Bahat M (2007b) Autofluorescence ductoscopy: a new imaging technique for intraductal breast endoscopy. Clin Breast Cancer 7:619–623

Kapenhas-Valdes E, Feldman SM, Boolbol SK (2008) The role of mammary ductoscopy in breast cancer: a review of the literature. Ann Surg Oncol 15:3350–3360

Khan SA, Baird C, Staradub VL, Morrow M (2002) Ductal lavage and ductoscopy: the opportunities and the limitations. Clin Breast Cancer 3:185–191

Kim JA, Crowe JP, Woletz J, Dinunzio A, Kelly T, Dietz JR (2004) Prospective study of intraoperative mammary ductoscopy in patients undergoing partial mastectomy for breast cancer. Am J Surg 188:411–414

Louie LD, Crowe JP, Dawson AE, Lee KB, Baynes DL, Dowdy T, Kim JA (2006) Identification of breast cancer in patients with pathologic nipple discharge: does ductoscopy predict malignancy? Am J Surg 192:530–533

Love SM, Barsky SH (1996) Brest-duct endoscopy to study stages of cancerous breast disease. Lancet 348:997–999

Love SM, Barsky SH (2004) Anatomy of the nipple and breast ducts revisited. Cancer 101:1947–1957

Matsunaga T, Ohta D, Misaka T, Hosokawa K, Fujii M, Kaise H, Kusama M, Koyanagi Y (2001) Mammary ductoscopy for diagnosis and treatment of intraductal lesions of the breast. Breast Cancer 8:213–221

Moncrief RM, Nayar R, Diaz LK, Staradub VL, Morrow M, Khan SA (2005) A comparison of ductoscopy-guided and conventional surgical excision in women with spontaneous nipple discharge. Ann Surg 241:575–581

Okazaki A, Okazaki M, Asaishi K, Satoh H, Watanabe Y, Mikami T, Toda K, Okazaki Y, Nabeta K, Hirata K, Narimatsu E (1991) Fiberoptic ductoscopy of the breast: a new diagnostic procedure for nipple discharge. Jpn J Clin Oncol 21:188–193

Okazaki A, Okazaki M, Watanabe Y, Hirata K (2007) Diagnostic significance of mammary ductoscopy for early breast cancer. Nippon Rinsho 65(Suppl6):295–297

Sauter E (2005) Breast cancer detection using mammary ductoscopy. Future Oncol 1:385–393

Sauter ER, Ehya H, Klein-Szanto AJ, Wagner-Mann C, MacGibbon B (2005) Fiberoptic ductoscopy findings in women with and without spontaneous nipple discharge. Cancer 103:914–921

Shao ZM, Nguyen M (2001) Nipple aspiration in diagnosis of breast cancer. Semin Surg Oncol 20:175–180

Shen K, Lu J, Yuan J, Wu G, Zhang J, Han Q, Shen Z (2000) Fiberoptic ductoscopy for patients with intraductal papillary lesions. Zhonghua Wai Ke Za Zhi 38:275–277

Valdes EK, Feldman SM, Balassanian R, Cohen JM, Boolbol SK (2005) Diagnosis of recurrent breast cancer by ductoscopy. Breast J 11:506

Yamamoto D, Shoji T, Kawanishi H, Nakagawa H, Haijima H, Gondo H, Tanaka K (2001a) A utility of ductography and fiberoptic ductoscopy for patients with nipple discharge. Breast Cancer Res Treat 70:103–108

Yamamoto D, Ueda S, Senzaki H, Shoji T, Haijima H, Gondo H, Tanaka K (2001b) New diagnostic approach to intracystic lesions of the breast by fiberoptic ductoscopy. Anticancer Res 21:4113–4116

Stop Breast Cancer Now! Imagining Imaging Pathways Toward Search, Destroy, Cure, and Watchful Waiting of Premetastasis Breast Cancer

10

Richard Gordon

"Progress in breast cancer… usually occurs by 'gilding the lily' – generating incremental improvements – as opposed to the introduction of dramatic new innovations (Freya Schnabel, personal communication, 1998)" (Lerner 2001).

10.1 Introduction

Tibor Tot has given me an unusual opportunity via his request to summarize my work in computed tomography (CT), which indeed since 1977 has been directed toward eliminating the scourge of breast cancer via search and destroy of premetastasis tumors, instead of the predominant, century-old magic bullet approach (Strebhardt and Ullrich 2008). I have had the strange career of a theoretical biologist (Fig. 10.1) on a continent where theoretical biology as a paid discipline died with James F. Danielli, discoverer of the bilayer structure of the cell membrane, and once Director of the Center for Theoretical Biology at the State University of New York at Buffalo and founding editor of the *Journal of Theoretical Biology* (JTB) (Danielli 1961; Rosen 1985; Stein 1986). Danielli became part of my story, which I will tell in the spirit of the wonderful biography of Louis Pasteur written by his lifetime laboratory assistant (Duclaux 1920). Lacking such a long-term companion to my train of thought, this shall have to be unabashedly

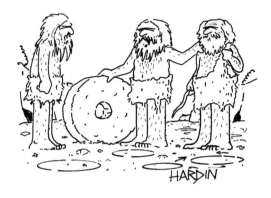

"To be honest, I would have never invented the wheel if not for Urg's ground breaking theoretical work with the circle."

Fig. 10.1 The fate of the theoretical biologist (Hardin 2003) (Reproduced with paid permission of CartoonStock)

autobiographical, with all the risks attendant to that form of literature. I shall try to be honest to you, the reader, and true to myself. If we consider the vast gossamer of activity in science, and CT in particular, my own path is but one thread through that web, but the one I know best. Nevertheless, when I use "I," please take it as shorthand for "I and my cited collaborators" where appropriate. My world line has crossed that of many others, who have enriched my journey, and made it possible. This includes George Gamow, Mr. World Line himself (Gamow 1970), both of us sitting in on a meteorology course in Boulder, Colorado about 1968, and later his son Igor at Woods Hole and Boulder regarding trying to model the growth of *Phycomyces* (Ortega et al. 1974).

R. Gordon
Department of Radiology, University of Manitoba,
Winnipeg, Manitoba, Canada
e-mail: gordonr@cc.umanitoba.ca

T. Tot (ed.), *Breast Cancer*, DOI: 10.1007/978-1-84996-314-5_10,
© Springer-Verlag London Limited 2011

10.2 3D Electron Microscopy

I was introduced to the problem of "reconstruction from projections" when I met Cyrus Levinthal (Levinthal 1968), my future postdoctoral supervisor (Department of Biological Sciences, Columbia University), at the Marine Biological Laboratory, Woods Hole, Massachusetts, in 1968, where I took the Embryology Course the following summer, a year later. Cyrus very wisely posed the problem of getting the 3D structure of a protein molecule from a tilt series of electron microscope images, without telling me that anyone else was working on it. The intersection of embryology, my first career (Gordon 1966), with breast cancer and Tot, is told in the Epilogue to this book (Gordon 2010). Let me just say that Woods Hole is a cauldron of intellectual activity every summer. While there in 1969, I also heard a talk by Albert Szent-Györgyi (Szent-Györgyi 1960, 1972) on banana peels, redox reactions and cancer, whose story of being turned down by NIH for a one-line grant application "I want to find a cure for cancer," *after* he received the Nobel prize, was conveyed to me on a long walk with Shinya Inoué (Inoué et al. 1986). This was seminal in my long and continuing battle to democratize science and prevent peer review from suppressing innovation (Gordon 1993; Poulin and Gordon 2001; Gordon and Poulin 2009a, b) as a member of the Canadian Association for Responsible Research Funding (Forsdyke 2009). Indeed, peer review is what has slowed my work on detection of breast cancer more than any other factor, and forced most of it to be theory rather than testing of that theory with real equipment and patients. This accounts for the word "imagining" in my title.

To reduce the selectiveness of my memory of events and my own thought process, I will go through my relevant papers in roughly chronological order, using them to weave this story, commenting on them in retrospect.

The work with Cyrus Levinthal, 1968-1969, was done on an expensive computer that would probably not stand up to any later handheld electronic calculator in speed, the latter device long since absorbed itself into laptop computers and cell phones. Thus, I had to be satisfied with attempting to reconstruct an array of numbers that could barely portray an image: 10×10 pixels. I worked with parallel projections, and came to think of the rows of parallel rays as if they were tracks for the tongs of a rake pulling pebbles across a Japanese rock garden (Fig. 10.2). This conception may have come to me before or during a seminar by Aaron Klug

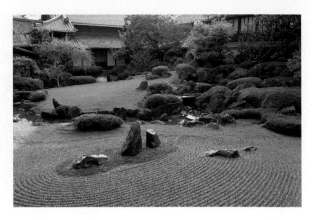

Fig. 10.2 A Japanese rock garden with the pebbles raked into rows that, if parallel, would correspond to a projection (From Wikipedia Contributors (2009), with permission under GFDL (GNU Free Documentation License) + creative commons 2.5)

that Levinthal sponsored, in which Klug talked about his Fourier approach to reconstruction from projections. That was the first time I knew anyone else was working on the problem. As Klug was much my senior, this created some sense of competition and importance of the problem beyond its intrinsic interest. We were to cross swords later.

At the time, few proteins could be crystallized, a necessary step for 3D reconstruction by the Fourier methods of x-ray crystallography championed by Max Perutz with his determination of the 3D structure of hemoglobin (Perutz 1990, 1998). Levinthal's goal was to open all proteins to structural determination via 3D electron microscopy, without the need for crystallization. Klug's approach to reconstruction from projections clearly grew out of the crystallography tradition, as did that of Ramachandran (Ramachandran and Lakshminarayanan 1971), but mine did not (Fig. 10.2). Perhaps the visit of a Japanese artist to the Art Institute of Chicago, where I took lessons when I was in my early teens, was in the back of my mind.

10.3 In Search of Phantoms

In CT, we have always been faced with the problem of suitable phantoms, that is, images of precisely known structure that nevertheless reasonably represent the real problem of determining the unknown structure (barring vivisection) of tissues within an individual person. There were no algorithms for generating complex pictures in those days, such as we now take for granted in 3D animation, rendering, and fractals. In New York, I did manage to get access to some of the first satellite pictures of clouds, whose textures I imagined might roughly represent that of cloud-like electron micrographs of 30-nm wide protein images, which were themselves generally casts in uranyl acetate stained with osmium tetroxide (a fixative I learned to handle with respect in Levinthal's lab). During that brief academic year I also learned about nuclear emulsions and their ability to track single emitted particles when used for autoradiography, and tried to visualize vitamin B_6 with a field ion emission microscope, a wonderful instrument in which He ions create the image one by one of all the activity on the tip of a metal needle on a phosphorescent screen, in the laboratory of Eugene S. Machlin (Machlin et al. 1975). Individual tip atoms, magnified a million times without optics, could be seen in real time using a photomultiplier tube. Earlier I had viewed the electron microscopy images of single uranium atoms and evidence of their diffusion in the lab of Albert V. Crewe (Wall et al. 1974; Isaacson et al. 1977) when I was an undergraduate at the University of Chicago. He later cited my CT work (Crewe and Crewe 1984). In retrospect, I can see that these "hands on" experiences, watching single atoms move, got me used to the idea of building up images from one quantum (particle or photon) at a time.

I did not solve the raking problem until I moved on to the Center for Theoretical Biology in Buffalo, where I postdoced with Robert Rosen because of a mutual interest in morphogenesis (Goel et al. 1970). Rosen gave me the academic freedom to pursue whatever I wanted. Confused about the difference between "computer center" and the new field of "computer science," I asked Computer Science Assistant Professor Gabor Herman about how to get computer time, and told him about the reconstruction problem I wanted to continue working on. A week later he was working on it, so I decided to collaborate with him.

In this computer science milieu, the raked pebbles were replaced by raked bits, whose sums had to add up to given projections, and thus we soon submitted our first paper on a Monte Carlo approach to reconstruction from projections that actually worked (Gordon and Herman 1971).

For a test pattern (phantom), in the spirit of the American civil rights movement of the time, I took a photographic print of a young black girl named "Judy,"

taken by Judith Carmichael, whose husband Jack was my host for a 1968 summer postdoc (Gordon et al. 1972), and found a lab with a photometer. I moved the print to 2,500 positions and read the voltmeter 2,500 times to produce a 50×50 pixel image. This was my first satisfactory phantom. Faces make good phantoms because we are so attuned to seeing distortions in them, making artifacts stand out.

While a number of increasingly sophisticated computer-simulated breast phantoms have been produced (Taylor and Owens 2001; Bakic et al. 2002a, b, 2003; Bliznakova et al. 2002, 2003, 2006; Taylor 2002; Hoeschen et al. 2005; Reiser et al. 2006; Zhou et al. 2006; Shorey 2007; Han et al. 2008; Li et al. 2009), I prefer the real thing (O'Connor et al. 2008). Perhaps the best x-ray phantom, the ultimate in "ground truth," would be a 3D map of the atomic composition of a breast, because x-ray absorption and scattering are primarily atomic and not molecular quantum phenomena. For the same reason, such a phantom would serve almost as well for magnetic resonance imaging (MRI), but not for ultrasound or electrical impedance tomography (EIT) or magnetic resonance spectroscopy (MRS), which measure molecular properties. I would like to propose that we create such "atomic breast phantoms" with petrographic methods. If we sectioned a cadaver breast, removing or etching away one planar slice after another, and imaged the exposed face of the remaining specimen, then we could get 3D data. Cooling or freezing might be needed during sectioning to have sufficient tissue rigidity. This would also preserve the tissue from bacterial degradation. To get atomic composition and do the etching, the ideal would be to put the open face in a large secondary ion mass spectrometer (SIMS), and get the full atomic composition at each voxel over the whole face (Hallégot et al. 2006). Voxel size should be chosen to be below the target resolution of any future 3D breast imaging modality (see below).

10.4 The Origin of ART

Robert Bender (Bender and Duck 1982) joined the Center for Theoretical Biology as a graduate student, and we became close friends. I had long been aware of the outstanding problem of protein synthesis from the University of Chicago work of Victor Fried (Haselkorn and Fried 1964) when we were both undergraduate students there in the Department of Biophysics, and later graduate students together at the University of Oregon. The problem boiled down to the questions of what are ribosomes and how do they work? I had done a Monte Carlo simulation of ribosomes moving along messenger RNA (Gordon 1969). Bender contacted David Sabatini (Sabatini 2005) and obtained a tilt series of electron micrographs of ribosomes from him. In the meantime, I had realized, probably because of my thesis work with Terrell L. Hill in statistical mechanics, that the Monte Carlo approach to reconstruction from projections (Gordon and Herman 1971) had a deterministic average, which could be expressed by a set of simultaneous linear equations. This new approach needed a name.

Bender and I loved to pun incessantly. He came up with Fast Algebraic Reconstruction Technique, which I toned down to ART, pleased with that acronym because I had been reared by an artist (Gordon 1979a). Boris K. Vainshtein (1972, personal communication) (Vainshtein 1971) later told me with delight that the acronym ART works in Russian too (and that he too was Jewish, while I used my opportunity in the Soviet Union to attend a Refusnik seminar with other members of the Committee of Concerned Scientists). ART Intended for Storage Tubes (ARTIST) later became the name of my first PET (positron emission tomography) algorithm (Gordon 1975c, 1983a). ARTIST used coincidence events (pairs of simultaneously emitted gamma rays traveling in opposite directions) and was my first published foray into imaging with single quantum events, producing a plausible reconstruction of a phantom with only 1,000 events. It was later made more sophisticated, using density estimation methods, by Barbara Pawlak (Pawlak and Gordon 2005, 2010). See below.

10.5 Youth Pursuing a Nobel Prize

There was urgency to our work, because we felt we were about to crack the problem of ribosome structure and function, the big molecular biology prize of the day. Being in my 20s, a bit more full of myself than I think I am now, I rehearsed my Nobel Prize speech in my head, or considered the chutzpah of declining it for long forgotten reasons associated with my opposition to and joining protests against the Vietnam War. In fact, Hill and I, earlier, had an escape route to Sweden

planned for me, to work with physical chemist Hugo Theorell, in case I got drafted. I had already just escaped the draft with the aid of my first graduate advisor, Aaron Novick (Novick and Szilard 1950).

But Bender and I had a problem: how to display our results? I had mastered overprinting to the point of once slicing across a half-meter-wide ink ribbon (cf. Gordon et al. 1976). Overprinting is the long forgotten skill of halting a chain printer so that more than one character struck the same spot. But the results were poor in terms of image quality. Bender located a prototype computer image printer at Xerox headquarters in Rochester, New York, which unfortunately only read paper tapes. So we drove from Buffalo to Ottawa with magnetic tapes, in Bender's car with a broken radiator that required frequent refilling with water, converted it to paper tapes at the National Research Council, and then drove to Xerox, where they allowed us to stay overnight reading in the paper tapes and printing our pictures.

The result was two papers, back to back, on the theory of ART and its application to ribosomes, in Danielli's JTB (Bender et al. 1970; Gordon et al. 1970), and the images for the earlier Monte Carlo work, which appeared subsequently (Gordon and Herman 1971). In the course of writing these I came to realize that the same method should work for x-rays, and thus included the naive "… and x-ray photography" in the title of the theory paper, as "radiography" was not yet in my active vocabulary. That was the beginning of my medical career:

"In body-section radiography (Kane 1953) the X-ray source and the film are moved in a coordinated fashion so that only one plane in the patient in between does not blur out. If our methods were used instead, the X-rays need only go across the plane of interest. The tissues above and below need not be exposed. By photometric reading of a fluorescent screen, the intensities could be passed directly to a small computer, and the reconstructed section displayed on a television screen within a minute or so. In effect, our methods provide rapid cross-sectioning of an object, without cutting…. The new method is easily generalized to nonparallel rays, which may occur in X-ray photography" (Gordon et al. 1970).

We did not attract the attention of the electron microscopists working on ribosomes. For example, we knew we could have reconstructed the structure of various subsets of ribosome components (Nomura 1987), to build a 3D map of where each was located. But divorces, collapse of the Center for Theoretical Biology, and dispersion of my collaborators killed the project. I moved on to NIH (U.S. National Institutes of

Health), with the help of Hill, who had moved there himself, and in 1972 became an "Expert" in the Mathematical Research Branch, National Institute of Arthritis, Metabolism and Digestive Diseases. While I made an attempt to deal with arrays of ribosomes with Marcello Barbieri (Barbieri et al. 1970), my request to set up a densitometer facility at NIH just led to hostility, as a proper flatbed scanner (now $50) cost a good fraction of a million dollars at that time. Although in my early 30s (born 1943), with a hiring freeze in long effect, I was a mere impudent youngster at NIH.

10.6 Dose Reduction in CT

Important lessons for radiology came out of this work from the electron microscopy. The electron beam damaged the ribosomes, which was apparent from the decreasing contrast in a tilt series (Bender et al. 1970). Thus, I learned directly about the consequences of dose, though my attitudes toward ionizing radiation had also been set by a high school essay on the first nuclear bomb (Gordon 1960).

For reconstruction from tomography, the fewer views the better, in terms of dose. On the other hand, for a given total dose, this meant that there is an optimization problem to be solved, as:

$$\text{Total dose} = \text{dose per view} \times \text{number of views}$$

This brings us right back to the quantum imaging problem, as a large number of noisy views, with few photons per view (in the limit, just one photon or quantum event per view, as in the ARTIST algorithm, Gordon 1975c, 1983a), might prove optimal. But this requires an algorithm that is less noise sensitive than either ART or filtered back projection (FBP). So finding the optimal number of views is still an open problem. Nowadays, this is seen as a subset of the more general compressive imaging or compressive sensing problem (Candes and Wakin 2008; Ramlau et al. 2008; Romberg 2008; Sidky and Pan 2008; Carron 2009; Pan et al. 2009; Yu et al. 2009).

The idea that CT dose reduction could be achieved through better algorithms (Gordon 1976b) rather than just adjusting patient positioning, exposure, and collimation parameters (Vock 2005), with the onus placed on the radiologist (Imhof et al. 2003), has yet to have any impact in medical practice, perhaps because the

CT algorithm (including raw data correction (Pan et al. 2009)) is regarded as a proprietary and mathematically obscure black box. The only company secret that CT manufacturers may have is that they have not done due diligence for dose reduction. Governments' approach seems to be to legislate the laws of physics (Krotz 1999).

Most of my work has focused on a few low noise views, a regime in which the ART algorithm does well, and much better than FBP (Herman and Rowland 1973; Barbieri 1974; Gordon and Herman 1974, Barbieri 1987). I have done CT with as few as three views. This was forced by our simple design of the first nevoscope to measure the depth of nevi (Dhawan et al. 1984b), the major prognostic factor for melanoma. While using just three views is undoubtedly suboptimal, my intuition suggests that for mammography we may find that 10–30 views do just fine (Wu et al. 2003; Sidky et al. 2006; Herman and Davidi 2008; Pan et al. 2009; Qian et al. 2009; Jia et al. 2010). If correct, this leads to the possibility of a CT scanner configuration consisting of a fixed array of a few x-ray sources aimed at detector arrays (Gordon 1985b), such as has been prototyped for breast tomosynthesis (Qian et al. 2009). The Mayo Clinic Dynamic Spatial Reconstructor consisted of 28 rotating x-ray sources (Altschuler et al. 1980), so these numbers are plausible. The extra cost of the x-ray sources might be more than offset by the scanner having no moving parts.

Another lesson came from the limited tilt range then available for the tilt stage in electron microscopes: images could indeed be reconstructed without a full 180° angle range, but they had anisotropic resolution that perhaps could be corrected for. The answer of how to do this came some time later, from the nevoscopy work, as described below.

10.7 More Equations than Data

It became clear, with the CT problem seen as solving simultaneous linear equations, that we had far fewer equations than unknowns, yet could still get reasonable reconstructed images, as judged by their comparison with the original phantom. In other words, when reconstructing n^2 pixels for an $n \times n$ picture, we could use m projections, where $m \ll n$ ($\ll$ means "much less than"). In contrast, Klug's Fourier approach was to interpolate in Fourier space, which required uniform sampling of views around the specimen at closely spaced angular intervals. The ground was set for conflict:

"DeRosier & Klug (DeRosier and Klug 1968) have given a Fourier method for the reconstruction of three-dimensional objects from electron micrographs. Unfortunately, there are limitations on their method, which make it practical only for highly symmetrical objects [for which one view provides data for many]. They estimate that in order to obtain a 30 Å reconstruction of a 250 Å ribosome, electron micrographs would have to be taken at approximately 30 different angles, on a stage capable of tilting ±90°. This number of pictures, if taken by ordinary electron microscopy, would destroy the ribosome and cover it with a thick layer of dirt from the microscope chamber. We will present an entirely new, direct method, an Algebraic Reconstruction Technique (ART), which has the following advantages over the Fourier method: (1) the ART method works readily for completely asymmetric objects; (2) it produces considerable detail of such objects with only 5 to 10 views; (3) ordinary tilting stages may be used, since the views may be taken over a relatively small range of angles (±30°); (4) computing time is approximately 30 seconds per section on a Control Data 6400; (5) small computers may be used, since little storage is required; (6) ART is directly applicable to macroscopic X-ray photography, and should require considerably less radiation than present methods of body-section radiography (Kane 1953).... 30 views over a 180° span would... correspond to solving for the ρ_{ij}'s on an 8×8 grid. It is clear that we are doing considerably better than this with only five views over a 60° span [on a 50×50 pixel image]" (Gordon et al. 1970).

Klug attacked with a long rebuttal of our work submitted to Danielli for publication, but also widely distributed as a preprint around the world. Danielli had been upset by how his friend, Maurice H.F. Wilkins (Wade 2004), had been sidelined in the hoopla over the structure of DNA (even though he received the Nobel Prize with James Watson and Francis Crick), and Klug was from the same community. But Danielli's only action was to delay publication of Klug's letter long enough to give us a month to respond in the same issue of JTB. In the meantime, Klug submitted a much toned down version. We responded by quoting from the original, because of the preprint distribution. To Klug's "ART and science" (Crowther and Klug 1971) we argued forcibly that "ART is science" (Bellman et al. 1971). We included a few nonverbal jabs, reconstructing an image of Klug taken from a *Time Magazine* issue, one of a fashion model who had accompanied Bender on a visit to Klug before this episode, who had unnerved him, and mitochondria in the shape of a star of David, as Bender, Klug, and I are all Jewish. Finally, S.H. Bellman, our lead author, was the bellman in Lewis Carroll's epic poem "The Hunting of the Snark." He

had been our mascot, as computer programming errors in our SNARK program, of which I wrote the early versions in Fortran II (Herman 2009), often produced images that were "a perfect and absolute blank" (Carroll 1876; Bellman 1970). In retrospect, we may have delayed Klug's Nobel Prize (Klug 1983), which was well deserved for much fine structural work on viruses, and I think we gained his respect, despite our young age, as he was cordial when we finally met years later. Klug even published a variant on ART (Crowther and Klug 1974). His complicated and dose hungry Fourier algorithm was apparently not used beyond his own laboratory, and ART was established as one way to solve the reconstruction problem.

10.8 Putting ART in Its Place

In the face of our chutzpah, we were to be humbled a bit too, when mathematicians later pointed out that ART, at least in its linear form, was a special case of Kaczmarz's general method for solving simultaneous linear equations (Kaczmarz 1937; Groetsch 1999), its publication predating our births. However, the nonlinear positivity constraint (equivalent to saying that a patient does not emit x-rays) has proven to be of paramount importance, including in the parallel field of deconvolution of spectra (Jansson 1984, 1997). Furthermore, Geoffrey Hounsfield came up with an ART-like algorithm independently, which was used in the first commercial head scanner by his company, EMI (Hounsfield 1973, 1976).

Computers were very slow in the 1970s, and computing time was one roadblock to patient throughput, which, given the $1 million price tag on what came to be known as computerized axial tomography (CAT) or later CT scanners, was of major concern. The ART algorithm at that time took 10× as much computer time as the FBP algorithm, and furthermore a high-speed special purpose computer could be built for the FBP, hard wired for the recently discovered fast Fourier transform (FFT) (Cooley and Tukey 1965).

The history of FBP went back to physicist Allan Cormack (Cormack 1963, 1964) and x-ray crystallographer G.N. Ramachandran (Ramachandran and Lakshminarayanan 1971; Subramanian 2001). This algorithm is a numerical solution to Radon's equation (Radon 1917), which itself is a generalization of Abelian integration conceived around 1830 by Niels Henrik Abel (Houzel 2004). We can now think of Abel's integral equation (Gorenflo and Vessella 1991) as the math for CT of a cylindrically symmetric object, and indeed it has long been used in the investigation of the structure of cylindrical flames (Daun et al. 2006), though it is now being replaced by CT (Chen et al. 1997). Cormack (1980) got the Nobel Prize along with Hounsfield (1980). One group that was overlooked designed and built a CT scanner much earlier than Hounsfield (Kalos et al. 1961) (Fig. 10.3).

ART was used in the first paper on MRI (Lauterbur 1973), which led to the Nobel Prize for Paul Lauterbur, but it was later dropped for Fourier methods. It is used inside of medicine for cardiac imaging (Nielsen et al. 2005), ultrasonic diffraction tomography (Ladas and Devaney 1991, 1993), metal artifact reduction and local region reconstruction (Wang et al. 1996, 1999),

PET (Matej et al. 1994), and nevoscopy (Maganti and Dhawan 1997), and outside of medicine for the solar corona (Saez et al. 2007), the ionosphere (Cornely 2003; Wen et al. 2008), plasma physics (Kazantsev and Pickalov 1999; Wan et al. 2003), proton tomography (Li et al. 2006), crystal grain boundaries (Markussen et al. 2004), Bénard patterns (Subbarao et al. 1997a), thermally nonuniform fluids (Mishra et al. 1999), nondestructive testing (Subbarao et al. 1997b), spectroscopy (Song et al. 2006a, b), tracer gas concentration profiles (Park et al. 2000), electron microscopy of thick sections (Jonges et al. 1999), etc. Process tomography, in which one images complex flows possibly changing over time, also makes use of ART (Fellholter and Mewes 1994; Lee et al. 2009; Zhang et al. 2009). In answer to the mathematical

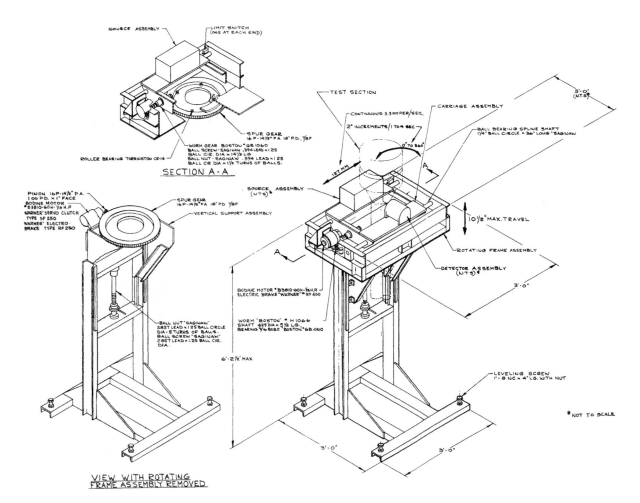

Fig. 10.3 The first CT scanner (Kalos et al. 1961), predating the conception of the EMI scanner (With permission of Malvin H. Kalos and the Office of Scientific and Technical Information, U.S. Department of Energy). The actual prototype, unfortunately, was not kept

purist, one could at least suggest that ART brought the Kaczmarz method into wide use.

I never gave up on ART, even as it faded from medical practice due to the speed of FBP, because of its versatility and demonstrated superiority with small numbers of views (Herman and Rowland 1973; Barbieri 1974, 1987; Gordon and Herman 1974). These properties of the algorithm may be the key to dose reduction and thus breast screening by CT, which later became my primary goal. ART persisted mostly as an academic exercise for many others, who have generated a literature of over 700 papers and some books (such as Marti 1979; Herman 1980; Eggermont et al. 1981; Trummer 1981, 1983; Andersen and Kak 1984; Byrne 1993, 2004; Watt 1994; Garcia et al. 1996; Mueller et al. 1997, 1998; Marabini et al. 1998; Guan et al. 1999; Mishra et al. 1999; Kak and Slaney 2001; Donaire and Garcia 2002; Kaipio and Somersalo 2004), many honestly mathematically over my head. It made a comeback as "cone beam ART" (Donaire and Garcia 1999; Nielsen et al. 2005), because of the failure of the Feldkamp FBP algorithm (Feldkamp et al. 1984) to handle the increasing cone angles between x-ray source and the array of detectors, as the number of rows of detectors kept increasing from 2 (Hounsfield 1973) to 320 (Pan et al. 2009). This is because ART can handle any geometry whatsoever (Gordon 1974). It can also be run on parallel computers, and my 1970s dream (Gordon et al. 1975) of running it on the harbinger 64 processor Illiac computer has been far exceeded on later parallel machines (Fitchett 1993; Garcia et al. 1996; Rajan and Patnaik 2001), backed by much new theory (Byrne 1996; Censor and Zenios 1997), including some I influenced (Martin et al. 2005).

10.9 Selling ART and Proselytizing CT

Bender and I presented our results to electron microscopists (Gordon and Bender 1971a) and started flogging our ideas for medical imaging to companies like Raytheon, Optronics, and Xerox, but with no takers. In retrospect, Hounsfield's success came about because he (Hounsfield 1973) was teamed up with a neurosurgeon (Ambrose 1973, 1974) (and did not have to seek grant support), whereas we and the earlier group of mathematicians (Kalos et al. 1961) were not then in medical circles. While we knew that "looking inside" the body was important, we had little depth of understanding why. But we learned.

While at NIH I had opportunities to travel to Switzerland (Gordon and Bender 1971b; Gordon 1972), Vienna (Gordon et al. 1971), and Moscow (Gordon and Kane 1972), where I visited crystallographer Boris K. Vainshtein. Vainshtein had devised simple optical additive reconstruction methods using film, mathematically identical to classical tomography and rotation tomography (Takahashi 1969), but made one crucial observation that has yet to be deliberately applied in CT: the point spread function (PSF) of fully 3D CT is much sharper than that of 2D (Vainshtein 1971): $1/r^2$ versus $1/r$, where r is the distance from any given point in the image (making deconvolution that much easier) (see Fig. 10.4). Any CT where the data is reconstructed plane by plane or slice by slice is therefore using far more x-ray dose than necessary (Gordon 1976b).

I was involved in two premature attempts to give a course on CT (Gordon and Bender 1971c; one with Z.H. Cho): no one registered. (Shortly thereafter courses proliferated, as the EMI scanner caught on.) So instead I published a tutorial (Gordon 1974), a full review of algorithms (Gordon and Herman 1974), a popular article (Gordon et al. 1975), and organized a session (Gordon and Lauterbur 1974) and then a conference (Gordon 1975b) on the wide range of applications of CT that were developing. The latter included the first comprehensive (and perhaps last such possible) bibliography on reconstruction from projections (Gordon 1975a). Because I was once an amateur astronomer, I was especially delighted to end up with a world tour of radio

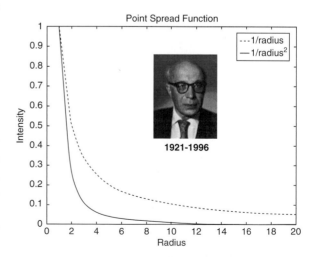

Fig. 10.4 Vainshtein's observation (Vainshtein 1971) that the point spread function of 3D reconstruction is sharper than that of 2D reconstruction (prepared by Michael J.A. Potter). Radius units are arbitrary, but the ratio of the two curves is not

astronomy observatories, a field that used much the same math to reconstruct its images (Gordon 1978b). Radio astronomers also contributed to medical CT (Bracewell 1977). I extended CT to the functioning of the brain itself, with visual receptive fields acting like rays in mental reconstruction of the image that falls on the retina (Gordon and Hirsch 1977; Gordon and Tweed 1983), and reached out to people interested in any and all applications of CT (Gordon and Rangaraj 1981).

My own presentation at the "Reconstruction from Projections" meeting (Gordon 1975c) introduced the idea of reconstructing an image from one photon or particle at a time; that is, a scanner would record one quantum event, and alter the image, before going to the next. The context was PET. The ordinary approach at that time was to place PET on the Procrustean bed of ordinary CT algorithms, define a ray as a strip through the patient between two detectors, and count the number of coincidence events falling into that strip. The result was a noisy, streaked reconstruction, due to the huge Poisson statistical fluctuations in these counts and the sensitivity of ordinary CT algorithms to noise. The detector widths had to be large (1-2 cm), reducing spatial resolution, not simply because they were expensive, but also because smaller detectors would produce noisy data well beyond the capacity of the CT algorithms. But in the ARTIST algorithm for PET, I envisaged the problem as one of estimating the location of the annihilation event along the coincidence line, an approach very much closer to the physics. The location chosen was influenced by the locations of the previously placed points, in a bootstrap manner. Barbara Pawlak later formalized and improved this approach using the now matured branch of statistics called density estimation (Pawlak and Gordon 2005, 2010; Pawlak 2007). New depth-of-interaction (DOI) detectors make it possible to localize each gamma ray within the detector (Shao et al. 2008), so that the coincidence line is much more sharply defined than the detector width.

The ARTIST concept also indirectly inspired a new approach to x-ray CT in which the scattered photons are additional sources of 3D and tissue composition data instead of being discarded (Bradford et al. 2002), potentially recorded one by one by energy discriminating detectors (as I learned was being done in x-ray astronomy (Garmire et al. 2003; Porter 2004)), permitting reconstruction of two images: absorption coefficient and electron density (Van Uytven et al. 2007, 2008), and further work is in progress on using scattered photons rather than discarding them by collimation or filtering (Alpuche Avilés et al. 2010).

10.10 The Challenge from Classical Tomography

It is worthwhile at this point to take a look back at classical tomography. Based on film, it always had superior and exquisite spatial resolution compared to CT. In fact, Hounsfield and Ambrose's first brain section CTs (Ambrose 1973; Hounsfield 1973) were inferior to rotational tomography brain sections produced in the 1940s (Takahashi 1969). The first prototype breast CT scanner (Chang et al. 1977, 1978) washed out the images of microcalcifications by a factor of 24,000 because of its large volume elements (1.56 mm×1.56 mm×10 mm) compared to their 0.1 mm diameter. Despite claims that it does not matter (Nab et al. 1992; Karssemeijer et al. 1993; Pachoud et al. 2005), we still have not achieved the resolution of film in digital mammography let alone CT (Chan et al. 1987; Nickoloff et al. 1990; Brettle et al. 1994; Kuzmiak et al. 2005; Yaffe et al. 2008) except in microCT for small animals, that is, with scanners far too small for the human body to fit in, and subjects for whom total radiation dose is a secondary consideration. In the late 1970s, attempts were made to overcome this spatial resolution limitation by doing CT from sinograms recorded directly onto film (Gmitro et al. 1980), but film scanner technology, then called microdensitometry, was itself then very expensive and labor intensive, so this step backward in instrumentation did not bring us forward. I have thus formulated a simple rule: if you can see a structure in a projection mammogram, there is no excuse not to see it in 3D CTM. No CT scanner has yet achieved this goal.

10.11 Underdetermined Equations

My undergraduate degree was in Mathematics from the University of Chicago, where I had taken a course on linear algebra from Alberto P. Calderón (Christ et al. 1998). Thus, I was keenly aware that in CT with ART we were taking the unusual step of solving for many more unknowns than we had equations. It may have been his belief that this was "impossible" (1974, personal communication) that constrained Hounsfield's use of his ART-like algorithm (Hounsfield 1975) to the overdetermined case, that is, many more projections than necessary, and this attitude may be the original cause of the high dose of CT to patients, because commercial medical scanners until recently have not deviated in concept from EMI's lead in turning away from

ART to FBP. In terms of dose for equivalent image quality: ART with fewer views « (is much less than) overdetermined ART which is about the same as FBP.

The consequences have been a significant increase in dose to populations due to CT (Huda 2002; Linton and Mettler 2003; Dawson 2004; Prokop 2005; Bertell et al. 2007; Colang et al. 2007). I did my own "back of the envelope" calculation a few years ago, given below. Breast CT may end up being the leader in correcting this situation, because no one has advocated any higher dose for 3D screening than the 2 mGy that has become the practice in ordinary mammography (Spelic 2009). (However, if we kept women with ataxia-telangiectasia (Hall et al. 1992; Ramsay et al. 1996, 1998) away from x-rays, the mean dose for the rest could be raised.) For example, Boone demonstrated that high-quality, high-resolution ($0.3 \times 0.3 \times 1.2$ mm^3 voxel) CT images of the pendant breast could be acquired at a mean glandular dose (MGD) equivalent to two-view mammography for women with breasts compressed to 5 cm (Boone et al. 2003), when using a very high energy x-ray beam typical of that of a body CT (120–140 kVp) (Chen and Ning 2002), so we have a hopeful, if not yet optimal, example. Synchrotron radiation, with the promise of future 10× dose reduction, has yielded diffraction-enhanced imaging CT (DEI-CT) slices with voxels $0.047 \times 0.047 \times 0.3$ mm^3 (Fiedler et al. 2004).

The problem with "underdetermined" equations is not that they have no solution, but on the contrary, that they have an infinity of solutions. This provides a potential source of error and consequences to the patient, if we generate or select the "wrong" solution. This may not be the esoteric problem it seems, for the CT/pathology correlation is not perfect (Turunen et al. 1986; Zwirewich et al. 1990; March et al. 1991; Murata et al. 1992; Bravin et al. 2007), and we do not yet understand why and when CT misses some features. In fact, Kennan Smith (1980, personal communication) began his work on CT when a neurologist friend had a patient who he was sure had a tumor, but none was revealed by CT (cf. Herman and Davidi 2008). This observation led to Smith's Indeterminacy Theorem (Smith et al. 1977; Gordon 1979c; Leahy et al. 1979; Hamaker et al. 1980; Gordon 1985b): "A finite set of radiographs tells nothing at all" (Smith et al. 1977), which he thought could be overcome by the positivity and other a priori constraints (Smith et al. 1978), which was later proven (Clarkson and Barrett 1997; Clarkson and Barrett 1998). This idea has recently been echoed: "It is fine to have an under-determined system of equations as long as there are some other constraints to help select a 'good' image out of the possibly large nullspace of an imaging equation" (Pan et al. 2009).

The behavior of EMI, which brought it from a monopoly in commercial CT to a total collapse of its market, was part of my personal experience. Hounsfield met with me to sign an agreement letting me have access to the raw data from the head scanner at George Washington University, where I was an Adjunct Professor of Radiology 1974–1978 while working at NIH. I found a systematic error in the data, by noting that, for parallel rays, the back projections of the centroids of the projection data should intersect at the centroid of a head section. They did not, but instead formed a circular envelope a few millimeters in diameter. When I told Hounsfield that I had a simple software correction and wanted to put the corrected data back into their computer, to see if the image improved, I never heard from him again. Later I was involved in defending the Technicare division of Johnson & Johnson (formerly Ohio Nuclear Corporation) against the 1976 patent infringement suit by EMI (Strong and Hurst 1994). Despite a simple to prove case that some of the claims were patenting linear algebra itself, and the fact that a complete scanner design had long been in the public domain (Kalos et al. 1961) (Fig. 10.3), to the disappointment of their Chicago patent attorneys, Johnson & Johnson settled out of court. Cormack concluded:

> "The genius of EMI's strategy against those it charged with infringing its patents in the US lay in its use of the legal system to push its suits as far and for as long as it could without their coming to trial, and so avoiding the possibility that the patents would be declared invalid. There are those of us who regret that the great success of this strategy was not matched by equal successes in engineering and marketing which would have kept the UK a leader in the production of CT scanners" (Cormack 1994).

10.12 Walking in Hyperspace

My earlier approach to dealing with underdetermined equations (Gordon 1973) harkened back to my electron microscopy experience. If we knew a priori that we were looking at examples of single protein molecules, then any image made of two disconnected parts was a priori an artifact. Now, I have generally eschewed the field of pattern recognition, leaving the interpretation of images to radiologists, and specified my job as giving them the best possible image to look at. Thus, I created an approach that would let a radiologist explore a CT image to test, to some extent, whether lesions in a CT image reconstructed from underdetermined equations were potential artifacts or real. The multiple solutions to the ART equations lie in what a mathematician calls a hyperplane, so I set off to do what I called "an intelligent walk in the hyperplane." This would allow the radiologist to bring to bear knowledge of anatomy and pathology of any sort, that is, a priori information well beyond the simple positivity constraint. I started with the ART image, and then erased one feature in it. The resulting image was no longer a solution to the equations, but it could be used as the initial image for restarting the ART algorithm, which would then converge back to the solution hyperplane, but to a different place in it. If the feature disappeared, then we could deem it a possible artifact, because the x-ray data was consistent with it being there or not. In other words, we would discover that there are two solutions, one containing the feature, and one not, solution undermining our confidence that the feature might be real. On the other hand, if the feature reappeared, that fact would increase our confidence that it might be real. While this may seem to be a lot of work, modern pattern recognition programs (Gavrielides et al. 2002; Nandi et al. 2006) could be used to automate the process, creating a "confidence map" for each feature seen in a CT image. It will be interesting to compare this highly nonlinear pattern recognition approach with recently developed statistical inverse methods that generate alternative solutions to the equations from different samplings of matrices containing white noise (Kaipio and Somersalo 2004).

10.13 Population Dose of CT

The main disadvantage of x-rays is that they cause cancer. Thus, screening must be done with at least the guideline that we detect and cure more cancers than we cause (Bailar 1976). It is therefore mandatory that we find every means to maximize the image quality to x-ray dose ratio (Gordon 1976b) while staying within acceptable limits to total dose and skin dose. Whether this prevents us from attaining the target size of 2–4 mm (see below) can only be determined by making the attempt, by pushing x-ray CT to its limits.

To appreciate the seriousness of the problem of maximizing the image quality to x-ray dose ratio, consider what is happening in general radiology. About 15% of the population exposure to ionizing radiation comes from the practice of medicine (Ron 2003). CT accounted for 5% of radiological

examinations in Germany in 1999, but was already responsible for 40% of the x-ray dose (Kalender 2000). US figures rose from 4% of procedures with 40% dose due to CT in the mid-1990s to 15% with 75% of the dose due to CT in 2002 (Wiest et al. 2002). This means that the average CT study delivers 16 times the dose of the average non-CT x-ray procedure and that the total x-ray dose to the population had by 2002 already increased four times per person over that before CT came into significant use.

The calculation proceeds as follows. Let

D_i = CT dose at time i

N_i = the number of CT studies at time i

d = non - CT dose

n = the number of non - CT studies

T_i = total population dose at time i

From Wiest et al. (2002) we have:

$$D_1 / (D_1 + d) = 0.4 \text{ at time } 1 (\text{mid} - 1990\text{s})$$

$$N_1 / (N_1 + n) = 0.04$$

$$D_2 / (D_2 + d) = 0.75 \text{ at time } 2 (2002)$$

$$N_2 / (N_2 + n) = 0.15$$

These lead to:

$$D_1 / N_1 = 16 \, d / n$$

$$D_2 / N_2 = 17 \, d / n$$

which are quite consistent, where we are assuming no change in the number n or dose d of non-CT studies. We also obtain:

$$D_2 = 3d$$

so that

$$T_2 = D_2 + d = 4d$$

One might anticipate that CT is reducing the use of non-CT procedures, making these figures slight overestimates. However, there was actually a slight increase in non-CT procedures (Rehani 2000).

This rapid increase in the use of x-ray CT (Prokop 2005) ("CT has become the major source of population exposure to diagnostic X-ray" (Hatziioannou et al. 2003)) is of particular concern in pediatric CT (Linton and Mettler 2003), since children are more sensitive than adults to induction of cancer by radiation (Brenner et al.

2001), especially breast cancer (Li et al. 1983; Rosenfield et al. 1989; Donnelly and Frush 2001; Berdon and Slovis 2002; Brenner 2002; Linton and Mettler 2003). The same reservations may apply specifically to the breasts of premenstrual women, which contain proliferating cells (Ferguson and Anderson 1981; Vogel et al. 1981; Going et al. 1988; Dabrosin et al. 1997; Dzendrowskyj et al. 1997), suggesting that x-ray imaging should be done at a time in the menstrual cycle of minimal cell proliferation (Bjarnason 1996). On the other hand, the claim that breast surgery should be timed to the menstrual cycle has been disproved (Kroman 2008; Thorpe et al. 2008; Grant et al. 2009). Other reasons to gate imaging to the menstrual cycle are to minimize the effects of changing volume (Malini et al. 1985; Fowler et al. 1990; Graham et al. 1995; Kato et al. 1995; White et al. 1998; Hussain et al. 1999) and tissue properties (Ferguson and Anderson 1981; Vogel et al. 1981; Nelson et al. 1985; Malberger et al. 1987; Going et al. 1988; Ferguson et al. 1990, 1992; Graham et al. 1995; Simpson et al. 1996; Dabrosin et al. 1997; Dzendrowskyj et al. 1997; Zarghami et al. 1997; Cubeddu et al. 2000).

10.14 Focus on Breast Cancer Detection

I do not recall exactly what got me started on the application of CT to breast imaging, but when I proposed to a large NIH audience of 500 or so people that we could screen women to detect small tumors, and it would take only a week of computing time per exam, I was greeted with derisive laughter (Gordon 1976a). One must have a thick skin. I suppose that I responded in my characteristic way (as I did later (Gordon 1989) when shunned for my calculations on the effectiveness of condoms to halt the spread of HIV/AIDS (Gordon 1987)), with the first attempt at an algorithm that tried to deal head on with the very high resolution needed for breast CT, while keeping the computer time plausible (Gordon 1977) and with the first lesson on dose reduction in CT for the medical community (Gordon 1976b). I did verbal battle with physicists over what resolution CT could achieve (Gordon 1978a, 1979c). I was thus bitten by the bug of how to catch breast cancer early, and by that awful burden of being certain that, if only people would listen, so many lives could be saved. One must have a skin that is not too thick.

Mammography unfortunately seems to have more than its share of opinionated hot heads, who in the long run impede the health of the women they serve:

"During my presentation, I described the tough issues of balancing the benefits for the few versus the harms for the many, and I suggested that maybe screening does not benefit the premenopausal woman at all. Despite my role in establishing the National Screening Programme when I was Chief of Surgery at King's College London in 1988, my comments were not well received, and, as the audience stormed out on me in a paroxysm of pique, I learned a painful lesson that day that some topics, particularly breast cancer screening, do not lend themselves to polite and rational scientific debate" (Baum 2004).

I moved to the University of Manitoba in 1978 and got wound up in the local issue, common also in developing countries, of radiologists being in urban centers and the need for teleradiology to serve remote and rural communities. As this was well before the Internet, transmission of images over phone lines using acoustic couplers was quite a feat. I upped the ante by proposing we could do CT remotely, even of breast, by transmitting just the projection data (mammograms acquired over a few angles), and doing the reconstructions and diagnoses centrally (Rangayyan and Gordon 1982a). We actually set up transmission from Brandon to Winnipeg (about 200 km) and tried it out (Gordon and Rangaraj 1982). Failing further local support, I took the project to China, where it collapsed when my collaborators there disbursed after the Tiananmen Square massacre. With the vidicon TV cameras and 512×512 8-bit digitization that we could afford then (digital cameras started at $50,000), this effort would never have been clinically significant. The vain attempt was closed out just before the Internet started (Gordon 1990). In retrospect, I had taken my own step backward in an attempt to create proof of principle for the unconvinced with inadequate technology.

10.15 Combining Imaging Modalities

One step forward that was "in the air" was that of combining imaging modalities in one scanner. At first people worked on registering, say, an MRI image with the CT image of the same slice, but it was obvious that the mechanical rigidity of a coaxial or simultaneous scanner was superior. I had proposed such to a visiting group of PET/nuclear medicine clinicians while at NIH, and we have, for instance, PET/CT scanners nowadays.

I later proposed that, however done mechanically, the data itself be taken into a "higher space" (Gordon and Coumans 1984). The example I gave was dual-energy CT, yielding two absorption coefficients for each pixel, (X_1, X_2), combined with MRI, say yielding the two relaxation coefficients (T_1, T_2). Tissue signatures from each modality might be sufficient to identify the tissue or tumor in the image. However, the cross product of the two 2D spaces is a 4D space, (X_1, X_2, T_1, T_2), in which we could anticipate additional correlations that would allow finer discriminations. By analogy with 2D versus 3D mammography itself, the 2D data spaces are projections from a higher 4D data space, and as such contain overlaps of clusterings that obscure detail. These correlations have to be worked out empirically, a research project for the future of image/pathology correlation of a higher order.

10.16   Deconvolution of CT Images and Adaptive Neighborhoods

Rangaraj Rangayyan, my postdoc on the teleradiology project, and I had two other adventures that have proved seminal. First, we tackled the problem of anisotropy in CT done from a limited angle range, by deconvolution methods (Gordon and Rangayyan 1983; Gordon et al. 1985; Soble et al. 1985); second, we invented adaptive neighborhood image processing for suppression of streaking artifacts in CT caused by high contrast objects (metal implants, bones, or microcalcifications) (Rangayyan and Gordon 1982b) and created a similar method to imitate the high-dose xeromammogram from a digitized image of a mammogram, that is, at no additional dose (Gordon and Rangayyan 1984a, b; Dhawan et al. 1986a, b; Dhawan and Gordon 1986). Adaptive neighborhoods became a subfield of image processing (Jiang et al. 1992; Sivaramakrishna et al. 2000; Rangayyan et al. 2001; Vasile et al. 2004).

10.17   Wiener Deconvolution

Deconvolution proved most successful in Atam Dhawan's hands, in which he deconvoluted the PSF of a CT algorithm itself. This is the blur function that Vainshtein clarified (Vainshtein 1971) (Fig. 10.4), but now made specific to the algorithm and geometry (set of views) at hand. For example, a circular disk phantom reconstructed with a limited angle range of views comes out as an ellipse, which it seemed one could just "pat" back together into a circle. We made the bold (i.e., mathematically false) assumption that the image

produced by a CT algorithm could be thought of as an anisotropic blurring of a single PSF (of the pixel in the middle of the image) applied to the whole of the real image we sought. We therefore used Wiener filtration to deconvolute the PSF from the CT image (Dhawan et al. 1984a, 1985). The result was spectacular: Dhawan's wife's face (Fig. 10.5a), not even recognizable as such in the limited range ART reconstruction (Fig. 10.5b), sprang forth after Wiener deconvolution (Fig. 10.5c) (Dhawan et al. 1985). We had achieved a major improvement over ART, itself an improvement over FBP, with no increase in patient dose. The algorithm was applied to extremely limited projection data using light microscopy, for estimating the thickness of a nevus (Gordon 1983b; Dhawan et al. 1984a, b, c). No one has worked on this algorithmic approach since, and I am still waiting to find someone to build a robotic skin scanner for screening for early melanomas, which should be simpler than breast, because tumors that are premetastasis are not obscured by overlying tissue.

There are three problems with our Wiener deconvolution that need further research. First, the PSF is not actually spatially invariant, as we had assumed. This could be tackled by Toeplitz matrix methods designed to correct aberrations in optics (Nagy 1993), such as occurred when one component in the Hubble orbiting telescope was put in backward, or by other approaches (Baker et al. 1992; Beekman et al. 1996). Second, ringing artifacts were introduced into the image, which could be suppressed (Ruttimann et al. 1989; Hu et al. 1991; Zhou et al. 1993; Schlueter et al. 1994; Sijbers and Postnov 2004). Third, the deconvolved image is not a solution to the projection equations, but perhaps by using it as a starting image for an iterative CT algorithm such as ART, convergence to an image that is both deconvolved and satisfies the equations may be possible (Gordon 1973).

Empirically, all CT algorithms based on solving simultaneous equations usually produce images that look similar. The Wiener solution is startlingly different. ART has been shown to produce the solution that minimizes the Euclidean distance between the unknown image and the reconstruction (Kaipio and Somersalo 2004), while multiplicative ART (MART) yields an image of maximum entropy (Lent 1977; Dusaussoy and Abdou 1991; Lent and Censor 1991). They thus fall into the category of what mathematicians call regularization algorithms (Bertero and Boccacci 1998; Engl et al. 2000). Yet Wiener deconvolution shows that regularization actually produces the wrong solution. Thus, CT may pay back to mathematics some new insights.

Fig. 10.5 The image of a face (**a**) was reconstructed by multiplicative ART (**b**) using only five views at viewing angles 45°, 67.5°, 90°, 112.5°, and 135° (0° is horizontal). Deconvolution of the point spread function by Wiener filtration produced (**c**) (Dhawan 1985)

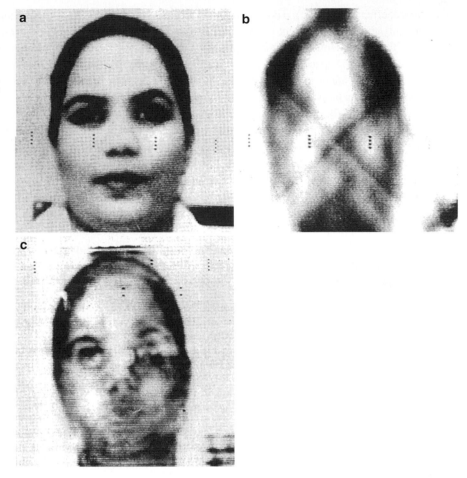

10.18 Registration of Longitudinal Images

Our Wiener filtration work was presented (Dhawan et al. 1985) at a workshop on industrial CT that I organized (Gordon 1985a), which gave me a chance to summarize my thoughts about limited view CT (Rangayyan et al. 1985) and how to get to detection of small breast tumors (Gordon 1985b). It was becoming clear that a 3D breast image might have many false-positive "lesions," and a bit later we learned that some small tumors regress (Nielsen et al. 1987; Nielsen 1989). Furthermore, especially because most are not vascularized, one could assume that the signature of small tumors might not be much different from that of the adjacent normal tissue. So the only signature that we could rely on is consistent growth. To spot this, we must accurately register two longitudinal images of the breast (taken some time apart, at the "screening interval"), a "soft object" that one cannot put into a rigid scanner the same way each time, and then digitally subtract the images one from the other. I proposed a complex registration algorithm based on iterative use of a hardware geometric warper, a special purpose computer that had recently been marketed (Gordon 1985b).

I set off on a long search for a robust 3D image registration algorithm that would work for breast using only internal, local, 3D texture, which should be unique at each neighborhood of a voxel. This involved the Ph.D. thesis work of three consecutive students. Xiaohua (now Albert) Zhou and I reviewed the field (Zhou and Gordon 1989) and then proceeded to develop a method to create fiducial marks using Zernicke polynomials, which could then be used to generate the geometric warping for a pair of 3D breast images from multiple fiducial points (Zhou 1991).

Andrzej Mazur, looking over Xiaohua's shoulder, decided he could do away with fiducial marks, with a simulated annealing approach (Mazur 1992; Mazur et al. 1993). Radhika Sivaramakrishna used what we called the starbyte transformation to segment a breast image into regions that could be matched between longitudinal images (Sivaramakrishna and Gordon 1997b; Sivaramakrishna 1998). We produced a vivid photographic demonstration, by using the cartoon character Waldo, of how registering and subtracting images could make a tumor stand out, but only if we dropped 2D mammography and imaged in 3D (Gordon and Sivaramakrishna 1999). Some of this work was carried out with Anthony (Tony) Miller as co-investigator on the only major grant I ever received for breast cancer research. Without such senior support, the general impression I had of the peer review process for breast cancer imaging was: "show us the pictures, then we'll fund you to produce them," that is, a Catch-22 (Heller 1961). Parliamentary testimony (Gordon 1992) had no impact on this situation.

By the time I was satisfied that 3D registration of longitudinal breast images was practical, we were "also rans" (Sivaramakrishna et al. 1999; Sivaramakrishna 2005a; Guo et al. 2006). But there is still registration work to do. It is "plausible to compare the two images *during* data collection, so that a difference-image is acquired at considerably lower dose than the original. If the patient's digital image records were preserved, she or he could be subject to such incremental radiology from then on" (Gordon 1979b). This is analogous to efficient transmission of video (Burg 2003) or compression of serial sections (Lee et al. 1993), in which only the parts of the image that have changed from one frame to the next are sent. Methods for reduction of structural registration noise in the difference image (Knoll and Delp 1986; Gong et al. 1992; Bruzzone and Cossu 2003) could also be useful during such incremental radiography.

Longitudinal registration might make it possible (Mazur et al. 1993; Liu et al. 2006) to detect zero contrast tumors by the local distortion of breast tissue texture (Chang et al. 1982; Shaw de Paredes 1994; Stomper et al. 1994; Goldberg and Dwyer 1995; Maes et al. 1997) of normal tissue that they cause. This 4D (four dimensional: 3D+time) approach might extend the detection of architectural distortion, which has been shown to be an often missed sign of early breast tumors using longitudinal pairs of unregisterable 2D

mammograms (Ayres and Rangayyan 2007; Rangayyan et al. 2007; Banik et al. 2009).

One curiosity of the period up through the early 1990s was a resistance to 3D imaging for breast from the biggest protagonists of standard projection mammography. Their publication records demonstrate their late awakening to 3D, with the zeal of new discovery, though most breast imaging investigators still genuflect to standard mammography by calling it the "gold standard." I call it the lead (Pb) standard (below silver and bronze). But the net result of the standard mammography enthusiasts' attitudes was to suppress funding for 3D imaging of breast for decades, not just for me but for others quite independent of my work, so that breast imaging joined the 3D world much later than just about any other branch of radiographic imaging, and is still in its infancy. For example, "No trials of screening average-risk women specifically evaluating the effectiveness of [2D] digital mammography [let alone of 3D x-ray CT] or [3D] MRI have been published" even though they "have become widely used" (Nelson et al. 2009). Two mass delusion phenomena, of stasis in the flatland (Abbott 1899) of standard 2D mammography, and the role of women's breast cancer activist groups in ignoring the delay in 3D breast imaging, are worthy of study by the sociologist of science:

> "To the extent that current methods of detection and treatment fail or fall short, America's breast-cancer cult can be judged as an outbreak of mass delusion, celebrating survivorhood by downplaying mortality and promoting obedience to medical protocols known to have limited efficacy" (Ehrenreich 2001).

As image quality of standard mammography has saturated, apparently reaching its limits (Spelic 2009) (Fig. 10.6), we can anticipate that further progress in image quality per x-ray dose requires a switch to 3D CT.

I used to support and help out at "runs for the cure" but stopped when I realized that most of the money goes for the status quo, and tried to suggest to women that they have to do the research themselves. Those few who understood what I was saying soon died of their breast cancers. The other trouble with such "runs" is that they focus on women with advanced breast cancer. Few get excited about prevention or screening, because those who need these approaches have no symptoms, nor have they generally had to deal with breast cancer in their lives. Yet "the cure" may lie in focusing on asymptomatic women.

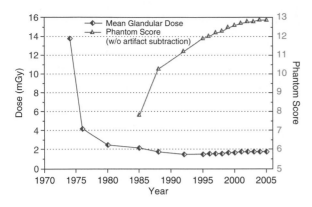

Fig. 10.6 "This graphic displays average values for mean glandular dose [decreasing curve] and estimates of image quality in [standard] mammography [increasing curve] for the period from the early 1970's to 2005" (Spelic 2009) (With permission of the U.S. Food and Drug Administration)

10.19 Faster and Better ART

We learned how to speed the ART algorithm itself, so that it almost converges in three or so iterations (Guan and Gordon 1994, 1996; Guan et al. 1998; Colquhoun and Gordon 2005b). It is amazing how many decades it took to discover the simple trick of reordering the projections so that consecutive ones were nearly perpendicular, instead of processing them sequentially by angle, and so FBP was unchallenged for decades in speed. Now, in a twist of the tale, my collaborator Glen D. Colquhoun has preliminary evidence that full 3D ART does not require any analogous trick.

Elzbieta Mazur found that rotating each pixel so that its projection was a simple rectangle rather than a trapezoid surprisingly improved ART reconstructions. This of course had to be done to a different angle for each projection (Mazur and Gordon 1995). Our blatant disregard for the usual assumption of rigidity of a pixel led to the notion that, as in pointillism (Düchting 2001), the exact shape, size, orientation, and position of a pixel hardly matter when an image is viewed from a far enough distance. We plan to put this concept to work.

We also found that MART images could be sharpened by raising the correction to a power (PMART=Power MART), which to our surprise had a critical value at which the computation became chaotic (Badea and Gordon 2004). This effect was later explained, leading to an "extended PMART" algorithm (Yoshinaga et al. 2008).

10.20 Extrapolating Epidemiology to Take Aim at Small Breast Cancers

Watching Miller's battle defending the results of the Canadian National Breast Screening Study (Baines et al. 1986; Burhenne and Burhenne 1993; Mettlin and Smart 1993; Miller 1993; Baines 1994; Tarone 1995; Bailar and MacMahon 1997) made me aware of the importance of epidemiology to solving the breast cancer problem. I was also aware of the huge impact on the practice of standard mammography made by epidemiologist John Bailar in the 1970s (Bailar 1976; Lerner 2001), resulting in a sevenfold reduction in dose (Spelic 2009) (Fig. 10.6). I thus came to use epidemiological data, extrapolated to smaller breast tumor sizes than were observable, to try to understand how small a tumor we should aim at imaging to have an impact on the disease. The result was startling: detecting 4 mm tumors with 100% efficiency and destroying them should halt breast cancer 99.6% of the time (Sivaramakrishna and Gordon 1997a). As commercial x-ray CT was approaching 0.5 mm resolution, and detectors at 0.05–0.1 mm were becoming common in digital radiography, this seemed an attainable goal. To bolster my confidence in the result, as extrapolations of data are always dangerous, I collaborated with epidemiologists to check it against alternative data sets (Sun et al. 1998; Chapman et al. 1999; Sun et al. 2002; Verschraegen et al. 2005; Vinh-Hung and Gordon 2005). The result held: if we could search for and destroy breast tumors in the 2-4 mm size range, we would, in effect, eliminate the disease as a major killer. Most such tumors have not yet, or not yet successfully, metastasized.

10.21 Planning a Race Between Imaging Modalities

I conceived of a race between imaging modalities to target premetastasis tumors, and got involved in MRI (Tomanek et al. 2000) and EIT (Murugan 2000). While the cost of breast MRI and the poor resolution of breast EIT (which I think may be due to using orders of magnitude too few electrodes, recently only 128 (Ye et al. 2008) to 256 (Cherepenin et al. 2002)) are obstacles to their adoption for 3D screening mammography, as both are harmless compared to x-ray CT, I believe they should be pursued to their physical limits. Here is a sampling (cf. Suri et al. 2006) of mostly recent references to an undoubtedly incomplete list of the incredible variety of physics being (or perhaps that should be) applied to breast imaging:

- CT laser mammography (Yee 2009)
- EIT (Cherepenin et al. 2002; Prasad and Houserkova 2007; Chen et al. 2008; Halter et al. 2008; Steiner et al. 2008; Ye et al. 2008), including current reconstruction magnetic resonance EIT (Gao and He 2008; Ng et al. 2008) and EIT spectroscopy (EIS) (Choi et al. 2007; Kim et al. 2007a; Poplack et al. 2007; Karellas and Vedantham 2008)
- Microwave imaging (Fang et al. 2004; Chen et al. 2007, 2008; Hand 2008; Kanj and Popovic 2008; Karellas and Vedantham 2008; Pramanik et al. 2008), radar (Poyvasi et al. 2005; Flores-Tapia et al. 2008), microwave imaging spectroscopy (MIS) (Poplack et al. 2007; Lazebnik et al. 2008), and dual polarization methods (Woten and El-Shenawee 2008)
- Microwave-induced thermoacoustic scanning CT (Nie et al. 2008)
- Molecular and nanoparticle imaging (Rayavarapu et al. 2007), including quantum dots (Park and Ikeda 2006; Chang et al. 2008)
- MRI (Kuhl et al. 2005; Park and Ikeda 2006; Brenner and Parisky 2007; Kim et al. 2007b; Hand 2008; Karellas and Vedantham 2008; Yee 2009) and MRS (Smith and Andreopoulou 2004)
- Multi-frequency transadmittance scanning (TAS) (Oh et al. 2007)
- Near-infrared spectral tomography (NIR) (Poplack et al. 2007)
- Neutron-stimulated emission computed tomography (Bender et al. 2007)
- Optical imaging (Huang and Zhu 2004; Park and Ikeda 2006; Karellas and Vedantham 2008; Konovalov et al. 2008; Lazebnik et al. 2008; Fang et al. 2009) including transillumination (Blyschak et al. 2004; Simick et al. 2004)
- PET or positron emission mammography (PEM) and PET/CT (Pawlak and Gordon 2005; Jan et al. 2006; Park and Ikeda 2006; Aliaga et al. 2007; Brenner and Parisky 2007; Prasad and Houserkova 2007; Shibata et al. 2007; Tafra 2007; Thie 2007; Yang et al. 2007; Zhang et al. 2007; Karellas and Vedantham 2008; Bowen et al. 2009; Wu et al. 2009; Yee 2009), perhaps combined in MagPET with strong magnetic

fields to constrain the range of the positrons before annihilation (Iida et al. 1986; Rickey et al. 1992; Hammer et al. 1994; Burdette et al. 2009), which could be used to increase the resolution of PET/MRI (Cherry et al. 2008; Judenhofer et al. 2008)

- Photoacoustic tomography (Pramanik et al. 2008)
- Proton and heavy ion CT (IonCT) (Holley et al. 1981a, b; Muraishi et al. 2009)
- Single photon emission CT (SPECT) (More et al. 2007; Karellas and Vedantham 2008) and scintimammography (McKinley et al. 2006; Li et al. 2007; Prasad and Houserkova 2007; Spanu et al. 2007; Thie 2007)
- Superconducting Quantum Interference Device (SQUID) (Anninos et al. 2000) and SQUID MRI (Clarke et al. 2007)
- Thermoacoustic tomography (Pramanik et al. 2008)
- Tomosynthesis (Karellas et al. 2008; Karellas and Vedantham 2008; Dobbins 2009; Gur et al. 2009; Yee 2009)
- Ultrasound (US) (Huang and Zhu 2004; Brenner and Parisky 2007; Karellas and Vedantham 2008; Yee 2009)
- Ultrasound elasticity imaging (elastography) (Bagchi 2007; Garra 2007) and vibro-acoustography (Alizad et al. 2005; Silva et al. 2006)
- Ultrasound reflection tomography (Steiner et al. 2008)
- X-ray CT by diffraction-enhanced or phase-sensitive imaging (Bravin et al. 2007; Karellas and Vedantham 2008; Zhou and Brahme 2008; Kao et al. 2009; Parham et al. 2009)
- X-ray CT using scattered photons with energy discrimination (Van Uytven et al. 2007, 2008)
- X-ray CT (Chen and Ning 2003; McKinley et al. 2006; Kalender and Kyriakou 2007; Kwan et al. 2007; Li et al. 2007; Karellas et al. 2008; Karellas and Vedantham 2008; Lindfors et al. 2008; Nelsona et al. 2008; Yang et al. 2008; Yee 2009), potentially with monochromatic (McKinley et al. 2004) or dual energy imaging (Kappadath and Shaw 2005; Bliznakova et al. 2006), especially using synchrotron radiation (Fabbri et al. 2002; Pani et al. 2004)

These references include many dual imaging techniques, some of them iterative with interlacing of two modalities to improve the images from each. A matrix of methods would reveal that only a few potential pairs of imaging modalities have been considered so far. Combining three or more modalities at once would also be technically feasible, though a challenge (Cherry 2006).

Some researchers are inhibited by the current costs of these novel methods. On the one hand, such worries come from a lack of historical perspective, in that all high technologies cost much to develop, after which the unit cost plunges. But even if, for example, an MRI screening continues to cost $1,000, the argument boils down to: what's a woman's life worth?

With the motivation of establishing a race between breast imaging modalities (the real "run for the cure"), I organized what I hoped would be a series of conferences, the Workshops on Alternatives to Mammography (WAM), that would terminate when the scourge of breast cancer ended. Unfortunately only two were held, in Winnipeg in 2004 (Colquhoun and Gordon 2005a; Sivaramakrishna 2005b, c) and Copenhagen in 2005, the latter led by Tibor Tot. Perhaps a professional society with a focus on breast cancer, prepared to take aim at search and destroy of premetastasis tumors, should take this on.

10.22 Future 0: Foxels and Seventh Generation CT for Breast Screening

At WAM2 Colquhoun and I introduced what we called "reverse cone beam" imaging (Colquhoun et al. 2004; Colquhoun and Gordon 2005a). This is based on the observation that over the past decades, while the focal spot of an x-ray tube has not decreased much, the size of the detector elements has fallen precipitously. Thus, while x-ray imaging is generally conceived of as a cone of radiation coming from a point source spreading over the patient, from the point of view of a detector pixel, it "sees" a focal spot often 10× wider than itself. The ray shape is thus that of a reverse cone beam. To take advantage of this situation, we divided the focal spot into an array of emitting pixels, about the same size as the detector elements, called them foxels, and our current research is to write computer code to carry out this very fine deconvolution during iterative reconstruction, which promises to substantially increase the spatial resolution, with no increase in dose. Michael J.A. Potter has joined us as a collaborator on this problem (Potter

et al. 2009). Note that reverse cone beam CT is distinct from "inverse-geometry CT" (Schmidt et al. 2006; Mazin and Pelc 2008; Bhagtani and Schmidt 2009) in that the latter uses multiple, widely spaced positions of the x-ray beam to image onto a small detector array, with no attempt to deconvolute the focal spot image.

We have also gone back to my old approach of the intelligent walk in the hyperplane of solutions (Gordon 1973), and conceive of CT as a meta-algorithm, in which standard CT algorithms (ART, MART, perhaps even FBP, etc.) are interleaved between iterations with each other and various image processing and pattern recognition operations. This metaprogramming approach may permit us to combine Wiener filtration, alternative ART and other algorithms, image enhancements, image segmentation, foxel deconvolution, determination of feature reliability, etc., for optimal search and eventual destruction of premetastasis tumors. Finally, in order to come as close as possible to Vainshtein's ideal of isotropic imaging with $1/r^2$ PSF (not quite achievable for breast because of the chest wall), our code allows arbitrary positioning of the x-ray source and a 2D detector array. Until we settle on the optimal set or program of positionings (including alternate data space subsets or "partitions" (Pan et al. 2009)), the gantry may be thought of as independent robot arms carrying the source (with its possibly dynamic and/or encoded collimation (Pan et al. 2009)) and the detector array. Our computer coding work on this has been greatly simplified by the use of homogeneous coordinates (Schaller et al. 1998; Karolczak et al. 2001; Alpuche Avilés 2004).

Note that this approach to improving CT imaging is opposite to the "plug-and-play" cooperation with industry that has been recommended, in which algorithm developers are exhorted to "take actual CT-scanner data and produce useful images" (Pan et al. 2009), though they do look forward to the day "…when engineers have real experience with advanced image-reconstruction algorithms and can use this knowledge to design more efficient and effective CT scanners. This development will likely occur first in dedicated CT systems such as head/neck CT, dental CT and breast CT."

We call our approach seventh-generation CT, then, because it incorporates four novelties: (1) a geometrically accurate 3D reconstruction algorithm that exploits foxels and handles any 3D x-ray source/detector array positioning; (2) metaprogramming that allows choice of different CT algorithms and image processing and pattern recognition steps in the course of image calculation; (3) feedback between the reconstruction algorithm and the scanning system to plan the next positioning of x-ray source and detector array based on the 3D image obtained so far; (4) distinction between the 3D computer memory array used for a particular gantry position and a master computer memory array containing the 3D picture being reconstructed, with appropriate 3D transformations to go between them.

I have labeled seventh-generation CT "Future 0" because every component needed for it can be built now or written in computer code, given the will and a little cash.

10.23 Future 1: The Intelligently Steered X-Ray Microbeam

There are more generations of x-ray CT that can be conceived, but require breakthroughs in technology or physics. One is the intelligently steered x-ray microbeam. Richard L. Webber organized a workshop on this approach 3 decades ago (Webber 1979):

> "An aimed beam allows one to attain a uniform signal-to-noise ratio by holding the beam at each point for an appropriate length of time. If the peak of the x-ray spectrum could also be dynamically tuned to the optimum energy for each local optical thickness [cf. Kalender et al. 2009], further dose reduction could be achieved" (Gordon 1979b).

The original invention dates back to 1950 (Moon 1950), and was tried for CT by Hitachi, using electron microscope technology to steer an electron beam, which produced a moving x-ray focal spot (Tateno and Tanaka 1976; Tateno et al. 1976). The x-rays were in turn steered by blocking all emitted x-rays except for those going through a pinhole.

One way to reduce dose via intelligently steered x-ray microbeams is to incorporate that pattern recognition that I originally eschewed, but in retrospect have always been drawn back to. All present-day x-ray imaging modalities splatter x-ray photons at all angles through the patient, except where constrained by collimators. Features are struck by photons

indiscriminately. Suppose that we do this with a light sprinkling of photons, to obtain a 3D "scout" image. That image would contain real features and spurious ones due to noise fluctuations. We then aim the beam at features of possible interest (defined by image characteristics or a priori criteria). They should either fade away if they are actually due to noise fluctuations, or sharpen up if real. The x-ray microbeam is thus "intelligently" guided to where it is needed, and the overall dose greatly reduced. This method awaits development of a compact steerable x-ray laser (Fill 1992) or refracted and focused x-ray beam (Cederstroem et al. 1999; Jorgensen et al. 1999; Gorenstein 2007) or an x-ray beam steered by grazing incidence reflection (Signorato et al. 1997; Harvey et al. 2001) of sufficient energy per photon and intensity to be of use for body or breast imaging. While synchrotrons (Burattini et al. 1995), now in experimental use for x-ray diffraction imaging of breast (Bravin et al. 2007), have the beam intensity needed to test these ideas, they are rather large (typically 600 m), requiring 3D 2-axis rotation of the patient for full 3D imaging. Even the "compact" versions of synchrotrons under development are "room size" (Lyncean Technologies 2009) (cf. Yamada et al. 2004; Hirai et al. 2006) (Fig. 10.7), but given the precedent of the 5-m diameter Mayo Clinic CT scanner (Altschuler et al. 1980), it is not absurd to think of rotating a whole room of equipment around a woman's pendent breast.

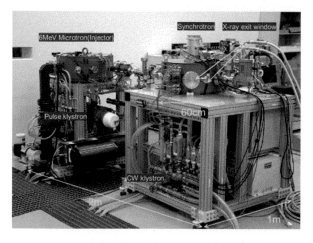

Fig. 10.7 A "compact" synchrotron x-ray source (From Yamada et al. (2004), with permission of Elsevier)

10.24 Future 2: Turnstile and Entangled Photons: Breast Imaging as a Game of Battleship

Primary x-ray photons are randomized twice, by the Poisson statistics of their emission from the anode, and then by the Poisson statistics of their scattering or absorption. For visible light photons ways have been invented to emit them on command, so-called turnstile photons, on changing a voltage, for quantum level communications and optical computing, where each bit is one photon (Imamoglu and Yamamoto 1994; Law and Kimble 1997; Kim et al. 1998, 1999; Benjamin 2000; Michler et al. 2000; McKeever 2004; Oxborrow and Sinclair 2005; Dayan et al. 2008), and aim them in a particular direction (Taminiau et al. 2008), even polarized (Lukishova et al. 2007). If we could do this for x-ray photons, then the photon statistics would be significantly improved, because we would be dealing with one Poisson process rather than the convolution of two of them (Melvin et al. 2002). X-ray imaging would then be analogous to the game of Battleship (Hasbro 2004) in which one drops a "bomb" (photon) onto the unseen opponent's board (a breast) and is told whether or not a "ship" (tumor) was hit (Foo 1999). Better statistics implies reduced dose. The challenge here is to construct a nanostructured material that would emit turnstile x-ray photons.

There is an alternative to turnstile photons that gives the equivalent effect (Edward H. Sargent, personal communication) (Sargent 2005). A method called parametric downconversion, a nonlinear optical process, could produce a pair of time-correlated, entangled photons (Abouraddy et al. 2001). One could be an x-ray photon and the other could be a visible photon. When a visible light photon is detected, we would know that an x-ray photon had been simultaneously launched toward the breast.

10.25 Stop Breast Cancer Now!

The ultimate breast screening scanner would detect all premetastasis tumors by comparing the current image with previous 3D images of the same breast, and then automatically destroy any suspicious lesions by any of a wide variety of ablation techniques presently under development (Noguchi 2003; Simmons 2003; Singletary 2003; O'Neal et al. 2004; Roubidoux et al. 2004; Vargas et al. 2004; Agnese and Burak 2005; Glaiberman et al. 2005; Huston and Simmons 2005; Lobo et al. 2005; Morrison et al. 2005; Nields 2005; Bao et al. 2008; Barnett et al. 2009), with thresholds for whether or not to ablate perhaps determined by therapy operating characteristic (TOC) curves (Barrett et al. 2010). My model is that used by dermatologists in handling suspicious nevi: first cut them out, and then ask questions (such as whether the resection margin was adequate). This attitude would eliminate breast biopsies, the major cost in present-day 2D mammography. Any device that automatically finds and destroys small potential tumors can also be set to pay special attention to the region of any previously ablated tumor, to look for recurrences. This is an effective form of watchful waiting, but one that does not wait too long. Watchful waiting replaces the pathology report.

I am well aware that what I am proposing, if it proves successful, would eliminate the radiologist, the radiology technologist, the surgeon, the medical physicist planning radiation treatment, the oncologist, the pathologist, the breast cancer molecular biologist, and ultimately the theoretical biologist. We have had enough of breast cancer wars (Lerner 2001), and should all disband when we succeed in making breast cancer a manageable problem. The components to attempt this now are all in existence: quantitatively predicted tumor target size that we need to detect and destroy (2-4 mm), many imaging modalities that singly or in combination would seem capable of reaching that target, and ablation techniques able to destroy them with small resection margins. The small proportion of recurrences expected could almost all be caught before metastasis by the same protocol. Research could switch to how to achieve compliance, whether we can safely and effectively extend the protocol to younger women with radiographically dense breasts (Law et al. 2007), whether "surgery-driven escape from dormancy" (Retsky et al. 2008) applies to partially ablated premetastasis tumors, honing of the protocol with experience, the search for induced tumors (Heyes et al. 2009; Shuryak et al. 2009), and further reduction of x-ray dose.

The difficult questions of prevention of the initiation of breast tumors, presumed by many to be due to artificial environmental toxins or lifestyle choices, or improving the immune response to nascent tumors, or intervening in the genetics of aberrant oncogenic or radiation sensitivity genes, such as women with ataxia-telangiectasia, a radiation-sensitive genetic condition (Hall et al. 1992; Ramsay et al. 1996, 1998), could be pursued in subsequent decades, with a firm data set from the search and destroy approach of how many small tumors are being detected across populations. If, in the interim, the magic bullet for breast cancer is found (Hubbard 1986; Strebhardt and Ullrich 2008), we might choose to pack up the whole search and destroy protocol, but that may be in the distant future, if ever: "...despite an avalanche of knowledge in molecular biology in recent years, not a single cancer-specific cell surface antigen has yet been discovered" (Gonenne 2009), though the author now claims:

> "MabCure has successfully generated hybridoma libraries for three different cancers that produce, respectively, antibodies to melanoma, to an aggressive form of prostate cancer and to ovarian carcinoma. These antibodies have been shown to be specific and 'universal' to each cancer respectively, i.e. they recognize every cancer from different individuals having that particular disease and do not react with any normal antigen tested so far. These Mabs [monoclonal antibodies] are the first candidates for the development of novel diagnostic tools, imaging agents and drugs to treat the corresponding cancers" (Mabcure 2009).

The contrast of this magic bullet approach to search and destroy is startling. For search and destroy we do not want specificity, diagnosis, or treatment, but rather to detect all cancers at early stages, destroying any suspicious lesion without confirming whether or not it had malignant potential. But nevertheless, through molecular imaging, they may prove complementary.

Will my message "Stop Breast Cancer Now!" be taken seriously? One could take the cynical view that each of us involved in breast cancer research has a vested interest in not seeing the problem solved. But I think the difficulty lies elsewhere, in how scientific and medical research is organized, and how we police each other through innovation suppressing peer review. Perhaps we need the old approach of the Longitude Prize offered by the British Parliament in 1714 (Sobel 1995), this time for solving breast cancer once and for all. While this might seem winner take all, the real winner would be the women (and a few men) who would no longer anticipate a life shortened by breast cancer.

The idea of prizes rather than grants has been renewed by the USA National Aeronautics & Space Administration:

> "In December 1903, Wilbur and Orville Wright, two bicycle mechanics working with no government support, initiated the age of powered flight with their success at Kitty Hawk. NASA's Prize Program honors the spirit of the Wright Brothers and other independent inventors by acknowledging the centennial of the first powered flight in 2003. The NASA Centennial Challenges program also recognizes that the rapid and dramatic progress in aeronautics in the early years of the first century of flight was often driven by prize competitions" (NASA 2009a).

But the present cash prize is not big enough: "...the resources that are expended in research and development by competitors are typically many times the value of the prize itself" (NASA 2009b).

10.26 The Sick Lobe: "A paradox, a paradox, a most ingenious paradox" (Gilbert and Sullivan 1879)

Except for our collaboration on the second Workshop on Alternatives to Mammography, Tibor Tot and I have not worked together. So when he asked me to say a few words about his sick lobe hypothesis in this chapter, I was suddenly confronted by what my collaborator Vincent Vinh-Hung recognized as a paradox:

> *One the one hand*: extrapolation of epidemiological data suggests that killing one small primary premetastasis breast tumor should be able to cure breast cancer.

> *On the other hand*: premetastasis tumors are frequently mulifocal, perhaps all in one sick lobe.

This is a universal predicament, as noted in *Fiddler on the Roof*:

> "Avram: (gestures at Perchik and Mordcha) He's right, and he's right? They can't both be right.

> "Tevye: You know... you are also right" (United Artists Corporation 1971).

At this point we can only speculate. Here I record our first thoughts as a dialogue extracted from e-mail:

> *Tibor Tot:*

> The 'lobar disease' theory means, in its simplified form, that breast cancer develops not on a single point in the breast, but within a several cm large area, often on several places in this area at the same time. In fact, according to our studies, carcinomas <10 mm are unifocal in 37%, multifocal in the rest and in about 50% of the cases foci

are seen in an area larger than or equal to 40 mm ('extensive cases'). It means that you will need to ablate not a 2–3 mm large lesion but several such lesions together with their genetically altered environment. I believe that one should ablate a sick lobe, but it can also be called the 'field of cancerization.'

Richard Gordon:

I would like to see an extrapolation of the probability of metastasis to smaller sizes for each # of foci found, and perhaps versus their distances apart. At least that is my first guess as to a proper analysis of the relationship between our previous extrapolations to obtain target size and your sick lobe hypothesis.

I would also like to see the evidence that multiple foci are actually in the same lobe. While I'm fully aware of your hypothesis, it is now time for a detailed understanding of exactly what you measured, and how you drew your conclusions.

It is also not clear to me how many of our target foci (<4 mm) must be found (and where) to conclude that one is dealing with a sick lobe, and whether, given >99% (predicted) success rate, it would be advisable to surgically or by ablation remove a lobe, or just do watchful waiting of it? The uncertainty is compounded by the fact that, for now, none of our imaging methods can reliably outline the breast lobes. For x-ray CT in particular, this might require increased dose, and therefore be counterproductive.

Tibor Tot:

While the [sick lobe] hypothesis is a hypothesis, the multifocal nature of the majority of breast carcinomas, also at the beginning of their development, is a morphological fact. I have studied and published this fact several times, and people before me using similar histology technique have reported similar results. This multifocality is evident already in the *in situ* phase, before the cancer invades and before it gives the metastases.

Now to my main point. We have a practical problem here: if a surgeon will read the first chapters of this book, he or she will get the impression that the correct surgery at early stage breast cancer is to cut big, remove a several cm area. Reading your chapter, they will have the impression that it is sufficient to cut small, 4 mm with a minimal margin. I am convinced, looking at early breast carcinomas every day, that the limited approach is not sufficient for the majority of the cases, but may be sufficient for a about 30–40%, the unifocals. I still believe that one should cut big even in these cases as small multiple foci are often missed on radiology.

Vincent Vinh-Hung:

I'm not sure how modeling could be handled. But I like paradoxes. The concept of lobe disease or field cancer-

ization, and that of very early detection, are not necessarily mutually exclusive.

Richard Gordon

I think that Vincent has hit the nail on the head, by calling this a paradox:

1. The extrapolated epidemiological data suggests that search and destroy of single premetastasis tumors should cure breast cancer.
2. The mutifocal data suggests that more tissue should be removed or ablated than one would ordinarily think for a <4 mm tumor.

So let's see if we can formulate some hypotheses consistent with both results, and then ways of testing them. Let me throw these out for your consideration:

1. The extrapolation is correct, but larger resection margins (perhaps the whole sick lobe) would decrease the chance of later disease (not just recurrence) even more. This is logically consistent with the extreme action: total mastectomy (Mokbel 2003). (This is in essence a refinement of the old battle between total mastectomy and lumpectomy, Lerner 2001.)
2. Removal of a single premetastasis tumor delays the occurrence of additional tumors in the same lobe. But if it's not removed, multifocal disease occurs.
3. The reason that premetastasis tumors can be multifocal, yet be consistent with the extrapolations, is that most of them regress (Nielsen et al. 1987; Nielsen 1989). In this case, since we don't know which will regress and which won't, we should ablate them all. This also suggests a possible competition between multifocal tumors, perhaps the larger one(s) actively suppressing the smaller.

I realize, and perhaps Vincent now agrees, that there is some serious new research to be done to resolve this paradox.

Vincent Vinh-Hung

Thinking aloud, can a tumor grow without some kind of cooperation from the host? There has been more attention given to the stroma/microenvironment where the tumor is growing (Hu and Polyak 2008). The concept of a lobe might be appropriate. It would make sense (Ellsworth et al. 2004). A lobe in which a first tumor appeared that grew beyond a few millimeters would be more permissive to additional tumors (cascade and/or recruitment of host facilities by the tumors). Removing the first tumor early enough would reduce the propensity of multifocality, rejoining your point #2B.

This is a terribly challenging topic that would take years.

So, we three have agreed to take on the challenge (Vinh-Hung et al. 2010).

10.27 Conclusion

The century-old magic bullet approach to cancer has not served us well. It became part of the hegemony of biochemistry and later molecular biology, genomics, and a massive pharmaceuticals industry with an attitude that there is a drug for every malady. In parallel, over the past century, x-ray and other forms of imaging developed and improved. These are now ready to overtake magic bullets precisely because they are nonspecific, that is, potentially capable of detecting all tumors. The target size for >99% of premetastasis breast tumors has been estimated at 2–4 mm diameter by extrapolation of three independent sets of epidemiological data. High-resolution, possibly multimodal imaging, perhaps combined with magic bullet molecular imaging, followed by co-registered ablation immediately after and in the same gantry as the screening, should be able to search and destroy most breast cancers at this early stage, with small resection margins. We need only the collective will to make it so. The sick lobe hypothesis is at first glance seemingly at odds with this epidemiological extrapolation, presenting a paradox that we will have to resolve.

Acknowledgments   Supported in part by the Organ Imaging Fund of the Department of Radiology, University of Manitoba. As a lifetime of work is covered, I would also like to thank the following agencies for support of my medical imaging work over the years: Atomic Energy Canada (1984: $5,000), CancerCare Manitoba (2002: $49,311), Friends… You Can Count On (2002: $40,000), Human Resources Development Canada (1995: $1,740), Manitoba Careerstart (1987: $1,418), Manitoba Institute of Child Health (2003: $5,000), Manitoba Medical Service Foundation (1982: $31,293; 1984: $50,000), Ministry for Industry, Trade and Technology, Province of Manitoba (1984: $1,000), National Cancer Institute of Canada (1984: $4,410; 1987: $74,665; 1989: $14,338), NATO (1970: $6,000), Natural Sciences and Engineering Research Council Canada (NSERC) (1979: $104,923), Organ Imaging Fund of the Department of Radiology, University of Manitoba (1992: $14,500; 2000: $25,000; 2009: $10,000), Sanofi-Winthrop (1992: $12,000), Shell Development Company (1984: $500), TRLabs (2004: $5,000), University of Manitoba Deans of Engineering (1982: $1,500) and Medicine (2000: $25,000), University of Manitoba Research Board (1982: $2,000; 1983: $1,250), U.S. SBIR (2000: $17,500), and Winnipeg Regional Health Authority (2004: $5,000). The total of $508,348 has supported 8 Ph.D., 4 Masters, and 20 undergraduate thesis students, plus four conferences. While I have learned that research productivity is inversely proportional to funding, this formula may not be optimal for achieving impact on medical care. I would like to thank my colleagues in the Department of Radiology, University of Manitoba, for their steady support over the past 3 decades, Tibor Tot and Vincent Vinh-Hung for permission to include their dialogue, the Department of Radiology, University of Arizona, for the opportunity of giving a 2007 seminar in which I first pulled these thoughts together, and Harrison H. Barrett and William R. Buckley for critical readings. Malvin H. Kalos corrected me on some of the history of the first CT scanner. Finally, I would like to profusely thank Glen D. Colquhoun for hanging in as a volunteer for so many years, keeping this effort alive. Dedicated to the memory of Boris K. Vainshtein.

References

Abbott EA (1899) Flatland: a romance of many dimensions. Little, Brown, Boston

Abouraddy AF, Saleh BE, Sergienko AV, Teich MC (2001) Role of entanglement in two-photon imaging. Phys Rev Lett 87:123602

Agnese DM, Burak WE Jr (2005) Ablative approaches to the minimally invasive treatment of breast cancer. Cancer J 11:77–82

Aliaga A, Rousseau JA, Cadorette J, Croteau E, van Lier JE, Lecomte R, Benard F (2007) A small animal positron emission tomography study of the effect of chemotherapy and hormonal therapy on the uptake of 2-deoxy-2-[F-18]fluoro-D-glucose in murine models of breast cancer. Mol Imaging Biol 9:144–150

Alizad A, Whaley DH, Greenleaf JF, Fatemi M (2005) Potential applications of vibro-acoustography in breast imaging. Technol Cancer Res Treat 4:151–158

Alpuche Avilés JE (2004) Multiplicative Algebraic Reconstruction Techniques for 3D Cone Beam CT of the Breast [Undergraduate Thesis, Supervisor: R. Gordon]. Mérida, Yucatán, México: Facultad de Ingeniería de la Universidad Autónoma de Yucatán

Alpuche Avilés JE., Pistorius S, Gordon R, Elbakri, IA (2010) A novel hybrid reconstruction algorithm for first generation incoherent scatter CT (ISCT) of large objects with potential medical imaging applications. J X-ray Sci Technol: in press.

Altschuler MD, Censor Y, Eggermont PP, Herman GT, Kuo YH, Lewitt RM, McKay M, Tuy HK, Udupa JK, Yau MM (1980) Demonstration of a software package for the reconstruction of the dynamically changing structure of the human heart from cone beam x-ray projections. J Med Syst 4:289–304

Ambrose J (1973) Computerised transverse axial scanning (tomography). II Clinical application. Br J Radiol 46:1023–1047

Ambrose J (1974) Computerized x-ray scanning of brain. J Neurosurg 40:679–695

Andersen AH, Kak AC (1984) Simultaneous algebraic reconstruction technique (SART): a superior implementation of the ART algorithm. Ultrason Imaging 6:81–94

Anninos PA, Kotini A, Koutlaki N, Adamopoulos A, Galazios G, Anastasiadis P (2000) Differential diagnosis of breast lesions by use of biomagnetic activity and non-linear analysis. Eur J Gynaecol Oncol 21:591–595

Ayres FJ, Rangayyan RM (2007) Reduction of false positives in the detection of architectural distortion in mammograms by using a geometrically constrained phase portrait model. Int J Comput Assist Radiol Surg 1:361–369

Badea C, Gordon R (2004) Experiments with the nonlinear and chaotic behaviour of the multiplicative algebraic reconstruction technique (MART) algorithm for computed tomography. Phys Med Biol 49:1455–1474

Bagchi S (2007) New technique for detecting breast cancer. Lancet Oncol 8:12

Bailar JC III (1976) Mammography: a contrary view. Ann Intern Med 84:77–84

Bailar JC III, MacMahon B (1997) Randomization in the Canadian National Breast Screening Study: a review for evidence of subversion. CMAJ 156:193–199

Baines CJ (1994) The Canadian National Breast Screening Study: a perspective on criticisms. Ann Intern Med 120:326–334

Baines CJ, Miller AB, Wall C, McFarlane DV, Simor IS, Jong R, Shapiro BJ, Audet L, Petitclerc M, Ouimet-Oliva D, Ladouceur J, Hèbert G, Minuk T, Hardy G, Standing HK (1986) Sensitivity and specificity of first screen mammography in the Canadian National Breast Screening Study: a preliminary report from five centers. Radiology 160:295–298

Baker JR, Budinger TF, Huesman RH (1992) Generalized approach to inverse problems in tomography: image reconstruction for spatially variant systems using natural pixels. Crit Rev Biomed Eng 20:47–71

Bakic PR, Albert M, Brzakovic D, Maidment ADA (2002a) Mammogram synthesis using a 3D simulation. I. Breast tissue model and image acquisition simulation. Med Phys 29:2131–2139

Bakic PR, Albert M, Brzakovic D, Maidment ADA (2002b) Mammogram synthesis using a 3D simulation. II. Evaluation of synthetic mammogram texture. Med Phys 29:2140–2151

Bakic PR, Albert M, Brzakovic D, Maidment AD (2003) Mammogram synthesis using a three-dimensional simulation. III. Modeling and evaluation of the breast ductal network. Med Phys 30:1914–1925

Banik S, Rangayyan RM, Desautels JEL (2009) Detection of architectural distortion in prior mammograms of interval-cancer cases with neural networks. In: 31st annual international conference of the IEEE EMBS, Minneapolis, Minnesota, USA, 2–6 September 2009, pp 6667–6670

Bao A, Goins B, Dodd GD, Soundararajan A, Santoyo C, Otto RA, Davis MD, Phillips WT (2008) Real-time iterative monitoring of radiofrequency ablation tumor therapy with ^{15}O-water PET imaging. J Nucl Med 49:1723–1729

Barbieri M (1974) A criterion to evaluate three dimensional reconstructions from projections of unknown structures. J Theor Biol 48:451–467

Barbieri M (1987) Co-information: a new concept in theoretical biology. Riv Biol 80:101–126

Barbieri M, Pettazzoni P, Bersani F, Maraldi NM (1970) Isolation of ribosome microcrystals. J Mol Biol 54:121–124

Barnett GH, Sloan AE, Torchia MG (20091) Preliminary results of novel laser interstitial therapy system for treatment of recurrent glioblastoma. In: American Association of Neurological Surgeons annual meeting, San Diego, 2–6 May 2009, pp abstract #54756

Barrett HH, Müller S, Wilson DW (2010) Therapy operating characteristic (TOC) curves and their application to the evaluation of segmentation algorithms. Proceedings of SPIE 7627:76270Z

Baum M (2004) Breast cancer screening comes full circle. J Natl Cancer Inst 96:1490–1491

Beekman FJ, Kamphuis C, Viergever MA (1996) Improved SPECT quantitation using fully three-dimensional iterative spatially variant scatter response compensation. IEEE Trans Med Imaging 15:491–499

Bellman SH (1970) A perfect and absolute blank. J Theor Biol 29:482

Bellman SH, Bender R, Gordon R, Rowe JE Jr (1971) ART is science, being a defense of Algebraic Reconstruction Techniques for three-dimensional electron microscopy. J Theor Biol 32:205–216

Bender R, Duck PD (1982) Chemical synthesis apparatus for preparation of polynucleotides. US Patent 4,353,989

Bender R, Bellman SH, Gordon R (1970) ART and the ribosome: a preliminary report on the three-dimensional structure of individual ribosomes determined by an Algebraic Reconstruction Technique. J Theor Biol 29:483–488

Bender JE, Kapadia AJ, Sharma AC, Tourassi GD, Harrawood BP, Floyd CE Jr (2007) Breast cancer detection using neutron stimulated emission computed tomography: prominent elements and dose requirements. Med Phys 34:3866–3871

Benjamin S (2000) Quantum cryptography: single photons "on demand". Science 290:2273–2274

Berdon WE, Slovis TL (2002) Where we are since ALARA and the series of articles on CT dose in children and risk of long-term cancers: what has changed? Pediatr Radiol 32:699

Bertell R, Ehrle LH, Schmitz-Feuerhake I (2007) Pediatric CT research elevates public health concerns: low-dose radiation issues are highly politicized. Int J Health Serv 37:419–439

Bertero M, Boccacci P (1998) Introduction to inverse problems in imaging. Taylor & Francis, Oxford

Bhagtani R, Schmidt TG (2009) Simulated scatter performance of an inverse-geometry dedicated breast CT system. Med Phys 36:788–796

Bjarnason GA (1996) Menstrual cycle chronobiology: is it important in breast cancer screening and therapy? Lancet 347:345–346

Bliznakova K, Bliznakov Z, Pallikarakis N (2002) A 3D breast software phantom for tomosynthetic mammography. In: Third European symposium on BME and MP, Patras, 30 August–1 September 2002

Bliznakova K, Bliznakov Z, Bravou V, Kolitsi Z, Pallikarakis N (2003) A three-dimensional breast software phantom for mammography simulation. Phys Med Biol 48:3699–3719

Bliznakova K, Kolitsi Z, Pallikarakis N (2006) Dual-energy mammography: simulation studies. Phys Med Biol 51:4497–4515

Blyschak K, Simick M, Jong R, Lilge L (2004) Classification of breast tissue density by optical transillumination spectroscopy: optical and physiological effects governing predictive value. Med Phys 31:1398–1414

Boone JM, Lindfors KK, Seibert JA, Nelson TR (2003) Breast cancer screening using a dedicated breast CT scanner: a feasibility study. In: Peitgen H-O (ed) IWDM 2002. Sixth international workshop on digital mammography, Bremen, Germany, 22–25 June 2002. Springer, New York, pp 6–11

Bowen SL, Wu Y, Chaudhari AJ, Fu L, Packard NJ, Burkett GW, Yang K, Lindfors KK, Shelton DK, Hagge R, Borowsky AD, Martinez SR, Qi J, Boone JM, Cherry SR, Badawi RD (2009) Initial characterization of a dedicated breast PET/CT scanner during human imaging. J Nucl Med 50:1401–1408

Bracewell RN (1977) Correction for collimator width (restoration) in reconstructive x-ray tomography. J Comput Assist Tomogr 1:6–15

Bradford CD, Peppler WW, Ross RE (2002) Multitapered x-ray capillary optics for mammography. Med Phys 29:1097–1108

Bravin A, Keyriläinen J, Fernandez M, Fiedler S, Nemoz C, Karjalainen-Lindsberg ML, Tenhunen M, Virkkunen P, Leidenius M, von Smitten K, Sipila P, Suortti P (2007) High-resolution CT by diffraction-enhanced x-ray imaging: mapping of breast tissue samples and comparison with their histo-pathology. Phys Med Biol 52:2197–2211

Brenner DJ (2002) Estimating cancer risks from pediatric CT: going from the qualitative to the quantitative. Pediatr Radiol 32:228–244

Brenner RJ, Parisky Y (2007) Alternative breast-imaging approaches. Radiol Clin North Am 45:907–923

Brenner D, Elliston C, Hall E, Berdon W (2001) Estimated risks of radiation-induced fatal cancer from pediatric CT. AJR Am J Roentgenol 176:289–296

Brettle DS, Ward SC, Parkin GJ, Cowen AR, Sumsion HJ (1994) A clinical comparison between conventional and digital mammography utilizing computed radiography. Br J Radiol 67:464–468

Bruzzone L, Cossu R (2003) An adaptive approach to reducing registration noise effects in unsupervised change detection. IEEE Trans Geosci Remote Sens 41:2455–2465

Burattini E, Cossu E, Di Maggio C, Gambaccini M, Indovina PL, Marziani M, Pocek M, Simeoni S, Simonetti G (1995) Mammography with synchrotron radiation. Radiology 195:239–244

Burdette D, Albani D, Chesi E, Clinthorne NH, Cochran E, Honscheid K, Huh SS, Kagan H, Knopp M, Lacasta C, Mikuz M, Schmalbrock P, Studen A, Weilhammer P (2009) A device to measure the effects of strong magnetic fields on the image resolution of PET scanners. Nucl Instrum Methods Phys Res A 609:263–271

Burg A (2003) Image and video compression: the principles behind the technology. Curr Probl Dermatol 32:17–23

Burhenne LJ, Burhenne HJ (1993) The Canadian National Breast Screening Study: a Canadian critique. AJR Am J Roentgenol 161:761–763

Byrne CL (1993) Iterative image reconstruction algorithms based on cross-entropy minimization. IEEE Trans Image Process 2:96–103

Byrne CL (1996) Block-iterative methods for image reconstruction from projections. IEEE Trans Image Process 5:792–794

Byrne C (2004) A unified treatment of some iterative algorithms in signal processing and image reconstruction. Inverse Prob 20:103–120

Candes EJ, Wakin MB (2008) An introduction to compressive sampling. IEEE Signal Process Mag 25:21–30

Carroll L (1876) The hunting of the snark: an agony in eight fits. Macmillan, New York

Carron I (2009) CS: these technologies do not exist: random x-ray collectors in CT. http://nuit-blanche.blogspot.com/2009/11/cs-these-technologies-do-not-exist_28.html

Cederstroem B, Cahn RN, Danielsson M, Lundqvist M, Nygren DR (1999) Refractive x-ray focusing with modified phonograph records. Proc SPIE 3767:80–89

Censor Y, Zenios SA (1997) Parallel optimization: theory, algorithms, and applications. Oxford University Press, New York

Chan HP, Vyborny CJ, MacMahon H, Metz CE, Doi K, Sickles EA (1987) Digital mammography. ROC studies of the effects of pixel size and unsharp-mask filtering on the detection of subtle microcalcifications. Invest Radiol 22:581–589

Chang CH, Sibala JL, Gallagher JH, Riley RC, Templeton AW, Beasley PV, Porte RA (1977) Computed tomography of the breast. A preliminary report. Radiology 124:827–829

Chang C, Sibala J, Fritz S, Gallagher J, Dwyer S 3rd, Templeton A (1978) Computed tomographic evaluation of the breast. AJR Am J Roentgenol 131:459–464

Chang CH, Nesbit DE, Fisher DR, Fritz SL, Dwyer SJ 3rd, Templeton AW, Lin F, Jewell WR (1982) Computed tomographic mammography using a conventional body scanner. AJR Am J Roentgenol 138:553–558

Chang CF, Chen CY, Chang FH, Tai SP, Yu CH, Tseng YB, Tsai TH, Liu IS, Su WF, Sun CK (2008) Cell tracking and detection of molecular expression in live cells using lipid-enclosed CdSe quantum dots as contrast agents for epi-third harmonic generation microscopy. Opt Express 16:9534–9548

Chapman J-A, Gordon R, Link MA, Fish EB (1999) Infiltrating breast carcinoma smaller than 0.5 centimeters. Is lymph node dissection necessary? Cancer 86:2186–2188

Chen B, Ning R (2002) Cone-beam volume CT breast imaging: feasibility study. Med Phys 29:755–770

Chen ZK, Ning R (2003) Why should breast tumour detection go three dimensional? Phys Med Biol 48:2217–2228

Chen YM, Wu SJ, Wang YY (1997) Application of holographic tomography to the measurement of 3D flame temperature field. J Chin Inst Chem Eng 28:197–203

Chen YF, Gunawan E, Low KS, Wang SC, Soh CB, Thi LL (2007) Time of arrival data fusion method for two-dimensional ultrawideband breast cancer detection. IEEE Trans Antennas Propag 55:2852–2865

Chen YF, Gunawan E, Low KS, Wang SC, Soh CB, Putti TC (2008) Time-reversal ultrawideband breast imaging: pulse design criteria considering multiple tumors with unknown tissue properties. IEEE Trans Antennas Propag 56:3073–3077

Cherepenin VA, Karpov AY, Korjenevsky AV, Kornienko VN, Kultiasov YS, Ochapkin MB, Trochanova OV, Meister JD (2002) Three-dimensional EIT imaging of breast tissues: system design and clinical testing. IEEE Trans Med Imaging 21:662–667

Cherry SR (2006) Multimodality in vivo imaging systems: twice the power or double the trouble? Annu Rev Biomed Eng 8:35–62

Cherry SR, Louie AY, Jacobs RE (2008) The integration of positron emission tomography with magnetic resonance imaging. Proc IEEE 96:416–438

Choi MH, Kao TJ, Isaacson D, Saulnier GJ, Newell JC (2007) A reconstruction algorithm for breast cancer imaging with electrical impedance tomography in mammography geometry. IEEE Trans Biomed Eng 54:700–710

Christ M, Kenig CE, Sadosky C, Weiss G (1998) Alberto Pedro Calderón (1920–1998). Not Amer Math Soc 45:1148–1153

Clarke J, Hatridge M, Mössle M (2007) SQUID-detected magnetic resonance imaging in microtesla fields. Annu Rev Biomed Eng 9:389–413

Clarkson E, Barrett H (1997) A bound on null functions for digital imaging systems with positivity constraints. Opt Lett 22:814–815

Clarkson E, Barrett H (1998) Bounds on null functions of linear digital imaging systems. J Opt Soc Am A Opt Image Sci Vis 15:1355–1360

Colang JE, Killion JB, Vano E (2007) Patient dose from CT: a literature review. Radiol Technol 79:17–26

Colquhoun GD, Gordon R (2005a) A superresolution computed tomography algorithm for reverse cone beam 3D x-ray mammography. In: Tot T (ed) Workshop on alternatives to mammography, Copenhagen, 29–30 September 2005

Colquhoun GD, Gordon R (2005b) The use of control angles with MART (Multiplicative Algebraic Reconstruction Technique). Technol Cancer Res Treat 4:183–184

Colquhoun GD, Gordon R, Elbakri IA (2004) Reversed cone beam coded aperture mammography [Abstract 4408744]. RSNA (rejected)

Cooley JW, Tukey JW (1965) An algorithm for machine calculation of complex Fourier series. Math Comput 19:297–301

Cormack AM (1963) Representation of a function by its line integrals, with some radiological applications. J Appl Phys 34:2722–2727

Cormack AM (1964) Representation of a function by its line integrals, with some radiological applications. II. J Appl Phys 35:2908–2913

Cormack AM (1980) Nobel Award address. Early two-dimensional reconstruction and recent topics stemming from it. Med Phys 7:277–282

Cormack AM (1994) EMI patent litigation in the US. Br J Radiol 67:316–317

Cornely PRJ (2003) Flexible prior models: three-dimensional ionospheric tomography. Radio Sci 38. Article Number: 1087

Crewe AV, Crewe DA (1984) Inexact reconstructions from projections. Ultramicroscopy 12:293–298

Crowther RA, Klug A (1971) ART and science or conditions for three-dimensional reconstruction from electron microscope images. J Theor Biol 32:199–203

Crowther RA, Klug A (1974) Three dimensional image reconstruction on an extended field: fast, stable algorithm. Nature 251:490–492

Cubeddu R, D'Andrea C, Pifferi A, Taroni P, Torricelli A, Valentini G (2000) Effects of the menstrual cycle on the red and near-infrared optical properties of the human breast. Photochem Photobiol 72:383–391

Dabrosin C, Hallstrom A, Ungerstedt U, Hammar M (1997) Microdialysis of human breast tissue during the menstrual cycle. Clin Sci 92:493–496

Danielli JF (1961) Preface. J Theor Biol 1:i

Daun KJ, Thomson KA, Liu F, Smallwood GJ (2006) Deconvolution of axisymmetric flame properties using Tikhonov regularization. Appl Opt 45:4638–4646

Dawson P (2004) Patient dose in multislice CT: why is it increasing and does it matter? Br J Radiol 77(Spec No 1): S10–S13

Dayan B, Parkins AS, Aoki T, Ostby EP, Vahala KJ, Kimble HJ (2008) A photon turnstile dynamically regulated by one atom. Science 319:1062–1065

DeRosier DJ, Klug A (1968) Reconstruction of three dimensional structures from electron micrographs. Nature 217:130

Dhawan AP (1985) Nevoscopy: three-dimensional computed tomography of nevi and melanomas in situ by transillumination to detect early cutaneous malignant melanomas. Ph.D. thesis, Supervisor: R. Gordon, Department of Electrical Engineering, University of Manitoba, Winnipeg

Dhawan AP, Gordon R (1986) Reply to comments on "Enhancement of mammographic features by optimal adaptive neighborhood image processing". IEEE Trans Med Imaging MI-6:82–83

Dhawan AP, Rangayyan RM, Gordon R (1984a) Wiener filtering for deconvolution of geometric artifacts in limited-view image reconstruction. Proc SPIE 515:168–172

Dhawan AP, Gordon R, Rangayyan RM (1984b) Computed tomography by transillumination to detect early melanoma. IEEE Trans Biomed Eng BME-31:574

Dhawan AP, Gordon R, Rangayyan RM (1984c) Nevoscopy: three-dimensional computed tomography for nevi and melanomas in situ by transillumination. IEEE Trans Med Imaging MI-3(2):54–61

Dhawan AP, Rangayyan RM, Gordon R (1985) Image restoration by Wiener deconvolution in limited-view computed tomography. Appl Opt 24:4013–4020

Dhawan AP, Buelloni G, Gordon R (1986a) Enhancement of mammographic features by optimal adaptive neighborhood image processing. IEEE Trans Med Imaging MI-5:8–15

Dhawan AP, Buelloni G, Gordon R (1986b) Errata: enhancement of mammographic features by optimal adaptive neighborhood image processing. IEEE Trans Med Imaging MI-5:120

Dobbins JT (2009) Tomosynthesis imaging: at a translational crossroads. Med Phys 36:1956–1967

Donaire JG, Garcia I (1999) On improving the performance of ART in 3D cone beam transmission tomography. In: Proceedings of the 1999 international meeting on fully 3D image reconstruction in radiology and nuclear medicine, pp 73–76

Donaire JG, Garcia I (2002) On using global optimization to obtain a better performance of a MART algorithm in 3D x-ray tomography. J Imaging Sci Technol 46:247–256

Donnelly LF, Frush DP (2001) Fallout from recent articles on radiation dose and pediatric CT. Pediatr Radiol 31:388–391

Düchting H (2001) Georges Seurat, 1859–1891: the master of pointillism. Taschen, Köln

Duclaux É (1920) Pasteur, the history of a mind. W.B. Saunders, Philadelphia

Dusaussoy NJ, Abdou IE (1991) The extended MENT algorithm: a maximum-entropy type algorithm using prior knowledge for computerized-tomography. IEEE Trans Signal Process 39: 1164–1180

Dzendrowskyj TE, Noyszewski EA, Beers J, Bolinger L (1997) Lipid composition changes in normal breast throughout the menstrual cycle. Magn Reson Mater Phys, Biol Med 5: 105–110

Eggermont PPB, Herman GT, Lent A (1981) Iterative algorithms for large partitioned linear systems, with applications to image reconstruction. Linear Algebra Appl 40:37–67

Ehrenreich B (2001) Welcome to Cancerland. Harper's Magazine November. http://www.barbaraehrenreich.com/cancerland.htm.

Ellsworth DL, Ellsworth RE, Love B, Deyarmin B, Lubert SM, Mittal V, Shriver CD (2004) Genomic patterns of allelic imbalance in disease free tissue adjacent to primary breast carcinomas. Breast Cancer Res Treat 88:131–139

Engl HW, Hanke M, Neubauer A (2000) Regularization of inverse problems. Springer, Dordrecht

Fabbri S, Taibi A, Longo R, Marziani M, Olivo A, Pani S, Tuffanelli A, Gambaccini M (2002) Signal-to-noise ratio evaluation in dual-energy radiography with synchrotron radiation. Phys Med Biol 47:4093–4105

Fang Q, Meaney PM, Geimer SD, Streltsov AV, Paulsen KD (2004) Microwave image reconstruction from 3-D fields coupled to 2-D parameter estimation. IEEE Trans Med Imaging 23:475–484

Fang QQ, Carp SA, Selb J, Boverman G, Zhang Q, Kopans DB, Moore RH, Miller EL, Brooks DH, Boas DA (2009) Combined optical imaging and mammography of the healthy breast: optical contrast derived from breast structure and compression. IEEE Trans Med Imaging 28:30–42

Feldkamp LA, Davis LC, Kress JW (1984) Practical cone-beam algorithm. J Opt Soc Am A 1:612–619

Fellholter A, Mewes D (1994) Mixing of large-volume gas-flows in pipes and ducts: visualization of concentration profiles. Chem Eng Technol 17:227–234

Ferguson DJ, Anderson TJ (1981) Morphological evaluation of cell turnover in relation to the menstrual cycle in the "resting" human breast. Br J Cancer 44:177–181

Ferguson JE, Schor AM, Howell A, Ferguson MW (1990) Tenascin distribution in the normal human breast is altered during the menstrual cycle and in carcinoma. Differentiation 42:199–207

Ferguson JE, Schor AM, Howell A, Ferguson MW (1992) Changes in the extracellular matrix of the normal human breast during the menstrual cycle. Cell Tissue Res 268:167–177

Fiedler S, Bravin A, Keyrilainen J, Fernández M, Suortti P, Thomlinson W, Tenhunen M, Virkkunen P, Karjalainen-Lindsberg M (2004) Imaging lobular breast carcinoma: comparison of synchrotron radiation DEI-CT technique with clinical CT, mammography and histology. Phys Med Biol 49:175–188

Fill EE (ed) (1992) X-ray lasers 1992: proceedings of the third international colloquium on x-ray lasers held at Schliersee. IOP, London

Fitchett JW (1993) A locally synchronous globally asynchronous vertex-8 processing element for image reconstruction on a mesh. Masters thesis. Department of Electrical and Computer Engineering, University of Manitoba, Winnipeg

Flores-Tapia D, Thomas G, Pistorius S (2008) A wavefront reconstruction method for 3-D cylindrical subsurface radar imaging. IEEE Trans Image Process 17:1908–1925

Foo C (1999) X-ray imaging via intelligently steered x-ray microbeams. B.Sc. thesis, Supervisor: R. Gordon. Department of Electrical & Computer Engineering, University of Manitoba, Winnipeg

Forsdyke DR (2009) Canadian Association for Responsible Research Funding. http://post.queensu.ca/~forsdyke/peer-rev.htm#PEER%20REVIEW

Fowler PA, Casey CE, Cameron GG, Foster MA, Knight CH (1990) Cyclic changes in composition and volume of the breast during the menstrual cycle, measured by magnetic resonance imaging. Br J Obstet Gynaecol 97:595–602

Gamow G (1970) My world line: an informal autobiography. Viking Adult, New York

Gao N, He B (2008) Noninvasive imaging of bioimpedance distribution by means of current reconstruction magnetic resonance electrical impedance tomography. IEEE Trans Biomed Eng 55:1530–1538

Garcia I, Roca J, Sanjurjo J, Carazo JM, Zapata EL (1996) Implementation and experimental evaluation of the constrained ART algorithm on a multicomputer system. Signal Process 51:69–76

Garmire GP, Bautz MW, Ford PG, Nousek JA, Ricker GR Jr (2003) Advanced CCD imaging spectrometer (ACIS) instrument on the Chandra X-ray Observatory. In: Proceedings of SPIE, vol 4851, pp 28–44

Garra BS (2007) Imaging and estimation of tissue elasticity by ultrasound. Ultrasound Q 23:255–268

Gavrielides MA, Lo JY, Floyd CE Jr (2002) Parameter optimization of a computer-aided diagnosis scheme for the segmentation of microcalcification clusters in mammograms. Med Phys 29:475–483

Gilbert WS, Sullivan A (1879) The pirates of Penzance, or the slave of duty. http://math.boisestate.edu/GaS/pirates/web_op/pirates18.html

Glaiberman CB, Pilgram TK, Brown DB (2005) Patient factors affecting thermal lesion size with an impedance-based radiofrequency ablation system. J Vasc Interv Radiol 16:1341–1348

Gmitro AF, Greivenkamp JE, Swindell W, Barrett HH, Chiu MY, Gordon SK (1980) Optical computers for reconstructing objects from their x-ray projections. Opt Eng 19:260–272

Goel NS, Campbell RD, Gordon R, Rosen R, Martinez H, Ycas M (1970) Self-sorting of isotropic cells. J Theor Biol 28:423–468

Going JJ, Anderson TJ, Battersby S, MacIntyre CC (1988) Proliferative and secretory activity in human breast during natural and artificial menstrual cycles. Am J Pathol 130:193–204

Goldberg MA, Dwyer SJ 3rd (1995) Telemammography: implementation issues. Telemed J 1:215–226

Gonenne A (2009) Tumour-specific markers: the holy grail of cancer diagnostics. Biotechnol Focus 12:17–18, 27

Gong P, Ledrew EF, Miller JR (1992) Registration noise reduction in difference images for change detection. Int J Remote Sens 13:773–779

Gordon R (1960) Oh Dear What Can the Matter Be? Oh dear what can the matter be? University of Chicago Laboratory School, Chicago

Gordon R (1966) On stochastic growth and form. Proc Natl Acad Sci USA 56:1497–1504

Gordon R (1969) Polyribosome dynamics at steady state. J Theor Biol 22:515–532

Gordon R (1972) Steps in performing a 3-dimensional reconstruction of single asymmetric particles from a tilt series of electron micrographs. In: Workshop on information treatment in electron microscopy, Basel

Gordon R (1973) Artifacts in reconstructions made from a few projections. In: Fu KS (ed) Proceedings of the first international joint conference on pattern recognition, Washington, D.C., 30 October to 1 November 1973. IEEE Computer Society, Northridge, pp 275–285

Gordon R (1974) A tutorial on ART (Algebraic Reconstruction Techniques). IEEE Trans Nucl Sci NS-21:78–93, 95

Gordon R (1975a) A bibliography on reconstruction from projections. In: Digest of technical papers. Topical meeting on image processing for 2-D and 3-D reconstruction from projections: theory and practice in medicine and the physical sciences, Stanford University, 4–7 August 1975. Optical Society of America, Washington, D.C

Gordon R (1975b) Digest of technical papers. Topical meeting on image processing for 2-D and 3-D reconstruction from projections: theory and practice in medicine and the physical sciences. Optical Society of America, Washington, D.C

Gordon R (1975c) Maximal use of single photons and particles in reconstruction from projections by ARTIST, Algebraic Reconstruction Techniques Intended for Storage Tubes. In: Gordon R (ed) Technical digest. Topical meeting on image processing for 2-D and 3-D reconstruction from projections: theory and practice in medicine and the physical sciences. Optical Society of America, Washington, D.C, pp paper TuC4

Gordon R (1976a) Dose reduction in computed tomography. In: Di Chiro G, Brooks RA (eds) Book of abstracts of the international symposium on computer assisted tomography in nontumoral diseases of the brain, spinal cord and eye. National Institutes of Health, Bethesda, 2 pp

Gordon R (1976b) Dose reduction in computerized tomography [Guest Editorial]. Invest Radiol 111:508–517

Gordon R (1977) High-speed reconstruction of the finest details available in x-ray projections. In: Ter-Pogossian MM, Phelps ME, Brownell GL, Cox JR Jr, Davis DO, Evens RG (eds) Reconstruction tomography in diagnostic radiology and nuclear medicine. University Park Press, Baltimore, pp 77–83

Gordon R (1978a) Higher-resolution tomography. Phys Today 31:46

Gordon R (1978b) Reconstruction from projections in medicine and astronomy. In: van Schoonveld C, Holland D (eds) Image formation from coherence functions in astronomy. Reidel, Dordrecht, pp 317–325

Gordon D (1979a) Spring linocut. In: Yochim LD (ed) Role and impact: the Chicago Society of Artists. Chicago Society of Artists, Chicago, pp 138, 240–241

Gordon R (1979b) Feedback control of exposure geometry in dental radiography workshop, University of Connecticut, 16 May 1978. Appl Opt 18:1769, 1834

Gordon R (1979c) Questions of uniqueness and resolution in reconstruction from projections [Book Review]. Phys Today 32:52–56

Gordon R (1983a) One man's noise is another man's data: the ARTIST algorithm for positron tomography [postdeadline paper, 2 pp]. In: Topical meeting on signal recovery and synthesis with incomplete information and partial constraints. Optical Society of America, Washington, D.C

Gordon R (1983b) Three dimensional computed tomography of nevi in situ by transillumination. Anal Quant Cytol 5:208

Gordon R (1985a) Industrial applications of computed tomography and NMR imaging: an OSA topical meeting. (Invited). Appl Opt 24:3948–3949

Gordon R (1985b) Toward robotic x-ray vision: new directions for computed tomography. Appl Opt 24:4124–4133

Gordon R (1987) There is no such thing as safe sex: chance of AIDS infection increases with time. Winnipeg Free Press March 7:7

Gordon R (1989) A critical review of the physics and statistics of condoms and their role in individual versus societal survival of the AIDS epidemic. J Sex Marital Ther 15:5–30

Gordon R (1990) Inexpensive computed tomography for remote areas. In: SPIE Proceedings, vol 1355, pp 184–188

Gordon R (1992) Testimony on breast cancer and mammography. Canadian House of Commons Proceedings, Sub-Committee on the Status of Women (21):1–23

Gordon R (1993) Grant agencies versus the search for truth. Accountability Res: Policies Qual Assur 2(4):297–301

Gordon R (2011) Epilogue: the diseased breast lobe in the context of X-chromosome inactivation and differentiation waves. In: Tot T (ed) Breast cancer: a lobar disease, Springer, pp 205–210

Gordon R, Bender R (1971a) New three-dimensional algebraic reconstruction techniques (ART). In: Proceedings of 29th annual meeting of the Electron Microscopy Society of America, Boston, pp 82–83

Gordon R, Bender R (1971b) The ART of sectioning without cutting. In: Third international congress for stereology, Berne. Abstracts, 17 pp

Gordon R, Bender R (1971c) Three-dimensional algebraic reconstruction techniques: a preliminary course. J Theor Biol 32:217

Gordon R, Coumans J (1984) Combining multiple imaging techniques for in vivo pathology: a quantitative method for coupling new imaging modalities. Med Phys 11(1):79–80

Gordon R, Herman GT (1971) Reconstruction of pictures from their projections. Commun ACM 14:759–768

Gordon R, Herman GT (1974) Three dimensional reconstruction from projections: a review of algorithms. Int Rev Cytol 38:111–151

Gordon R, Hirsch HVB (1977) Vision begins with direct reconstruction of the retinal image, how the brain sees and stores pictures. In: Schallenberger H, Schrey H (eds) Gegenstrom, Für Helmut Hirsch zum Siebzigsten [Against the stream, for Helmut Hirsch on his 70th birthday]. Peter Hammer, Wuppertal, pp 201–214

Gordon R, Kane J (1972) Three-dimensional reconstruction: the state of the "ART". In: Fourth international biophysics congress, Moscow. Abstracts of Contributed Papers, 2, 37

Gordon R, Lauterbur PC (1974) Introduction to the session on experimental aspects of reconstruction from projections. In: Marr RB (ed) Techniques of three-dimensional reconstruction. Proceedings of an international workshop. Brookhaven National Laboratory, Upton, pp 17–19

Gordon R, Poulin BJ (2009a) Cost of the NSERC science grant peer review system exceeds the cost of giving every qualified researcher a baseline grant. Accountability Res: Policies Qual Assur 16:1–28

Gordon R, Poulin BJ (2009b) Indeed: cost of the NSERC science grant peer review system exceeds the cost of giving every qualified researcher a baseline grant. Accountability Res: Policies Qual Assur 16:232–233

Gordon R, Rangaraj MR (1981) The need for cross-fertilization between the fields of profile inversion and computed tomography. In: Best WG, Weselake SA (eds) Proceedings of the seventh Canadian symposium on remote sensing. Canadian Aeronautics and Space Institute, Ottawa, pp 538–540

Gordon R, Rangaraj MR (1982) Computed tomography from a few ordinary radiographs. In: Proceedings of IEEE, COMPMED-82, pp 54–58

Gordon R, Rangayyan RM (1983) Geometric deconvolution: a meta-algorithm for limited view computed tomography. IEEE Trans Biomed Eng 30:806–810

Gordon R, Rangayyan RM (1984a) Correction: feature enhancement of film mammograms using fixed and adaptive neighborhoods. Appl Opt 23:2055

Gordon R, Rangayyan RM (1984b) Feature enhancement of film mammograms using fixed and adaptive neighborhoods. Appl Opt 23:560–564

Gordon R, Sivaramakrishna R (1999) Mammograms are waldograms: why we need 3D longitudinal breast screening [Guest Editorial]. Appl Radiol 28:12–25

Gordon R, Tweed D (1983) Quantitative reconstruction of visual cortex receptive fields. Univ Manit Med J 53(2):75

Gordon R, Bender R, Herman GT (1970) Algebraic reconstruction techniques (ART) for three-dimensional electron microscopy and x-ray photography. J Theor Biol 29:471–481

Gordon R, Rowe JE Jr, Bender R (1971) ART: a possible replacement for x-ray crystallography at moderate resolution. In: Broda E, Locker A, Springer-Lederer H (eds) Proceedings of the first European biophysics congress, vol VI: Theoretical molecular biology, biomechanics, biomathematics, environmental biophysics, techniques, education. Verlag der Wiener Medizinischer Akademie, Vienna, pp 441–445

Gordon R, Carmichael JB, Isackson FJ (1972) Saltation of plastic balls in a 'one-dimensional' flume. Water Resour Res 8:444–459

Gordon R, Herman GT, Johnson SA (1975) Image reconstruction from projections. Sci Am 233:56–61, 64–68

Gordon R, Silver L, Rigel DS (1976) Halftone graphics on computer terminals with storage display tubes. Proc Soc Inf Disp 17:78–84

Gordon R, Dhawan AP, Rangayyan RM (1985) Reply to "Comments on geometric deconvolution: a meta-algorithm for limited view computed tomography". IEEE Trans Biomed Eng BME-32(3):242–244

Gorenflo R, Vessella S (1991) Abel integral equations: analysis and applications. Springer, Berlin

Gorenstein P (2007) Diffractive–refractive x-ray optics for very high angular resolution x-ray astronomy. Adv Space Res 40:1276–1280

Graham SJ, Stanchev PL, Lloydsmith JOA, Bronskill MJ, Plewes DB (1995) Changes in fibroglandular volume and water content of breast tissue during the menstrual cycle observed by MR imaging at 1.5 T. J Magn Reson Imaging 5:695–701

Grant CS, Ingle JN, Suman VJ, Dumesic DA, Wickerham DL, Gelber RD, Flynn PJ, Weir LM, Intra M, Jones WO, Perez EA, Hartmann LC (2009) Menstrual cycle and surgical treatment of breast cancer: findings from the NCCTG N9431 study. J Clin Oncol 27:3620–3626

Groetsch CW (1999) Inverse problems, activities for undergraduates. The Mathematical Association of America, Washington D.C.

Guan H, Gordon R (1994) A projection access order for speedy convergence of ART (Algebraic Reconstruction Technique): a multilevel scheme for computed tomography. Phys Med Biol 39:2005–2022

Guan H, Gordon R (1996) Computed tomography using Algebraic Reconstruction Techniques (ARTs) with different projection access schemes: a comparison study under practical situations. Phys Med Biol 41:1727–1743

Guan H, Gordon R, Zhu Y (1998) Combining various projection access schemes with the Algebraic Reconstruction Technique for low-contrast detection in computed tomography. Phys Med Biol 43:2413–2421

Guan H, Gaber MW, DiBianca FA, Zhu Y (1999) CT reconstruction by using the MLS-ART technique and the KCD imaging system – I: low-energy x-ray studies. IEEE Trans Med Imaging 18:355–358

Guo YJ, Sivaramakrishna R, Lu CC, Suri JS, Laxminarayan S (2006) Breast image registration techniques: a survey. Med Biol Eng Comput 44:15–26

Gur D, Abrams GS, Chough DM, Ganott MA, Hakim CM, Perrin RL, Rathfon GY, Sumkin JH, Zuley ML, Bandos AI (2009) Digital breast tomosynthesis: observer performance study. AJR Am J Roentgenol 193:586–591

Hall EJ, Geard CR, Brenner DJ (1992) Risk of breast cancer in ataxia-telangiectasia. N Engl J Med 326:1358–1361

Hallégot P, Audinot JN, Migeon HN (2006) Direct NanoSIMS imaging of diffusible elements in surfaced block of cryoprocessed biological samples. Appl Surf Sci 252:6706–6708

Halter RJ, Hartov A, Paulsen KD (2008) A broadband high-frequency electrical impedance tomography system for breast imaging. IEEE Trans Biomed Eng 55:650–659

Hamaker C, Smith KT, Solmon DC, Wagner SL (1980) The divergent beam x-ray transform. Rocky Mountain J Math 10:253–283

Hammer BE, Christensen NL, Heil BG (1994) Use of a magnetic field to increase the spatial resolution of positron emission tomography. Med Phys 21:1917–1920

Han T, Shaw CC, Chen L, Lai C, Wang T (2008) Simulation of mammograms and tomosynthesis imaging with cone beam breast CT images. Proc SPIE 6913:17.11–17.17

Hand JW (2008) Modelling the interaction of electromagnetic fields (10 MHz–10 GHz) with the human body: methods and applications. Phys Med Biol 53:R243–R286

Hardin P (2003) To be honest, I would have never invented the wheel if not for Urg's ground breaking theoretical work with the circle. Artist: Hardin, Patrick, Catalogue Ref: pha0045. http://www.cartoonstock.com/

Harvey JE, Krywonos A, Thompson PL, Saha TT (2001) Grazing-incidence hyperboloid–hyperboloid designs for wide-field x-ray imaging applications. Appl Opt 40:136–144

Hasbro 2004. Battleship Game, http://www.hasbro.com

Haselkorn R, Fried VA (1964) Cell-free protein synthesis: messenger competition for ribosomes. Proc Natl Acad Sci USA 51:1001–1007

Hatziioannou K, Papanastassiou E, Delichas M, Bousbouras P (2003) A contribution to the establishment of diagnostic reference levels in CT. Br J Radiol 76:541–545

Heller J (1961) Catch-22: a novel. Simon and Schuster, New York

Herman GT (1980) Image reconstruction from projections: the fundamentals of computerized tomography. Academic, San Francisco

Herman GT (2009) SNARK09 – a programming system for the reconstruction of 2D images from 1D projections. http://www.snark09.com/

Herman GT, Davidi R (2008) Image reconstruction from a small number of projections. Inverse Prob 24:17

Herman GT, Rowland S (1973) Three methods for reconstructing objects from x-rays: a comparative study. Comput Graphics Image Process 2:151–178

Heyes GJ, Mill AJ, Charles MW (2009) Mammography – oncogenecity at low doses. J Radiol Prot 29:A123–A132

Hirai T, Yamada H, Sasaki M, Hasegawa D, Morita M, Oda Y, Takaku J, Hanashima T, Nitta N, Takahashi M, Murata K (2006) Refraction contrast 11×-magnified x-ray imaging of large objects by MIRRORCLE-type table-top synchrotron. J Synchrotron Radiat 13:397–402

Hoeschen C, Fill U, Zankl M, Panzer W, Regulla D, Dohring W (2005) A high-resolution voxel phantom of the breast for dose calculations in mammography. Radiat Prot Dosimetry 114:406–409

Holley WR, Tobias CA, Fabrikant JI, Benton EV (1981a) Computerized heavy-ion tomography: phantom and tissue specimen studies. AJR Am J Roentgenol 136:1278

Holley WR, Tobias CA, Fabrikant JI, Llacer J, Chu WT, Benton EV (1981b) Computerized heavy-ion tomography. Proc SPIE 273:283–293

Hounsfield GN (1973) Computerized transverse axial scanning (tomography). 1. Description of system. Br J Radiol 46:1016–1022

Hounsfield GN (1975) Method of and apparatus for examining a body by radiation such as X or gamma radiation. US Patent 3,924,131. United States Patent Office, Washington, D.C.

Hounsfield GN (1976) Historical notes on computerized axial tomography. J Can Assoc Radiol 27:135–142

Hounsfield GN (1980) Nobel lecture, 8 December 1979. Computed medical imaging. J Radiol 61:459–468

Houzel C (2004) The work of Niels Henrik Abel. Springer, New York

Hu M, Polyak K (2008) Molecular characterisation of the tumour microenvironment in breast cancer. Eur J Cancer 44:2760–2765

Hu XP, Johnson V, Wong WH, Chen CT (1991) Bayesian image processing in magnetic resonance imaging. Magn Reson Imaging 9:611–620

Huang M, Zhu Q (2004) Dual-mesh optical tomography reconstruction method with a depth correction that uses a priori ultrasound information. Appl Opt 43:1654–1662

Hubbard D (1986) A magic bullet for breast cancer. J Nucl Med 27:305

Huda W (2002) Dose and image quality in CT. Pediatr Radiol 32:709–713, discussion 751–754

Hussain Z, Roberts N, Whitehouse GH, Garcia-Finana M, Percy D (1999) Estimation of breast volume and its variation during the menstrual cycle using MRI and stereology. Br J Radiol 72:236–245

Huston TL, Simmons RM (2005) Ablative therapies for the treatment of malignant diseases of the breast. Am J Surg 189:694–701

Iida H, Kanno I, Miura S, Murakami M, Takahashi K, Uemura K (1986) A simulation study of a method to reduce positron annihilation spread distributions using a strong magnetic field in positron emission tomography. IEEE Trans Nucl Sci 33:597–599

Imamoglu A, Yamamoto Y (1994) Turnstile device for heralded single photons: Coulomb blockade of electron and hole tunneling in quantum confined p–i–n heterojunctions. Phys Rev Lett 72:210–213

Imhof H, Schibany N, Ba-Ssalamah A, Czerny C, Hojreh A, Kainberger F, Krestan C, Kudler H, Nobauer I, Nowotny R (2003) Spiral CT and radiation dose. Eur J Radiol 47:29–37

Inoué S, Walter RJ Jr, Berns MW, Ellis GW, Hansen E (1986) Video microscopy. Plenum, New York

Isaacson M, Kopf D, Utlaut M, Parker NW, Crewe AV (1977) Direct observations of atomic diffusion by scanning transmission electron microscopy. Proc Natl Acad Sci USA 74:1802–1806

Jan ML, Ni YC, Chuang KS, Liang HC, Fu YK (2006) Detectionability evaluation of the PEImager for positron emission applications. Phys Med 21(Suppl 1):109–113

Jansson P (1984) Deconvolution, with applications in spectroscopy. Academic, Orlando

Jansson PA (ed) (1997) Deconvolution of images and spectra. Academic, San Diego

Jia X, Lou Y, Lewis J, Li R, Gu X, Men C, Jiang SB (2010) GPU-based cone beam CT reconstruction via total variation regularization. http://arxiv.org/ftp/arxiv/papers/1001/1001.0599.pdf

Jiang X, Guan H, Gordon R (1992) Contrast enhancement using "feature pixels" or "fixels" for pixel independent image processing. Radiology 185(Suppl):391

Jonges R, Boon PNM, van Marle J, Dietrich AJJ, Grimbergen CA (1999) CART: a controlled algebraic reconstruction technique for electron microscope tomography of embedded, sectioned specimen. Ultramicroscopy 76:203–219

Jorgensen SM, Reyes DA, MacDonald CA, Ritman EL (1999) Micro-CT scanner with a focusing polycapillary x-ray optic. Proc SPIE 3772:158–166

Judenhofer MS, Wehrl HF, Newport DF, Catana C, Siegel SB, Becker M, Thielscher A, Kneilling M, Lichy MP, Eichner M, Klingel K, Reischl G, Widmaier S, Rocken M, Nutt RE, Machulla HJ, Uludag K, Cherry SR, Claussen CD, Pichler BJ (2008) Simultaneous PET-MRI: a new approach for functional and morphological imaging. Nat Med 14:459–465

Kaczmarz S (1937) Angenäherte Auflösung von Systemen linearer Gleichungen. Bull Int Acad Pol Sci Let A 35:335–357

Kaipio J, Somersalo E (2004) Statistical and computational inverse problems. Springer, New York

Kak AC, Slaney M (2001) Principles of computerized tomographic imaging. Society of Industrial and Applied Mathematics, Philadelphia

Kalender W (2000) Computed tomography: fundamentals, system technology, image quality, applications. Publicis MCD, Munich

Kalender WA, Kyriakou Y (2007) Flat-detector computed tomography (FD-CT). Eur Radiol 17:2767–2779

Kalender WA, Deak P, Kellermeier M, van Straten M, Vollmar SV (2009) Application- and patient size-dependent optimization of x-ray spectra for CT. Med Phys 36:993–1007

Kalos MH, Davis DSA, Mittelman MPS, Mastras MP (1961) Conceptual design of a vapor fraction instrument. Nuclear Development Corporation of America, White Plains, http://www.osti.gov/energycitations/product.biblio.jsp?query_id=0&page=0&osti_id=4837780

Kane IJ (1953) Section radiography of the chest. Springer, New York

Kanj H, Popovic M (2008) Two-element T-array for cross-polarized breast tumor detection. Appl Computat Electromagnetics Soc 23:249–254

Kao T, Connor D, Dilmanian FA, Faulconer L, Liu T, Parham C, Pisano ED, Zhong Z (2009) Characterization of diffraction-enhanced imaging contrast in breast cancer. Phys Med Biol 54:3247–3256

Kappadath SC, Shaw CC (2005) Dual-energy digital mammography for calcification imaging: scatter and nonuniformity corrections. Med Phys 32:3395–3408

Karellas A, Vedantham S (2008) Breast cancer imaging: a perspective for the next decade. Med Phys 35:4878–4897

Karellas A, Lo JY, Orton CG (2008) Cone beam x-ray CT will be superior to digital x-ray tomosynthesis in imaging the breast and delineating cancer. Med Phys 35:409–411

Karolczak M, Schaller S, Engelke K, Lutz A, Taubenreuther U, Wiesent K, Kalender W (2001) Implementation of a cone-beam reconstruction algorithm for the single-circle source orbit with embedded misalignment correction using homogeneous coordinates. Med Phys 28:2050–2069

Karssemeijer N, Frieling JT, Hendriks JH (1993) Spatial resolution in digital mammography. Invest Radiol 28:413–419

Kato I, Beinart C, Bleich A, Su S, Kim M, Toniolo PG (1995) A nested case–control study of mammographic patterns, breast volume, and breast cancer (New York City, NY, United States). Cancer Causes Control 6:431–438

Kazantsev IG, Pickalov VV (1999) On the accuracy of line-, strip- and fan-based algebraic reconstruction from few projections. Signal Process 78:117–126

Kim J, Benson O, Kan H, Yamamoto Y (1998) Single-photon turnstile device: simultaneous Coulomb blockade for electrons and holes. Semicond Sci Technol 13(8A Suppl S):A127–A129

Kim J, Benson O, Kan H, Yamamoto Y (1999) A single-photon turnstile device. Nature 397:500–503

Kim BS, Isaacson D, Xia HJ, Kao TJ, Newell JC, Saulnier GJ (2007a) A method for analyzing electrical impedance spectroscopy data from breast cancer patients. Physiol Meas 28:S237–S246

Kim DY, Moon WK, Cho N, Ko ES, Yang SK, Park JS, Kim SM, Park IA, Cha JH, Lee EH (2007b) MRI of the breast for the detection and assessment of the size of ductal carcinoma in situ. Korean J Radiol 8:32–39

Klug A (1983) From macromolecules to biological assemblies. Nobel lecture, 8 December 1982. Biosci Rep 3:395–430

Knoll TF, Delp EJ (1986) Adaptive gray scale mapping to reduce registration noise in difference images. Comp Vis Graphics Image Proc 33:129–137

Konovalov AB, Vlasov VV, Mogilenskikh DV, Kravtsenyuk OV, Lyubimov VV (2008) Algebraic reconstruction and postprocessing in one-step diffuse optical tomography. Quantum Electron 38:588–596

Kroman N (2008) Timing of breast cancer surgery in relation to the menstrual cycle – the rise and fall of a hypothesis. Acta Oncol 47:576–579

Krotz D (1999) U.S. watches efforts in Europe to slash CT radiation load. Diagn Imaging (San Franc) 21:47–49

Kuhl CK, Schild HH, Morakkabati N (2005) Dynamic bilateral contrast-enhanced MR imaging of the breast: trade-off between spatial and temporal resolution. Radiology 236:789–800

Kuzmiak CM, Pisano ED, Cole EB, Zeng D, Burns CB, Roberto C, Pavic D, Lee Y, Seo BK, Koomen M, Washburn D (2005) Comparison of full-field digital mammography to screen-film mammography with respect to contrast and spatial resolution in tissue equivalent breast phantoms. Med Phys 32:3144–3150

Kwan ALC, Boone JM, Yang K, Huang SY (2007) Evaluation of the spatial resolution characteristics of a cone-beam breast CT scanner. Med Phys 34:275–281

Ladas KT, Devaney AJ (1991) Generalized ART algorithm for diffraction tomography. Inverse Prob 7:109–125

Ladas KT, Devaney AJ (1993) Application of an ART algorithm in an experimental study of ultrasonic diffraction tomography. Ultrason Imaging 15:48–58

Lauterbur PC (1973) Image formation by induced interactions: examples employing nuclear magnetic resonance. Nature 242:191–192

Law CK, Kimble HJ (1997) Deterministic generation of a bit-stream of single-photon pulses. J Mod Opt 44:2067–2074

Law J, Faulkner K, Young KC (2007) Risk factors for induction of breast cancer by x-rays and their implications for breast screening. Br J Radiol 80:261–266

Lazebnik M, Zhu CF, Palmer GM, Harter J, Sewall S, Ramanujam N, Hagness SC (2008) Electromagnetic spectroscopy of normal breast tissue specimens obtained from reduction surgeries: comparison of optical and microwave properties. IEEE Trans Biomed Eng 55:2444–2451

Leahy JV, Smith KT, Solmon DC (1979) Uniqueness, nonuniqueness, and inversion in the x-ray and Radon problems. In: Proceedings of the international symposium on ill-posed problems, University of Delaware, Newark

Lee H, Frank MS, Rowberg AH, Choi HS, Kim Y (1993) A new method for computed tomography image compression using adjacent slice data. Invest Radiol 28:678–685

Lee NY, Jung SH, Kim JB (2009) Evaluation of the measurement geometries and data processing algorithms for industrial gamma tomography technology. Appl Radiat Isot 67:1441–1444

Lent A (1977) A convergent algorithm for maximum entropy image restoration, with a medical x-ray application. In: Shaw R (ed) Image analysis and evaluation. Society of Photographic Scientists and Engineers, Washington, D.C., pp 249–257

Lent A, Censor Y (1991) The primal-dual algorithm as a constraint-set-manipulation device. Math Program 50:343–357

Lerner BH (2001) Breast cancer wars: hope, fear, and the pursuit of a cure in twentieth-century America. Oxford University Press, New York

Levinthal C (1968) Are there pathways for protein folding? J Chim Phys 65:44–45

Li FP, Corkery J, Vawter G, Fine W, Sallan SE (1983) Breast carcinoma after cancer therapy in childhood. Cancer 51:521–523

Li T, Liang Z, Singanallur JV, Satogata TJ, Williams DC, Schulte RW (2006) Reconstruction for proton computed tomography by tracing proton trajectories: a Monte Carlo study. Med Phys 33:699–706

Li H, Zheng YB, More MJ, Goodale PJ, Williams MB (2007) Lesion quantification in dual-modality mammotomography. IEEE Trans Nucl Sci 54:107–115

Li CM, Segars WP, Tourassi GD, Boone JM, Dobbins JT III (2009) Methodology for generating a 3D computerized breast phantom from empirical data. Med Phys 36:3122–3131

Lindfors KK, Boone JM, Nelson TR, Yang K, Kwan ALC, Miller DF (2008) Dedicated breast CT: initial clinical experience. Radiology 246:725–733

Linton OW, Mettler FA Jr (2003) National conference on dose reduction in CT, with an emphasis on pediatric patients. AJR Am J Roentgenol 181:321–329

Liu DS, Gong P, Kelly M, Guo QH (2006) Automatic registration of airborne images with complex local distortion. Photogramm Eng Remote Sens 72:1049–1059

Lobo SM, Liu ZJ, Yu NC, Humphries S, Ahmed M, Cosman ER, Lenkinski RE, Goldberg W, Goldberg SN (2005) RF tumour ablation: computer simulation and mathematical modelling of the effects of electrical and thermal conductivity. Int J Hyperthermia 21:199–213

Lukishova SG, Schmid AW, Knox R, Freivald P, Bissell LJ, Boyd RW, Stroud CR, Marshall KL (2007) Room temperature source of single photons of definite polarization. J Mod Opt 54:417–429

Lyncean Technologies (2009) Illuminating x-ray science. http://www.lynceantech.com/

Mabcure (2009) The technology. http://www.mabcure.com/technology.html

Machlin ES, Freilich A, Agrawal DC, Burton JJ, Briant CL (1975) Field ion microscopy of biomolecules. J Microsc 104:127–168

Maes RM, Dronkers DJ, Hendriks JH, Thijssen MA, Nab HW (1997) Do non-specific minimal signs in a biennial mammographic breast cancer screening programme need further diagnostic assessment? Br J Radiol 70:34–38

Maganti SS, Dhawan AP (1997) Three-dimensional Nevoscope image reconstruction using diverging ray ART. Proc SPIE 3032:340–348

Malberger E, Gutterman E, Bartfeld E, Zajicek G (1987) Cellular changes in the mammary gland epithelium during the menstrual cycle. A computer image analysis study. Acta Cytol 31:305–308

Malini S, Smith EO, Goldzieher JW (1985) Measurement of breast volume by ultrasound during normal menstrual cycles and with oral contraceptive use. Obstet Gynecol 66:538–541

Marabini R, Herman GT, Carazo JM (1998) 3D reconstruction in electron microscopy using ART with smooth spherically symmetric volume elements (blobs). Ultramicroscopy 72:53–65

March DE, Wechsler RJ, Kurtz AB, Rosenberg AL, Needleman L (1991) CT-pathologic correlation of axillary lymph nodes in breast carcinoma. J Comput Assist Tomogr 15:440–444

Markussen T, Fu XW, Margulies L, Lauridsen EM, Nielsen SF, Schmidt S, Poulsen HF (2004) An algebraic algorithm for generation of three-dimensional grain maps based on diffraction with a wide beam of hard x-rays. J Appl Crystallogr 37:96–102

Marti JT (1979) Convergence of the discrete ART algorithm for the reconstruction of digital pictures from their projections. Computing 21:105–111

Martin D, Thulasiraman P, Gordon R (2005) Local independence in computed tomography as a basis for parallel computing. Technol Cancer Res Treat 4:187–188

Matej S, Herman GT, Narayan TK, Furuie SS, Lewitt RM, Kinahan PE (1994) Evaluation of task-oriented performance of several fully 3D PET reconstruction algorithms. Phys Med Biol 39:355–367

Mazin SR, Pelc NJ (2008) Fourier rebinning algorithm for inverse geometry CT. Med Phys 35:4857–4862

Mazur AK (1992) Image correlation technique for recovering deformation fields from pictures. Ph.D. thesis, Supervisor: R. Gordon. Department of Electrical & Computer Engineering, University of Manitoba, Winnipeg

Mazur EJ, Gordon R (1995) Interpolative algebraic reconstruction techniques without beam partitioning for computed tomography. Med Biol Eng Comput 33:82–86

Mazur AK, Mazur EJ, Gordon R (1993) Digital differential radiography (DDR): a new diagnostic procedure for locating neoplasms, such as breast cancers, in soft, deformable tissues. SPIE 1905:443–455

McKeever WF (2004) An X-linked three allele model of hand preference and hand posture for writing. Laterality 9:149–173

McKinley RL, Tornai MP, Samei E, Bradshaw ML (2004) Simulation study of a quasi-monochromatic beam for x-ray computed mammotomography. Med Phys 31(4):800–813

McKinley RL, Tornai MP, Brzymialkiewicz C, Madhav P, Samei E, Bowsher JE (2006) Analysis of a novel offset cone-beam computed mammotomography system geometry for accommodating various breast sizes. Phys Med 21(Suppl 1):48–55

Melvin C, Abdel-Hadi K, Cenzano S, Gordon R (2002) A simulated comparison of turnstile and Poisson photons for x-ray imaging. In: Canadian conference on electrical and computer engineering, 2002. IEEE CCECE 2002, vol 2. IEEE, pp 1165–1170

Mettlin CJ, Smart CR (1993) The Canadian National Breast Screening Study. An appraisal and implications for early detection policy. Cancer 72(4 Suppl):1461–1465

Michler P, Kiraz A, Becher C, Schoenfeld WV, Petroff PM, Zhang L, Hu E, Imamolu A (2000) A quantum dot single-photon turnstile device. Science 290:2282–2285

Miller AB (1993) Canadian National Breast Screening Study: response. Can Med Assoc J 149:1374–1375

Mishra D, Muralidhar K, Munshi P (1999) A robust MART algorithm for tomographic applications. Num Heat Transf B – Fund 35:485–506

Mokbel K (2003) Risk-reducing strategies for breast cancer – a review of recent literature. Int J Fertil Womens Med 48:274–277

Moon RJ (1950) Amplifying and intensifying the fluoroscopic image by means of a scanning x-ray tube. Science 112:389–395

More MJ, Li H, Goodale PJ, Zheng YB, Majewski S, Popov V, Welch B, Williams MB (2007) Limited angle dual modality breast imaging. IEEE Trans Nucl Sci 54:504–513

Morrison PR, vanSonnenberg E, Shankar S, Godleski J, Silverman SG, Tuncali K, Jaklitsch MT, Jolesz FA (2005) Radiofrequency ablation of thoracic lesions: part 1, experiments in the normal porcine thorax. AJR Am J Roentgenol 184:375–380

Mueller K, Yagel R, Cornhill JF (1997) The weighted-distance scheme: a globally optimizing projection ordering method for ART. IEEE Trans Med Imaging 16:223–230

Mueller K, Yagel R, Wheller JJ (1998) A fast and accurate projection algorithm for the Algebraic Reconstruction Technique (ART). Proc SPIE 3336:724–732

Muraishi H, Nishimura K, Abe S, Satoh H, Hara S, Hara H, Takahashi Y, Mogaki T, Kawai R, Yokoyama K, Yasuda N, Tomida T, Ohno Y, Kanai T (2009) Evaluation of spatial resolution for heavy ion CT system based on the measurement of residual range distribution with HIMAC. IEEE Trans Nucl Sci 56:2714–2721

Murata K, Takahashi M, Mori M, Kawaguchi N, Furukawa A, Ohnaka Y, Itoh R, Kawakami K, Morioka Y, Morita R (1992) Pulmonary metastatic nodules: CT-pathologic correlation. Radiology 182:331–335

Murugan RM (2000) An improved electrical impedance tomography (EIT) algorithm for the detection of early stages of breast cancer. Ph.D. thesis, Supervisors: A. Wexler & R. Gordon. Department of Electrical & Computer Engineering, University of Manitoba, Winnipeg

Nab HW, Karssemeijer N, Van Erning LJ, Hendriks JH (1992) Comparison of digital and conventional mammography: a ROC study of 270 mammograms. Med Inform (Lond) 17:125–131

Nagy JG (1993) Fast inverse QR factorization for Toeplitz matrices. SIAM J Sci Stat Comput 14:1174–1193

Nandi RJ, Nandi AK, Rangayyan RM, Scutt D (2006) Classification of breast masses in mammograms using genetic programming and feature selection. Med Biol Eng Comput 44:683–694

NASA (2009a) Innovative Partnerships Program. http://www.nasa.gov/offices/ipp/innovation_incubator/cc_home.html

NASA (2009b) New NASA prize challenges: an opportunity to shape the prize challenges that NASA will offer to America's citizen inventors. External call for prize concepts. Innovative Partnerships Program, National Aeronautics and Space Administration, Washington, D.C

Nelson TR, Pretorius DH, Schiffer LM (1985) Menstrual variation of normal breast NMR relaxation parameters. J Comput Assist Tomogr 9:875–879

Nelson HD, Tyne K, Naik A, Bougatsos C, Chan B, Nygren P, Humphrey L (2009) Screening for breast cancer: systematic evidence review update for the U. S. Preventive Services Task Force. Evidence Review Update No. 74. AHRQ Publication No. 10-05142-EF-1. Agency for Healthcare Research and Quality, Rockville

Nelsona TR, Cervino LI, Boone JM, Lindfors KK (2008) Classification of breast computed tomography data. Med Phys 35:1078–1086

Ng EY, Sree SV, Ng KH, Kaw G (2008) The use of tissue electrical characteristics for breast cancer detection: a perspective review. Technol Cancer Res Treat 7:295–308

Nickoloff EL, Donnelly E, Eve L, Atherton JV, Asch T (1990) Mammographic resolution: influence of focal spot intensity distribution and geometry. Med Phys 17:436–447

Nie LM, Xing D, Zhou Q, Yang DW, Guo H (2008) Microwave-induced thermoacoustic scanning CT for high-contrast and noninvasive breast cancer imaging. Med Phys 35:4026–4032

Nields M (2005) Industry perspective: maximizing the benefit of improved detection with guided and monitored thermal ablation of small tumors. Technol Cancer Res Treat 4:123–130

Nielsen M (1989) Autopsy studies of the occurrence of cancerous, atypical and benign epithelial lesions in the female breast. APMIS 10(Suppl):1–56

Nielsen M, Thomsen JL, Primdahl S, Dyreborg U, Andersen JA (1987) Breast cancer and atypia among young and middle-aged women: a study of 110 medicolegal autopsies. Br J Cancer 56:814–819

Nielsen T, Manzke R, Proksa R, Grass M (2005) Cardiac cone-beam CT volume reconstruction using ART. Med Phys 32:851–860

Noguchi M (2003) Radiofrequency ablation treatment for breast cancer to meet the next challenge: how to treat primary breast tumor without surgery. Breast Cancer 10:1–3

Nomura M (1987) The role of RNA and protein in ribosome function: a review of early reconstitution studies and prospects for future studies. Cold Spring Harb Symp Quant Biol 52:653–663

Novick A, Szilard L (1950) Experiments with the chemostat on spontaneous mutations of bacteria. Proc Natl Acad Sci USA 36:708–719

O'Connor JM, Das M, Didier C, Mah'D M, Glick SJ (2008) Using mastectomy specimens to develop breast models for breast tomosynthesis and CT breast imaging. Proc SPIE 6913:15.11–15.16

Oh TI, Lee J, Seo JK, Kim SW, Woo EJ (2007) Feasibility of breast cancer lesion detection using a multi-frequency trans-admittance scanner (TAS) with 10 Hz to 500 kHz bandwidth. Physiol Meas 28:S71–S84

O'Neal DP, Hirsch LR, Halas NJ, Payne JD, West JL (2004) Photo-thermal tumor ablation in mice using near infrared-absorbing nanoparticles. Cancer Lett 209:171–176

Ortega JK, Harris JF, Gamow RI (1974) The analysis of spiral growth in *Phycomyces* using a novel optical method. Plant Physiol 53:485–490

Oxborrow M, Sinclair AG (2005) Single-photon sources. Contemp Phys 46:173–206

Pachoud M, Lepori D, Valley JF, Verdun FR (2005) Objective assessment of image quality in conventional and digital mammography taking into account dynamic range. Radiat Prot Dosimetry 114:380–382

Pan X, Sidky EY, Vannier M (2009) Why do commercial CT scanners still employ traditional, filtered back-projection for image reconstruction? Inverse Prob 25:1–36, #123009

Pani S, Longo R, Dreossi D, Montanari F, Olivo A, Arfelli F, Bergamaschi A, Poropat P, Rigon L, Zanconati F, Dalla Palma L, Castelli E (2004) Breast tomography with synchrotron radiation: preliminary results. Phys Med Biol 49:1739–1754

Parham C, Zhong Z, Connor DM, Chapman LD, Pisano ED (2009) Design and implementation of a compact low-dose diffraction enhanced medical imaging system. Acad Radiol 16:911–917

Park JM, Ikeda DM (2006) Promising techniques for breast cancer detection, diagnosis, and staging using non-ionizing radiation imaging techniques. Phys Med 21(Suppl 1):7–10

Park DY, Fessler JA, Yost MG, Levine SP (2000) Tomographic reconstruction of tracer gas concentration profiles in a room with the use of a single OP-FTIR and two iterative algorithms: ART and PWLS. J Air Waste Manag Assoc 50:357–370

Pawlak B (2007) Density estimation for positron emission tomography. Masters thesis, Supervisor: R. Gordon. Department of Electrical & Computer Engineering, University of Manitoba, Winnipeg

Pawlak B, Gordon R (2005) Density estimation for positron emission tomography. Technol Cancer Res Treat 4:131–142

Pawlak B, Gordon R (2010) Low dose positron emission tomography algorithm: kernel density estimation, in preparation

Perutz MF (1990) Haemoglobin. Nature 348:583–584

Perutz MF (1998) I wish I'd made you angry earlier. Essays on science, scientists and humanity. Cold Spring Harbor Laboratory Press, New York

Poplack SP, Tosteson TD, Wells WA, Pogue BW, Meaney PM, Hartov A, Kogel CA, Soho SK, Gibson JJ, Paulsen KD (2007) Electromagnetic breast imaging: results of a pilot study in women with abnormal mammograms. Radiology 243:350–359

Porter FS (2004) Low-temperature detectors in x-ray astronomy. Nucl Instrum Methods A 520:354–358

Potter MJA, Colquhoun G, Gordon R (2009) Design of a 3D microtumour breast scanner using 7th-generation CT (Computed Tomography). In: PowerPoint presentation, Department of Cell Biology & Anatomy/Faculty of Medicine, University of Calgary, 10 September 2009. Department of Radiology, University of Manitoba, Winnipeg

Poulin BJ, Gordon R (2001) How to organize science funding: the new Canadian Institutes for Health Research (CIHR), an opportunity to vastly increase innovation. Can Public Policy 27:95–112

Poyvasi M, Noghanian S, Thomas G, Flores D, Pistorius S (2005) Ultra-wide-band radar for early breast tumor detection. Technol Cancer Res Treat 4:190–191

Pramanik M, Ku G, Li CH, Wang LV (2008) Design and evaluation of a novel breast cancer detection system combining both thermoacoustic (TA) and photoacoustic (PA) tomography. Med Phys 35:2218–2223

Prasad SN, Houserkova D (2007) The role of various modalities in breast imaging. Biomed Pap Med Fac Univ Palacky Olomouc Czech Repub 151:209–218

Prokop M (2005) Cancer screening with CT: dose controversy. Eur Radiol 15(Suppl 4):D55–D61

Qian X, Rajaram R, Calderon-Colon X, Yang G, Phan T, Lalush DS, Lu JP, Zhou O (2009) Design and characterization of a spatially distributed multibeam field emission x-ray source for stationary digital breast tomosynthesis. Med Phys 36:4389–4399

Radon J (1917) Über die Bestimmung von Funktionen durch ihre integralwerte längs gewisser Mannigfaltigkeiten [On the determination of functions from their integrals along certain manifolds] [German]. Ber Sachs Akad Wiss Leipzig, Math-Phys Kl 69:262–277

Rajan K, Patnaik LM (2001) CBP and ART image reconstruction algorithms on media and DSP processors. Microprocess Microsyst 25:233–238

Ramachandran GN, Lakshminarayanan AV (1971) Three-dimensional reconstruction from radiographs and electron micrographs: application of convolutions instead of Fourier transforms. Proc Natl Acad Sci USA 68:2236–2240

Ramlau R, Teschke G, Zhariy M (2008) A compressive Landweber iteration for solving ill-posed inverse problems. Inverse Prob 24. Article Number: 065013

Ramsay J, Birrell G, Lavin M (1996) Breast cancer and radiotherapy in ataxia-telangiectasia heterozygote. Lancet 347:1627

Ramsay J, Birrell G, Lavin M (1998) Testing for mutations of the ataxia telangiectasia gene in radiosensitive breast cancer patients. Radiother Oncol 47:125–128

Rangayyan RM, Gordon R (1982a) Computed tomography for remote areas via teleradiology. Proc SPIE 318:182–185

Rangayyan RM, Gordon R (1982b) Streak preventive image reconstruction with ART and adaptive filtering. IEEE Trans Med Imaging MI-1:173–178

Rangayyan RM, Dhawan AP, Gordon R (1985) Algorithms for limited-view computed tomography: an annotated bibliography and a challenge. Appl Opt 24:4000–4012

Rangayyan RM, Alto H, Gavrilov D (2001) Parallel implementation of the adaptive neighborhood contrast enhancement technique using histogram-based image partitioning. J Electron Imaging 10:804–813

Rangayyan RM, Ayres FJ, Desautels JEL (2007) A review of computer-aided diagnosis of breast cancer: toward the detection of subtle signs. J Franklin Inst 344:312–348

Rayavarapu RG, Petersen W, Ungureanu C, Post JN, van Leeuwen TG, Manohar S (2007) Synthesis and bioconjugation of gold nanoparticles as potential molecular probes for light-based imaging techniques. Int J Biomed Imaging 2007:1–10, Article Number: 29817

Rehani MM (2000) CT: caution on radiation dose. Indian J Radiol Imaging 10:19–20

Reiser I, Sidky EY, Nishikawa RM, Pan X (2006) Development of an analytic breast phantom for quantitative comparison of reconstruction algorithms for digital breast tomosynthesis. In: Astley SM, Brady M, Rose C, Zwiggelaar R (eds) Proceedings, digital mammography, 8th international workshop, IWDM 2006, Manchester, UK, 18–21 June 2006. Springer, Berlin, pp 190–196

Retsky MW, Demicheli R, Hrushesky WJ, Baum M, Gukas ID (2008) Dormancy and surgery-driven escape from dormancy help explain some clinical features of breast cancer. APMIS 116:730–741

Rickey DW, Gordon R, Huda W (1992) On lifting the inherent limitations of positron emission tomography by using magnetic fields (MagPET). Automedica 14:355–369

Romberg J (2008) Imaging via compressive sampling. IEEE Signal Process Mag 25:14–20

Ron E (2003) Cancer risks from medical radiation. Health Phys 85:47–59

Rosen R (1985) James F. Danielli: 1911–1984. J Soc Biol Struct 8:1–11

Rosenfield NS, Haller JO, Berdon WE (1989) Failure of development of the growing breast after radiation therapy. Pediatr Radiol 19:124–127

Roubidoux MA, Sabel MS, Bailey JE, Kleer CG, Klein KA, Helvie MA (2004) Small (<2.0-cm) breast cancers: mammographic and US findings at US-guided cryoablation – initial experience. Radiology 233:857–867

Ruttimann UE, Qi XL, Webber RL (1989) An optimal synthetic aperture for circular tomosynthesis. Med Phys 16:398–405

Sabatini DD (2005) In awe of subcellular complexity: 50 years of trespassing boundaries within the cell. Annu Rev Cell Dev Biol 21:1–33

Saez F, Llebaria A, Lamy P, Vibert D (2007) Three-dimensional reconstruction of the streamer belt and other large-scale structures of the solar corona. Astron Astrophys 473: 265–277

Sargent EH (2005) The dance of molecules: how nanotechnology is changing our lives. Viking Canada, Toronto

Schaller S, Karolczak M, Engelke K, Wiesent K, Kalender WA (1998) Implementation of a fast cone-beam backprojection algorithm for microcomputed tomography (HCT) using homogeneous coordinates. Radiology 209P:433–434

Schlueter FJ, Wang G, Hsieh PS, Brink JA, Balfe DM, Vannier MW (1994) Longitudinal image deblurring in spiral CT. Radiology 193:413–418

Schmidt TG, Star-Lack J, Bennett NR, Mazin SR, Solomon EG, Fahrig R, Pelc NJ (2006) A prototype table-top inverse-geometry volumetric CT system. Med Phys 33: 1867–1878

Shao YP, Yao RT, Ma TY (2008) A novel method to calibrate DOI function of a PET detector with a dual-ended-scintillator readout. Med Phys 35:5829–5840

Shaw de Paredes E (1994) Evaluation of abnormal screening mammograms. Cancer 74(1 Suppl):342–349

Shibata K, Uno K, Wu J, Ko W (2007) Imaging of cancer activity and range of tumor involvement – applying to cancer. Rinsho Byori 55:648–655

Shorey J (2007) Stochastic simulations for the detection of objects in three dimensional volumes: applications in medical imaging and ocean acoustics. Ph.D. thesis, Duke University, Durham

Shuryak I, Hahnfeldt P, Hlatky L, Sachs RK, Brenner DJ (2009) A new view of radiation-induced cancer: integrating short- and long-term processes. Part II: second cancer risk estimation. Radiat Environ Biophys 48:275–286

Sidky EY, Pan XC (2008) Image reconstruction in circular cone-beam computed tomography by constrained, total-variation minimization. Phys Med Biol 53:4777–4807

Sidky EY, Kao CM, Pan XH (2006) Accurate image reconstruction from few-views and limited-angle data in divergent-beam CT. J Xray Sci Technol 14:119–139

Signorato R, Susini J, Goulon J, Gauthier C, Marion P (1997) Reflective optics for the ESRF beamline ID 26. J Phys IV 7(C2):331–332

Sijbers J, Postnov A (2004) Reduction of ring artefacts in high resolution micro-CT reconstructions. Phys Med Biol 49:N247–N253

Silva GT, Frery AC, Fatemi M (2006) Image formation in vibro-acoustography with depth-of-field effects. Comput Med Imaging Graph 30:321–327

Simick MK, Jong R, Wilson B, Lilge L (2004) Non-ionizing near-infrared radiation transillumination spectroscopy for breast tissue density and assessment of breast cancer risk. J Biomed Opt 9:794–803

Simmons RM (2003) Ablative techniques in the treatment of benign and malignant breast disease. J Am Coll Surg 197:334–338

Simpson HW, Griffiths K, McArdle C, Pauson AW, Hume P, Turkes A (1996) The luteal heat cycle of the breast in disease. Breast Cancer Res Treat 37:169–178

Singletary SE (2003) Radiofrequency ablation of breast cancer. Am Surg 69:37–40

Sivaramakrishna R (1998) Breast image registration using a textural transformation. Med Phys 25:2249

Sivaramakrishna R (2005a) 3D breast image registration – a review. Technol Cancer Res Treat 4:39–48

Sivaramakrishna R (2005b) Foreword: imaging techniques alternative to mammography for early detection of breast cancer. Technol Cancer Res Treat 4:1–4

Sivaramakrishna R (2005c) Foreword: workshop on alternatives to mammography II. Technol Cancer Res Treat 4:121–122

Sivaramakrishna R, Gordon R (1997a) Detection of breast cancer at a smaller size can reduce the likelihood of metastatic spread: a quantitative analysis. Acad Radiol 4:8–12

Sivaramakrishna R, Gordon R (1997b) Mammographic image registration using the Starbyte transformation. In: McLaren PG, Kinsner W (eds) WESCSANEX'97. IEEE, Winnipeg, pp 144–149

Sivaramakrishna R, Powell KA, Chilcote WA, Obuchowski NA, Barry MM, Coll DM (1999) Comparing the performance of image enhancement algorithms utilizing different methodologies in visualizing known lesions in digitized mammograms in a soft-copy display setting. Radiology 213P:969

Sivaramakrishna R, Obuchowski NA, Chilcote WA, Cardenosa G, Powell KA (2000) Comparing the performance of mammographic enhancement algorithms: a preference study. AJR Am J Roentgenol 175:45–51

Smith JA, Andreopoulou E (2004) An overview of the status of imaging screening technology for breast cancer. Ann Oncol 15(Suppl 1):I18–I26

Smith KT, Solmon DC, Wagner SL (1977) Practical and mathematical aspects of the problem of reconstructing objects from radiographs. Bull Am Math Soc 83:1227–1270

Smith KT, Solmon DC, Wagner SL, Hamaker C (1978) Mathematical aspects of divergent beam radiography. Proc Natl Acad Sci USA 75:2055–2058

Sobel D (1995) Longitude: the true story of a lone genius who solved the greatest scientific problem of his time. Walker, New York

Soble P, Rangayyan RM, Gordon R (1985) Quantitative and qualitative evaluation of geometric deconvolution of distortion in limited-view computed tomography. IEEE Trans Biomed Eng BME-32:330–335

Song YZ, Hu GY, He AZ (2006a) Simple self-correlative algebraic reconstruction technique. Spectroscop Spectral Anal 26:2364–2367

Song YZ, Sun T, Hu GY, He AZ (2006b) Analyzing the methods to smooth field reconstructed by algebraic reconstruction technique with spectroscopy. Spectroscop Spectral Anal 26:1411–1415

Spanu A, Cottu P, Manca A, Chessa F, Sanna D, Madeddu G (2007) Scintimammography with dedicated breast camera in unifocal and multifocal/multicentric primary breast cancer detection: a comparative study with SPECT. Int J Oncol 31:369–377

Spelic DC (2009) Updated trends in mammography dose and image quality. http://www.fda.gov/Radiation-EmittingProducts/MammographyQualityStandardsActandProgram/FacilityScorecard/ucm113352.htm

Stein WD (1986) James Frederic Danielli, 1911–1984, Elected F.R.S. 1957. Biogr Mem Fellows R Soc 32:115–135

Steiner G, Soleimani M, Watzenig D (2008) A bio-electromechanical imaging technique with combined electrical impedance and ultrasound tomography. Physiol Meas 29:S63–S75

Stomper PC, Mazurchuk RV, Tsangaris TN (1994) Breast MRI as an adjunct in the diagnosis of a carcinoma partially obscured on mammography. Clin Imaging 18:195–198

Strebhardt K, Ullrich A (2008) Paul Ehrlich's magic bullet concept: 100 years of progress. Nat Rev Cancer 8:473–480

Strong AB, Hurst RA (1994) EMI patents on computed tomography: history of legal actions. Br J Radiol 67:315–316

Subbarao PMV, Munshi P, Muralidhar K (1997a) Performance evaluation of iterative tomographic algorithms applied to reconstruction of a three-dimensional temperature field. Num Heat Transf B – Fund 31:347–372

Subbarao PMV, Munshi P, Muralidhar K (1997b) Performance of iterative tomographic algorithms applied to non-destructive evaluation with limited data. NDT and E Int 30: 359–370

Subramanian E (2001) G.N. Ramachandran [Obituary]. Nat Struct Biol 8:489–491

Sun J, Chapman JA, Gordon R, Sivaramakrishna R, Link MA, Fish EB (1998) Survival from primary breast cancer by tumour size for the age groups with different screening guidelines. Breast Cancer Res Treat 50:281

Sun J, Chapman JA, Gordon R, Sivaramakrishna R, Link MA, Fish EB (2002) Survival from primary breast cancer after routine clinical use of mammography. Breast J 8:199–208

Suri JS, Rangayyan R, Laxminarayan S (eds) (2006) Emerging technologies in breast and mammography imaging and its applications. ASP, Stevenson Ranch

Szent-Györgyi A (1960) Introduction to a submolecular biology. Academic, New York

Szent-Györgyi A (1972) The living state, with observations on cancer. Academic, New York

Tafra L (2007) Positron emission tomography (PET) and mammography (PEM) for breast cancer: importance to surgeons. Ann Surg Oncol 14:3–13

Takahashi S (1969) An atlas of axial transverse tomography and its clinical application. Springer, New York

Taminiau TH, Stefani FD, Segerink FB, Van Hulst NF (2008) Optical antennas direct single-molecule emission. Nat Photonics 2:234–237

Tarone RE (1995) The excess of patients with advanced breast cancer in young women screened with mammography in the Canadian National Breast Screening Study. Cancer 75: 997–1003

Tateno Y, Tanaka H (1976) Low-dosage x-ray imaging system employing flying spot x-ray microbeam (dynamic scanner). Radiology 121:189–195

Tateno Y, Tanaka H, Watanabe E (1976) Dynamic scanner, an imaging system employing flying spot x-ray microbeam. J Nucl Med 17:551–552

Taylor PHS (2002) Computational physiology of the human breast. Ph.D. thesis. Department of Computer Science, University of Western Australia, Perth, Australia

Taylor P, Owens R (2001) Simulated mammography of a three-dimensional breast model. In: Astley S, Fujita H, Gale A, Giger M, Karssemeijer N, Peitgen HO, Pisano E, Williams M, Yaffe M (eds) IWDM 2000. Abstracts of the 5th international conference on digital mammography, Toronto, June 2000. Medical Physics, Madison, 138 pp

Thie JA (2007) Optimizing dual-time and serial positron emission tomography and single photon emission computed tomography scans for diagnoses and therapy monitoring. Mol Imaging Biol 9:348–356

Thorpe H, Brown SR, Sainsbury JR, Perren TJ, Hiley V, Dowsett M, Nejim A, Brown JM (2008) Timing of breast cancer surgery in relation to menstrual cycle phase: no effect on 3-year prognosis: the ITS Study. Br J Cancer 98:39–44

Tomanek B, Hoult DI, Chen X, Gordon R (2000) A probe with chest shielding for improved breast MR imaging. Magn Reson Med 43:917–920

Trummer MR (1981) Reconstructing pictures from projections: on the convergence of the ART algorithm with relaxation. Computing 26(3):189–195

Trummer MR (1983) SMART: an algorithm for reconstructing pictures from projections. Z Angew Math Physik 34: 743–753

Turunen MJ, Huikuri K, Lempinen M (1986) Results of 32 major hepatic resections for primary and secondary malignancies of the liver. Ann Chir Gynaecol 75:209–214

United Artists Corporation (1971) Fiddler on the roof [Video]

Vainshtein BK (1971) The synthesis of projecting functions. Sov Physics Dokl 16:66–99

Van Uytven E, Pistorius S, Gordon R (2007) An iterative three-dimensional electron density imaging algorithm using uncollimated Compton scattered x rays from a polyenergetic primary pencil beam. Med Phys 34:256–274

Van Uytven E, Pistorius S, Gordon R (2008) A method for 3D electron density imaging using single scattered X rays with application to mammographic screening. Phys Med Biol 53:5445–5459

Vargas HI, Dooley WC, Gardner RA, Gonzalez KD, Venegas R, Heywang-Kobrunner SH, Fenn AJ (2004) Focused microwave phased array thermotherapy for ablation of early-stage breast cancer: results of thermal dose escalation. Ann Surg Oncol 11:139–146

Vasile G, Trouve E, Ciuc M, Buzuloiu V (2004) General adaptive-neighborhood technique for improving synthetic aperture radar interferometric coherence estimation. J Opt Soc Am A Opt Image Sci Vis 21:1455–1464

Verschraegen C, Vinh-Hung V, Cserni G, Gordon R, Royce ME, Vlastos G, Tai P, Storme G (2005) Modeling the effect of tumor size in early breast cancer. Ann Surg 241:309–318

Vinh-Hung V, Gordon R (2005) Quantitative target sizes for breast tumor detection prior to metastasis: a prerequisite to rational design of 4D scanners for breast screening. Technol Cancer Res Treat 4:11–21

Vinh-Hung V, Tot T, Gordon R (2010) One or many targets? Towards resolving the paradox of single versus multifocal breast cancer from epidemiological data, in preparation

Vock P (2005) CT dose reduction in children. Eur Radiol 15:2330–2340

Vogel PM, Georgiade NG, Fetter BF, Vogel FS, McCarty KS Jr (1981) The correlation of histologic changes in the human breast with the menstrual cycle. Am J Pathol 104:23–34

Wade N (2004) Maurice H. F. Wilkins, 87, a DNA Nobelist, Dies. NY Times October 7

Wall J, Langmore J, Isaacson M, Crewe AV (1974) Scanning transmission electron microscopy at high resolution. Proc Natl Acad Sci USA 71:1–5

Wan X, Gao YQ, Wang Q, Le SP, Yu SL (2003) Limited-angle optical computed tomography algorithms. Opt Eng 42: 2659–2669

Wang G, Snyder DL, O'Sullivan JA, Vannier MW (1996) Iterative deblurring for CT metal artifact reduction. IEEE Trans Med Imaging 15:657–664

Wang G, Vannier MW, Cheng PC (1999) Iterative x-ray cone-beam tomography for metal artifact reduction and local region reconstruction. Microsc Microanal 5:58–65

Watt DW (1994) Column relaxed algebraic reconstruction algorithm for tomography with noisy data. Appl Opt 33: 4420–4427

Webber RL (ed) (1979) Feedback control of exposure geometry in dental radiography. Publication No. 80-1954. National Institutes of Health, Bethesda

Wen DB, Yuan YB, Ou JK, Zhang KF, Liu K (2008) A hybrid reconstruction algorithm for 3-D ionospheric tomography. IEEE Trans Geosci Remote Sens 46:1733–1739

White E, Velentgas P, Mandelson MT, Lehman CD, Elmore JG, Porter P, Yasui Y, Taplin SH (1998) Variation in mammographic breast density by time in menstrual cycle among women aged 40–49 years. J Natl Cancer Inst 90:906–910

Wiest PW, Locken JA, Heintz PH, Mettler FA Jr (2002) CT scanning: a major source of radiation exposure. Semin Ultrasound CT MR 23:402–410

Wikipedia Contributors (2009) Japanese rock garden. Wikipedia, the free encyclopedia. Wikimedia Foundation, San Francisco. http://en.wikipedia.org/wiki/Japanese_rock_garden

Woten DA, El-Shenawee M (2008) Broadband dual linear polarized antenna for statistical detection of breast cancer. IEEE Trans Antennas Propag 56:3576–3580

Wu T, Stewart A, Stanton M, McCauley T, Phillips W, Kopans DB, Moore RH, Eberhard JW, Opsahl-Ong B, Niklason L, Williams MB (2003) Tomographic mammography using a limited number of low-dose cone-beam projection images. Med Phys 30:365–380

Wu YB, Bowen SL, Yang K, Packard N, Fu L, Burkett G, Qi JY, Boone JM, Cherry SR, Badawi RD (2009) PET characteristics of a dedicated breast PET/CT scanner prototype. Phys Med Biol 54:4273–4287

Yaffe MJ, Mainprize JG, Jong RA (2008) Technical developments in mammography. Health Phys 95:599–611

Yamada H, Saisho H, Hirai T, Hirano J (2004) X-ray fluorescence analysis of heavy elements with a portable synchrotron. Spectrochim Acta B 59:1323–1328

Yang SK, Cho N, Moon WK (2007) The role of PET/CT for evaluating breast cancer. Korean J Radiol 8:429–437

Yang K, Kwan ALC, Huang SY, Packard NJ, Boone JM (2008) Noise power properties of a cone-beam CT system for breast cancer detection. Med Phys 35:5317–5327

Ye G, Lim KH, George RT, Ybarra GA, Joines WT, Liu QH (2008) 3D EIT for breast cancer imaging: system, measure-

ments, and reconstruction. Microwave Opt Technol Lett 50:3261–3271

Yee KM (2009) Breast imaging: new technologies emerge. http://medicalphysicsweb.org/cws/article/research/40184

Yoshinaga T, Imakura Y, Fujimoto K, Ueta T (2008) Bifurcation analysis of iterative image reconstruction method for computed tomography. Int J Bifurcation Chaos 18:1219–1225

Yu HY, Cao GH, Burk L, Lee Y, Lu JP, Santago P, Zhou O, Wang G (2009) Compressive sampling based interior reconstruction for dynamic carbon nanotube micro-CT. J Xray Sci Technol 17:295–303

Zarghami N, Grass L, Sauter ER, Diamandis EP (1997) Prostate-specific antigen in serum during the menstrual cycle. Clin Chem 43:1862–1867

Zhang J, Olcott PD, Chinn G, Foudray AM, Levine CS (2007) Study of the performance of a novel 1 mm resolution dual-panel PET camera design dedicated to breast cancer imaging using Monte Carlo simulation. Med Phys 34:689–702

Zhang B, He Y, Song Y, He AZ (2009) Deflection tomographic reconstruction of a complex flow field from incomplete projection data. Opt Lasers Eng 47:1183–1188

Zhou X (1991) Digital subtraction mammography via geometric unwarping for detection of early breast cancer. Ph.D. thesis, Supervisor: R. Gordon. Department of Electrical & Computer Engineering, University of Manitoba, Winnipeg

Zhou SA, Brahme A (2008) Development of phase-contrast x-ray imaging techniques and potential medical applications. Phys Med 24:129–148

Zhou XH, Gordon R (1989) Detection of early breast cancer: an overview and future prospects. Crit Rev Biomed Eng 17:203–255

Zhou X, Liang ZP, Cofer GP, Beaulieu CF, Suddarth SA, Johnson GA (1993) Reduction of ringing and blurring artifacts in fast spin-echo imaging. J Magn Reson Imaging 3:803–807

Zhou L, Oldan J, Fisher P, Gindi G (2006) Low-contrast lesion detection in tomosynthetic breast imaging using a realistic breast phantom. Proc SPIE 6142:5A.1–5A.12

Zwirewich CV, Miller RR, Muller NL (1990) Multicentric adenocarcinoma of the lung: CT-pathologic correlation. Radiology 176:185–190

Epilogue: The Diseased Breast Lobe in the Context of X-Chromosome Inactivation and Differentiation Waves

11

Richard Gordon

The debate over whether cancer starts in a single cell (Hahn and Weinberg 2002) or is a multifocal disease (the latter variously referred to as the multicellular model [Attolini and Michor 2009] or field theory [Soto et al. 2008]) has a long history. This book, *Breast Cancer: A Lobar Disease*, may be a stepping stone toward trying to resolve this long-standing issue. My own work on breast cancer detection has been based on the assumption, at first sight contrary to Tibor Tot's sick lobe hypothesis, that targeting a single small lesion will halt breast cancer, and the epidemiological evidence would seem to point that way. And yet, as can be seen by the dialogue with Tot and Vincent Vinh-Hung at the end of my chapter (Gordon 2010), more subtle considerations may let us see breast cancer both ways, i.e., that they are not mutually exclusive. It may be that one could either stop breast cancer recurrence for an extended time by ablating a single small tumor, or for the remainder of a women's life by removing the whole of a sick lobe, difficult outcomes to distinguish. As in the debate over total mastectomy versus lumpectomy (Lerner 2001), both may prove clinically equivalent in terms of prolongation of life. At least, lobectomy is less disfiguring than mastectomy, so passions need not run as high. Much work remains ahead to determine the outcome of this debate, though we will see what we can tease out of retrospective epidemiological data (Vinh-Hung et al. 2010).

I was taught, by a physics high school teacher at John Dewey's Laboratory School of the University of Chicago, that the ideal in science controversies is for each protagonist to ride the other's horse. It's a tough thing to do, because so many of us get wrapped up in our own ideas and confuse them with the greater reality outside our own minds. Fortunately, in this case, I have also developed a tissue perspective on disease out of my work in embryology (Gordon 1999). Tibor Tot's request for me to write this Epilogue has thus jarred me into riding his horse, albeit with my own saddle.

If we look at variegated plants with green and white areas, we see clones of cells that do or do not synthesize functional chlorophyll (Yu et al. 2007). The cells all come from a single zygote, so something epigenetic occurs during plant development (Linn et al. 1990; Hoekenga et al. 2000; Iida et al. 2004). For a plant, partial lack of chlorophyll generally reduces its growth (except perhaps in bananas [Zaffari et al. 1998; TyTy Nursery 2010]) and presumably, therefore, fitness (Funayama et al. 1997; Funayama-Noguchi 2001), so we could regard each of those white areas as "sick lobes." Indeed, variegated plants are rare in nature, and survive long-term only as cultivars, their fitness restored by a symbiotic relationship with humans.

In variegated color phenotypes in mice (Lyon 1961, 2003) and calico cats (Davidson 1964; Osgood 1994), there is also an epigenetic effect that leads to spottiness in their pigmentation. This almost always (Lyon 2003) occurs only in females and is due to "random" inactivation of (all but) one X chromosome. We now understand that all XX women are mosaic organisms consisting of clones with one or the other X chromosome active, a selection that occurs around the 4 to 20 cell stage of embryogenesis (Puck et al. 1992; Monteiro et al. 1998; Chitnis et al. 1999; Brown and Robinson 2000).

Tot has hypothesized that each breast lobe is a clone starting from a single cell sometime between 8 and 25 weeks of gestational age (Tot 2010), which is well after X inactivation has occurred. This concept could thus be tested by ascertaining whether all cells in a

R. Gordon
Department of Radiology, University of Manitoba,
Winnipeg, MB, Canada
e-mail: gordonr@cc.umanitoba.ca

T. Tot (ed.), *Breast Cancer*, DOI: 10.1007/978-1-84996-314-5_11,

lobe have the same X inactivation (Brown and Robinson 2000), at least those cells that have not yet formed tumors as tumor cells can switch which X is inactivated (Vincent-Salomon et al. 2007). In such tests, one should also look for the possibility that healthy lobes in the same breast have the other X chromosome active (Kristiansen et al. 2005).

Skewness of X inactivation has been defined by various authors as 67–90% of the cells in a tissue having the same X chromosome inactivated, instead of 50% (Buller et al. 1999; Lose et al. 2008). The median number of breast lobes is 27 (Going and Moffat 2004). Suppose we were to entertain the hypothesis that an aberrant allele of some unknown gene on the X chromosome is involved in the causation of breast cancer, as some authors have claimed, though without age-matched controls (Lose et al. 2008) (cf. [Kristiansen et al. 2005]). Then we would expect, on average, that the number of sick lobes should be 50%, or about 14, rather than one or two. A caveat here is, of course, the large patches in skin coloration observed on white calico cats (smaller in tortoiseshell cats) (Vella and Robinson 1999) so that by analogy we might anticipate a bimodal distribution of skewness in a localized tissue such as breast. Nevertheless, preliminary evidence of uniformity of skewness between tissues has been claimed in humans (Buller et al. 1999). Three hypotheses have been suggested for skewed X inactivation: An X-linked allele confers a proliferative advantage to cells; it is due to a genetic predisposition; it is a protective mechanism to reduce expression of detrimental X-linked alleles (Lose et al. 2008). The unknown mechanism of skewing of X chromosome inactivation may occur in a tissue-specific manner at specific times in the course of embryogenesis, starting from a 50:50 proportion (Muers et al. 2007), with stochastic effects that accumulate, causing exponential deviations with age from 50:50 (Vickers et al. 2001; Kristiansen et al. 2003). Until these spatial, statistical, ageing and epidemiological aspects of skewed X inactivation are better worked out, we should just keep an eye on the possibility of a link between the sick lobe hypothesis and skewed X inactivation.

The assumption that a sick lobe is a clone of one cell is compatible with both the single cell and multifocal points of view. In fact, one could suggest that the whole sick lobe is actually a tumor somehow held in the earliest stage of cancer progression. Cases of stabilization of tumor cells by incorporation into normal embryogenesis, leading to whole normal looking tissues made of aberrant cells, are known (Mintz and Illmensee 1975; Pierce et al. 1982; Kulesa et al. 2006; Hendrix et al. 2007; Kasemeier-Kulesa et al. 2008), so this is a plausible scenario.

But outside of highly clonal, mosaic development, such as occurs in the early stages of snail (Raven 1966), ascidian (Nishida 2005), and nematode (Sulston et al. 1983) embryos, most other organisms use so-called regulative development. One consequence of this is that the cells in a given clone generally do not end up as the same differentiated cell type. A rarely asked question is how this happens, that clones can get split up? Something else is going on in embryogenesis, which may also be labeled "epigenetic," that allows cells in a clone to have different fates from one another.

I have written a rather large and overbearing book on this subject (Gordon 1999), based on my prediction (Gordon and Brodland 1987) that differentiation waves, observable as waves of expansion and contraction of epithelia in embryos, traverse subregions of the embryo (regardless of clonal origins of their cells) and trigger off a step of differentiation as they go. The prediction was found to be correct by Natalie K. Björklund (Brodland et al. 1994), and the waves proved easy to see (Gordon and Björklund 1996). Unfortunately, they were not popular with molecular developmental biologists, who for decades did not like the notion of physical phenomena organizing and triggering gene expression, presuming that "control" was always in the cell nucleus, not of it, as exemplified in this textbook:

> Some researchers have proposed that all cells in an embryo initially express the same genes until their physical interactions [such as differentiation waves] generate groups of cells with different mechanical states, which then secondarily cause these cells to express specific combinations of genes (Gordon and Brodland 1987). However, most researchers today assume that cells are first programmed to express certain master genes, which in turn coordinate other genes with more limited functions…. It is the latter approach that we will explore in this text (Kalthoff 2001).

This situation is turning around: "Biomechanical forces are emerging as critical regulators of embryogenesis…" (Adamo et al. 2009) (cf. [Beloussov and Gordon 2006]), as well as differentiation and tumorogenesis (Lopez et al. 2008; Tenney and Discher 2009; Wang et al. 2009). Thus, the work of relating these waves to the many so-called determinants of cell differentiation was never funded, and is left for the next generation. Such researchers are slowly being recruited through an online embryo physics course held in a virtual world (Gordon and Buckley 2010). Thus for now the job of relating differentiation waves to the molecular epigenetic correlates of differentiation (and perhaps dedifferentiation [Rossant 2009]) has hardly begun (Björklund and Gordon 2006).

Differentiation waves lead to a simple view of development: Each embryonic tissue is split into two new tissues by two waves. One is a wave of contraction, and the other is a wave of expansion. In epithelia, these waves seem to propagate via a cytoskeletal apparatus at the apical surface of each cell, that we call the "cell state splitter" (Gordon and Brodland 1987, Björklund and Gordon 1993; Martin and Gordon 1997). This device, somewhat akin to the spindle apparatus in its mechanical antagonism between microtubules and microfilaments, is constructed in a metastable state ready for a radial tug-of-war between its apical microtubules and apical microfilament ring (Gordon and Brodland 1987). The cell state splitter resolves this instability in one of two ways: Either the microfilaments win, greatly contracting the apical surface, or the microtubules win, flattening the cell (Gordon and Brodland 1987). We presume that a one-bit signal then proceeds to the nucleus by some sort of signal transduction, resulting in one of two readied gene cascades being triggered (Björklund and Gordon 1993). Cell differentiation is thereby conceived as a binary bifurcating process, i.e., each intermediate cell type during embryogenesis gives rise to exactly two new cell types.

What triggers the waves and what stops them are still matters of speculation, and detailed, quantitative investigations of live embryos, watching all the cells at once, are sorely needed (Gordon and Westfall 2009; Gordon 2009).

Perhaps breast lobes are carved out of a precursor tissue by differentiation waves instead of arising as clones of a single cell? If so, then we must ask what might be the initial event that differs between healthy and sick lobes? There are three obvious components of the process to consider: the cell state splitter, signal transduction from the cell state splitter to the nucleus, and the consequent change in gene expression. Differentiation waves do not provide the answer, only a working hypothesis that can direct our attention. However, if differentiation waves are the cause of breast lobes, then some lobes should consist of more than one clone, giving us at least one criterion for distinguishing this hypothesis from Tot's clonal hypothesis (Tot 2010).

If we consider the history of the development of an organism from the point of view of a single cell, it has its own history of what intermediate cell types it came from.

Considering all the cells in an organism, we can call their collective histories a "cell lineage tree." Except for striate muscle cells, which are multinucleate due to the fusion of myoblasts, this conceptual tree has no anastomoses, and due to cell division, branches in a strictly binary fashion.

Differentiation waves give us another tree, a "tissue lineage tree," where we define a tissue as all cells that have experienced the same sequence of contraction (C) and expansion (E) waves. This means that, if differentiation waves are the primary trigger of cell differentiation, every cell, at every stage of development, can be assigned a binary code, such as CEECECCEEE, etc., representing its history of participation in differentiation waves. This "differentiation code" (Björklund and Gordon 1994) may actually have some kind of representation in the cell, which would be its "memory" of what it has been and now is. The concept that every embryonic tissue gives rise to exactly two tissues further on in development is only implicit in the literature (Gordon 1999), and needs further investigation. Thus, the notion that the tissue lineage tree also branches in a strictly binary fashion awaits confirmation.

There is one major exception to differentiation waves, which leads to another way of looking at the origin of the sick lobe. At the boundaries of and between the expansion and contraction waves that traverse a given embryonic tissue, there are likely to be some cells that do not participate in either type of wave. This may be the origin of stem cells, cells that are stuck in an embryonic state, perhaps able to wait indefinitely for something to trigger them to the next stage(s) (Gordon 2006). The differentiation code of these stem cells, insofar as a cell acts on its past, or rather its stored memory of that past, may limit the kinds of cells it can differentiate into. This would explain why stem cells are generally pleuripotent rather than totipotent. Thus, differentiation waves may explain the origin of the many kinds of pleuripotent stem cells that have been discovered in recent years. Some cancer stem cells may derive from normal stem cells (Vermeulen et al. 2008). A clone of such cancer stem cells in a breast lobe (Howard and Ashworth 2006) may be what makes it a sick lobe:

An epidemiological link to fetal stages has been found for breast and prostate cancer (Fackelmann 1997)[(Trichopoulos 1990; Ekbom et al. 1992)]. One might wonder whether competent cells that somehow miss a differentiation wave are candidates for later tumor development (Gordon 1999).

The cell lineage tree is then a subset of the tissue lineage tree, and stem cells are termini of the cell lineage tree in suspended animation. To clarify this relationship, I have drawn one branch of a tissue lineage tree (i.e., "differentiation tree" [Gordon 1999]) with the branches of a few cells' contributions to the cell lineage tree shown within it (Fig. 11.1).

The interplay between X inactivation, cells, clones, tissues and differentiation waves is a rich source of ideas for untangling the relationship between single cell and multifocal hypotheses for cancer, in which we may find the fundamental basis for the sick lobe, and the aberrant cells that form within it. For example, the vague concept of a "morphogenetic field" (Waddington 1934; Beloussov et al. 1997) from which the "tissue organization field theory of carcinogenesis and neoplasia" derives its name (Soto et al. 2008) is replaced by the subset of cells covered by the trajectory of a specific, observable differentiation wave (Gordon 1999). What holds like cells together as a tissue in adults (Soto et al. 2008) is a mystery that may also involve some kind of persisting waves between them (Gordon 1999). There is much work ahead, but by combining cytogenetics, embryology, pathology, molecular biology, and modern methods of 4D microscopy, we may be able to unravel this puzzle.

Acknowledgments   I would like to thank William R. Buckley, Stephen A. Krawetz, and Natalie K. Björklund for critical comments and Stephen P. McGrew (New Light Industries, Spokane) and the Organ Imaging Fund of the Department of Radiology, University of Manitoba for support.

References

Adamo L, Naveiras O, Wenzel PL, McKinney-Freeman S, Mack PJ, Gracia-Sancho J, Suchy-Dicey A, Yoshimoto M, Lensch MW, Yoder MC, García-Cardeña G, Daley GQ (2009) Biomechanical forces promote embryonic haematopoiesis. Nature 459:1131–1135

Attolini CS, Michor F (2009) Evolutionary theory of cancer. Ann NY Acad Sci 1168:23–51

Beloussov LV, Gordon R (2006) Preface. Morphodynamics: bridging the gap between the genome and embryo physics. Int J Dev Biol 50:79–80

Beloussov LV, Opitz JM, Gilbert SF (1997) Life of Alexander G. Gurwitsch and his relevant contribution to the theory of morphogenetic fields. Int J Dev Biol 41:771–779

Björklund NK, Gordon R (1993) Nuclear state splitting: a working model for the mechanochemical coupling of differentiation waves to master genes. Russian J Dev Biol 24:79–95

Björklund NK, Gordon R (1994) Surface contraction and expansion waves correlated with differentiation in axolotl embryos. I. Prolegomenon and differentiation during the plunge through the blastopore, as shown by the fate map. Comput Chem 18:333–345

Björklund NK, Gordon R (2006) A hypothesis linking low folate intake to neural tube defects due to failure of post-translation methylations of the cytoskeleton. Int J Dev Biol 50: 135–141

Brodland GW, Gordon R, Scott MJ, Björklund NK, Luchka KB, Martin CC, Matuga C, Globus M, Vethamany-Globus S, Shu D (1994) Furrowing surface contraction wave coincident with primary neural induction in amphibian embryos. J Morphol 219:131–142

Brown CJ, Robinson WP (2000) The causes and consequences of random and non-random X chromosome inactivation in humans. Clin Genet 58:353–363

Buller RE, Sood AK, Lallas T, Buekers T, Skilling JS (1999) Association between nonrandom X-chromosome inactivation and BRCA1 mutation in germline DNA of patients with ovarian cancer. J Natl Cancer Inst 91:339–346

Chitnis S, Derom C, Vlietinck R, Derom R, Monteiro J, Gregersen PK (1999) X chromosome-inactivation patterns confirm the late timing of monoamniotic-MZ twinning. Am J Hum Genet 65:570–571

Davidson RG (1964) The Lyon hypothesis. J Pediatr 65:765–775

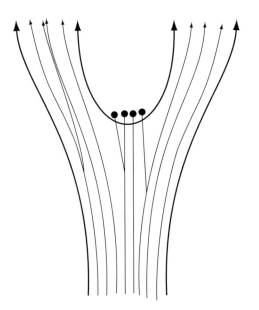

Fig. 11.1 The thicker arrows define a branch of a tissue lineage tree or "differentiation tree" (Gordon 1999). The vertical direction defines increasing developmental time. Inside is the cell lineage with the thin lines indicating individual cells. Those cells on the left experience a contraction wave while those on the right experience an expansion wave. Thus, cells at the earlier stage of development at the bottom, all of one type, become cells of two types. However, some cells are missed by both waves and become stem cells, as indicated by the dots now off the differentiation tree. Cell divisions are indicated by branch points of the cell lineage tree. Both trees, followed backward in time, would converge at the one-cell stage of the embryo, namely the zygote

Ekbom A, Trichopoulos D, Adami HO, Hsieh CC, Lan SJ (1992) Evidence of prenatal influences on breast cancer risk. Lancet 340:1015–1018

Fackelmann KA (1997) The birth of a breast cancer: do adult diseases start in the womb? Sci News 151:108–109

Funayama S, Hikosaka K, Yahara T (1997) Effects of virus infection and growth irradiance on fitness components and photosynthetic properties of *Eupatorium makinoi* (Compositae). Am J Bot 84:823–829

Funayama-Noguchi S (2001) Ecophysiology of virus-infected plants: a case study of *Eupatorium makinoi* infected by geminivirus. Plant Biol 3:251–262

Going JJ, Moffat DF (2004) Escaping from Flatland: clinical and biological aspects of human mammary duct anatomy in three dimensions. J Pathol 203:538–544

Gordon R (1999) The hierarchical genome and differentiation waves: novel unification of development, genetics and evolution. World Scientific & Imperial College Press, Singapore/London

Gordon R (2006) Mechanics in embryogenesis and embryonics: prime mover or epiphenomenon? Int J Dev Biol 50:245–253

Gordon R (2009) Google embryo for building quantitative understanding of an embryo as it builds itself: II. Progress towards an embryo surface microscope. Biol Theory 4:396–412

Gordon R (2010) Stop breast cancer now! Imagining imaging pathways towards search, destroy, cure and watchful waiting of premetastasis breast cancer [invited]. In: Tot T (ed) Breast cancer – a lobar disease. Springer, London, pp. 167–203

Gordon R, Björklund NK (1996) How to observe surface contraction waves on axolotl embryos. Int J Dev Biol 40:913–914

Gordon R, Brodland GW (1987) The cytoskeletal mechanics of brain morphogenesis. Cell state splitters cause primary neural induction. Cell Biophys 11:177–238

Gordon R, Westfall JE (2009) Google embryo for building quantitative understanding of an embryo as it builds itself: I. Lessons from Ganymede and Google earth. Biol Theory 4:390–395

Gordon R, Buckley WR (2010) International Embryo Physics Course – An Effort in Reverse Engineering, http://embryophysics.org/

Hahn WC, Weinberg RA (2002) Modelling the molecular circuitry of cancer. Nat Rev Cancer 2:331–341

Hendrix MJC, Seftor EA, Seftor REB, Kasemeier-Kulesa J, Kulesa PM, Postovit LM (2007) Reprogramming metastatic tumour cells with embryonic microenvironments. Nat Rev Cancer 7:246–255

Hoekenga OA, Muszynski MG, Cone KC (2000) Developmental patterns of chromatin structure and DNA methylation responsible for epigenetic expression of a maize regulatory gene. Genetics 155:1889–1902

Howard B, Ashworth A (2006) Signalling pathways implicated in early mammary gland morphogenesis and breast cancer. PLoS Genet 2(e112):1121–1130

Iida S, Morita Y, Choi JD, Park KI, Hoshino A (2004) Genetics and epigenetics in flower pigmentation associated with transposable elements in morning glories. Adv Biophys 38:141–159

Kalthoff KO (2001) Analysis of biological development. McGraw-Hill Higher Education, Columbus

Kasemeier-Kulesa JC, Teddy JM, Postovit LM, Seftor EA, Seftor REB, Hendrix MJC, Kulesa PM (2008) Reprogramming multipotent tumor cells with the embryonic neural crest microenvironment. Dev Dyn 237:2657–2666

Kristiansen M, Helland A, Kristensen GB, Olsen AO, Lønning PE, Borresen-Dale AL, Orstavik KH (2003) X chromosome inactivation in cervical cancer patients. Cancer Genet Cytogenet 146:73–76

Kristiansen M, Knudsen GP, Maguire P, Margolin S, Pedersen J, Lindblom A, Ørstavik KH (2005) High incidence of skewed X chromosome inactivation in young patients with familial non-BRCA1/BRCA2 breast cancer. J Med Genet 42:877–880

Kulesa PM, Kasemeier-Kulesa JC, Teddy JM, Margaryan NV, Seftor EA, Seftor REB, Hendrix MJC (2006) Reprogramming metastatic melanoma cells to assume a neural crest cell-like phenotype in an embryonic microenvironment. Proc Natl Acad Sci USA 103:3752–3757

Lerner BH (2001) breast cancer wars: hope, fear, and the pursuit of a cure in twentieth-century America. Oxford University Press, New York

Linn F, Heidmann I, Saedler H, Meyer P (1990) Epigenetic changes in the expression of the maize A1 gene in *Petunia hybrida*: role of numbers of integrated gene copies and state of methylation. Mol Gen Genet 222:329–336

Lopez JI, Mouw JK, Weaver VM (2008) Biomechanical regulation of cell orientation and fate. Oncogene 27:6981–6993

Lose F, Duffy DL, Kay GF, Kedda MA, Spurdle AB (2008) Skewed X chromosome inactivation and breast and ovarian cancer status: evidence for X-linked modifiers of *BRCA1*. J Natl Cancer Inst 100:1519–1529

Lyon MF (1961) Gene action in the X-chromosome of the mouse (*Mus musculus* L.). Nature 190:372–373

Lyon MF (2003) The Lyon and the LINE hypothesis. Semin Cell Dev Biol 14:313–318

Martin CC, Gordon R (1997) Ultrastructural analysis of the cell state splitter in ectoderm cells differentiating to neural plate and epidermis during gastrulation in embryos of the axolotl Ambystoma mexicanum. Russian J Dev Biol 28:71–80

Mintz B, Illmensee K (1975) Normal genetically mosaic mice produced from malignant teratocarcinoma cells. Proc Natl Acad Sci USA 72:3585–3589

Monteiro J, Derom C, Vlietinck R, Kohn N, Lesser M, Gregersen PK (1998) Commitment to X inactivation precedes the twinning event in monochorionic MZ twins. Am J Hum Genet 63:339–346

Muers MR, Sharpe JA, Garrick D, Sloane-Stanley J, Nolan PM, Hacker T, Wood WG, Higgs DR, Gibbons RJ (2007) Defining the cause of skewed X-chromosome inactivation in X-linked mental retardation by use of a mouse model. Am J Hum Genet 80:1138–1149

Nishida H (2005) Specification of embryonic axis and mosaic development in ascidians. Dev Dyn 233:1177–1193

Osgood MP (1994) X-chromosome inactivation: the case of the calico cat. Am J Pharm Educ 58:204–205

Pierce GB, Pantazis CG, Caldwell JE, Wells RS (1982) Specificity of the control of tumor formation by the blastocyst. Cancer Res 42:1082–1087

Puck JM, Stewart CC, Nussbaum RL (1992) Maximum-likelihood analysis of human T-cell X chromosome inactivation patterns: normal women versus carriers of X-linked severe combined immunodeficiency. Am J Hum Genet 50:742–748

Raven CP (1966) An outline of development physiology. Pergamon, Oxford

Rossant J (2009) Reprogramming to pluripotency: from frogs to stem cells. Cell 138:1047–1050

Soto AM, Maffini MV, Sonnenschein C (2008) Neoplasia as development gone awry: the role of endocrine disruptors. Int J Androl 31:288–293

Sulston JE, Schierenberg E, White JG, Thomson JN (1983) The embryonic cell lineage of the nematode *Caenorhabditis elegans*. Dev Biol 100:64–119

Tenney RM, Discher DE (2009) Stem cells, microenvironment mechanics, and growth factor activation. Curr Opin Cell Biol 21:630–635

Tot T (2011) The theory of the sick lobe. In: Tot T(ed) Breast cancer – a lobar disease. Springer, London, pp. 1–17

Trichopoulos D (1990) Hypothesis: does breast cancer originate in utero? Lancet 335:939–940

TyTy Nursery (2010) Variegated Banana Tree [*Musa aeae*]: the fast growth of this remarkable variegated plant ironically grows faster than most pure-green leafed banana plants, which is a shocking inconsistency to normally accepted biological principals. http://www.tytyga.com/product/Variegated+Banana+Tree

Vella CM, Robinson R (1999) Robinson's genetics for cat breeders and veterinarians, 4th edn. Amsterdam, Elsevier Health Sciences

Vermeulen L, Sprick MR, Kemper K, Stassi G, Medema JP (2008) Cancer stem cells–old concepts, new insights. Cell Death Differ 15:947–958

Vickers MA, McLeod E, Spector TD, Wilson IJ (2001) Assessment of mechanism of acquired skewed X inactivation by analysis of twins. Blood 97:1274–1281

Vincent-Salomon A, Ganem-Elbaz C, Manié E, Raynal V, Sastre-Garau X, Stoppa-Lyonnet D, Stern MH, Heard E (2007) X inactive-specific transcript RNA coating and genetic instability of the X chromosome in *BRCA1* breast tumors. Cancer Res 67:5134–5140

Vinh-Hung V, Tot T, Gordon R (2010) One or many targets? Towards resolving the paradox of single versus multifocal breast cancer from epidemiological data. In preparation

Waddington CH (1934) Morphogenetic fields. Sci Prog (Lond) 29:336–346

Wang N, Tytell JD, Ingber DE (2009) Mechanotransduction at a distance: mechanically coupling the sextracellular matrix with the nucleus. Nat Rev Mol Cell Biol 10:75–82

Yu F, Fu A, Aluru M, Park S, Xu Y, Liu H, Liu X, Foudree A, Nambogga M, Rodermel S (2007) Variegation mutants and mechanisms of chloroplast biogenesis. Plant Cell Environ 30:350–365

Zaffari GR, Peres LEP, Kerbauy GB (1998) Endogenous levels of cytokinins, indoleacetic acid, abscisic acid, and pigments in variegated somaclones of micropropagated banana leaves. J Plant Growth Regul 17:59–61

Index